Occupational Hazards to Dental Staff

Occupational Hazards to Dental Staff

Professor Crispian Scully, PhD, MD, MDS, FDS, FFD, MRCPath

Centre for the Study of Oral Disease, University Department of Oral Medicine, Surgery and Pathology, Bristol Dental Hospital and School, Lower Maudlin Street, Bristol BS1 2LY, UK

Professor Roderick A. Cawson, MD, BDS, FDS, FRCPath

Emeritus Professor of Oral Medicine and Pathology, University of London, UK

Dr Mark Griffiths, MB, BS, BDS, FDS

University Department of Oral Medicine, Surgery and Pathology, Bristol Dental Hospital and School, Lower Maudlin Street, Bristol BS1 2LY, UK

1990

Published by the British Dental Association
64 Wimpole Street, London W1M 8AL

ISBN 0 904588 27 0

Typeset by Latimer Trend and Company Ltd, Plymouth

Printed in Great Britain by
Eyre & Spottiswoode Ltd,
London and Margate

Preface

Some 10 years ago, an Editorial in the British Dental Journal pointed out that there was a need in dentistry for a 'list or index of risks and some guidance as to when to flap and when not'. The purpose of the present book is therefore to alert dental trainees, dental surgeons, dental surgery assistants, hygienists and other clinical, and laboratory dental staff, to some of the occupational hazards that may have to be faced, their prevention and the relevant legislation. The aim is not to spread alarm and despondency, but hazards are much diminished if one is aware of, and particularly if one is prepared for them.

Not so very long ago, the hazards to dental staff from their occupation were hardly considered. Radiation burns and tumours had been recognised, but little more than lip service was given to radiation safety. No one seemed greatly concerned about the toxicity of dental materials, mercury, or anaesthetic agents, which were used with remarkably little care. Serious transmissible infection was almost disregarded and the possibility of illness through occupational stress was only briefly considered. Furthermore, undergraduates and other trainees received little or no training in recognising or avoiding the occupational hazards of dentistry, and safe work practices were not defined or implemented, despite the fact that there were clear hazards.

Now, by contrast, the perceptions of risk by the dental profession, staff and the public at large, have been greatly sharpened, particularly by the AIDS epidemic. In the United Kingdom, governmental concern and the defining of safe work practices and measures for implementing them by the Health and Safety at Work etc Act (1974) and Regulations such as the Ionizing Radiations Regulations (1988) and Control of Substances Hazardous to Health Regulations (1988), have brought the matter of occupational hazards in dentistry into sharper focus. Even more recently, Family Practitioner Committees and Health Boards in Britain, as well as Dental Reference Officers, have been given powers to enter dental practices and check adherence to terms of service, including facilities, especially those related to cross-infection control, compressor maintenance, waste disposal, radiation safety and drug security. The Health and Safety Executive appear to be increasingly active and this factor already has implications for dentistry.

Overall, the major dangers now threatening clinical dental staff from the practice of dentistry are infections, particularly hepatitis B and probably non-A non-B hepatitis, and, to a much lesser extent as yet, human immunodeficiency viruses. There are also risks to dental staff in the form of accidents, eye damage, irradiation, dental materials and drugs, stress and from the rapidly growing level of drug abuse.

The importance of health and safety at work is highlighted by a recent case where a dentist was disciplined by the General Dental Council on charges as proved for failing:

(1) to ensure that appropriate precautions were taken to protect staff and patients from the risk of cross-infection;
(2) to provide adequate sterilisation facilities;
(3) to provide sufficient dental equipment and instruments to enable Associates adequately to treat patients;
(4) to ensure that appropriate radiation protection methods were adopted for the safety of staff and patients;
(5) notwithstanding the fact that the technique of intravenous sedation was used from time to time on patients, failure to have sufficient resuscitation equipment readily available.

Furthermore, increasing numbers of patients have acquired totally unrealistic expectations that every dental procedure or drug must be 100% risk-free and totally effective. Partly as a consequence of this, patients are now more prepared to initiate litigation, although, fortunately, this is as yet on a small scale in the UK in comparison with some other countries. Some occupational hazards are therefore directed at the practitioner's pocket, but can also cause considerable anxiety and loss of time.

Although for many years there has been the need to implement the requirements of various pieces of legislation, especially the Employment Act, and Health and Safety at Work Etc Act, there has been little attention to this in the dental curriculum and there is a dangerous ignorance of the legislation. At the very least, studying these regulations consumes working or leisure time, while at worst, a troublesome employee may be able to make life a burden. Staff and public are, rightly, increasingly aware of the laws and the General Dental Council has included in the Recommendations concerning the Dental Curriculum an indication that dental students 'should be aware of the requirements of the Health and Safety at Work Act and of their responsibilities for the health and welfare of patients and auxiliary staff'.

However, it is also essential to try to acquire a sense of proportion about the level of risks involved in dentistry and not to become overwhelmed by unjustified anxiety. Some of the hazards of dentistry are real, but at the same time remote; others are more imaginary than real. Clinical practice, particularly in hospitals and dental laboratory work, undoubtedly constitutes a greater occupational risk than general dental practice, but overall the risks are still low where there are good work practices. In fact, it is difficult to think of many occupations that are safer. All occupations are associated with some hazards and many are far more hazardous than dentistry. Oil rig workers are an obvious example and the Health Education Authority has recently emphasised the risks in the construction industry.

Accidents on the roads and in the home, or related to leisure activities, are undoubtedly a far greater risk to dental staff than dentistry. Life is a risk activity! Perhaps if dental staff appreciated more fully the dangers of smoking, and of drinking alcohol, the 30 or so illnesses they could contract from their pets, the innumerable dangers involved in travel at home and abroad, the frequency of accidents in the home, the hazards of sexual relationships (particularly those outside marriage), and the risks to life and limb from many sports, they might be happier about their profession. Indeed, undertaking virtually any human activity is based on the balancing of benefit or pleasure and possible costs or hazards.

This book comprises seven chapters covering the main hazards in dentistry, the means to minimise risks, and the relevant legislation. Inevitably, there is some overlap between chapters, but we hope few omissions or errors. The first section deals with morbidity and mortality of dental staff, the second with the more obvious specific hazards, and the last with legal aspects. We cannot *guarantee* accuracy, hard though we have tried, and readers must check the original literature and legislation if serious employment or medicolegal problems should arise in a practice or laboratory. The data have taken nearly 5 years to collect and we have presented the overall picture as up-to-date, as at early 1990, as we could manage. Details of suppliers of protective material are provided at the ends of each chapter. We have included selected and mostly recent references to help further reading. We would be most interested to hear any comments.

C. Scully
R. A. Cawson
M. J. Griffiths
Bristol and London
1990

'There is scarce any (folly) against which warnings are of less efficacy, than the neglect of health'

Samuel Johnson: *The Rambler*
1 September, 1750

This text is dedicated to Patrick Scully, dental technician, who succumbed in his early fifties to lung cancer.

Acknowledgements

We are most grateful to the following colleagues for advice, criticism and comments: Mr Christopher Bell (Bristol); Dr David Brown (London); Mr John Bunn (Bristol); Mr Terry Foad (Bristol); Mr J. O. Forrest (London); Mr Trevor Griffiths (Cardigan); Mr Colin Howard (Department of Health, London); Dr Robin Huggett (Bristol); Mr Joe Mee (High Wycombe); Dr Stephen Porter (Bristol); Dr Alan Preece (Bristol) and Mr Eric Whaite (London). We also wish to express our gratitude to the staff of the Medical Protection Society for their unfailing courtesy and helpfulness, but particularly to Dr R. N. Palmer, the Secretary, and Mr L. Walters, the Dental Secretary, for their invaluable comments on Chapter 7, and to Mr D. A. Phillips for other information. We are also grateful to Mr Norman Davies, Registrar, General Dental Council; Mr Norman Whitehouse, Secretary, British Dental Association; and the American Dental Association for permission to use and adapt material. We thank the Dental Laboratory Association, British Association of Dental Hygienists and the Association of British Dental Surgery Assistants for trying to help, despite the fact that their efforts revealed concern, but virtually no data on specific hazards.

We are also most grateful to Connie Blake and Alison Scott for their help and secretarial assistance, to Ni Fathers and Derek Coles for assistance with the illustrations and to Mr Sidney Luck for his indefatigable help with reference retrieval. Finally, we are grateful to Dr Sue Silver of the British Dental Journal for her expert help in publishing this book, and to Margaret Seward for her encouragement.

Contents

1

Mortality and Some Aspects of Morbidity

No occupation is without risk, but modern dentistry is probably among the least hazardous. Leisure activities are far more hazardous (fig. 1.1). In the past, dentistry was associated with some real hazards, not least from ionising radiation and physical damage from instruments and equipment. For example, there are occasional accounts of dentists damaging their eyes, ribs, and even their abdomens whilst performing tooth extraction, of fatal septicaemia following sharps injuries, and of injuries from naked flames or from exploding vulcanisers.[1] This century has seen dramatic improvements in dental equipment and work practices, yet only some 30 years ago, British dentists had higher mortality rates than most comparable professions.[2,3] Almost one half of American dentists who retired early, did so because of ill health.[3]

In westernised countries, dentists now have better work practices and they have high social status, a high level of education, and an above average income. They are therefore invariably in the upper socioeconomic groups, which have better health than groups of lower socioeconomic status. There is, for example, in upper socioeconomic groups, a lower mortality from cardiovascular disease, cancer, poisonings, accidents and violence. This is related to the lower smoking rates, better eating habits, better health education and better living and working conditions of the upper socioeconomic groups.[4] In contrast, dentists in some Third World countries may have poorer work practices, and are frequently exposed to, and may contract, contagious diseases such as tuberculosis.

Some other occupations are clearly associated with significant morbidity and mortality,[5] and it is remarkable that, despite the low risks in dentistry, dental staff clearly perceive that occupationally-

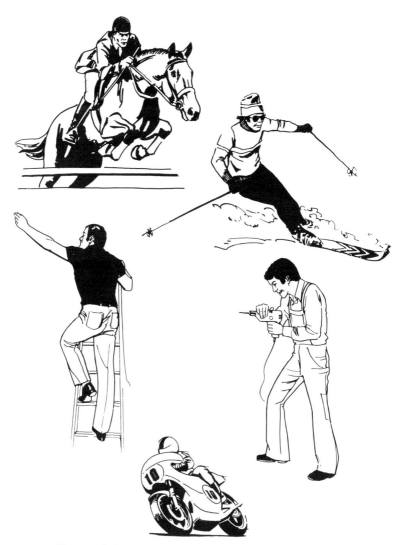

Fig. 1.1   Leisure activities can be more hazardous than dentistry.

related diseases, especially stress, are common. One survey of Finnish clinical dental staff revealed that nearly 30% of dentists and 10% of surgery assistants had been off work in the previous 2 years as a result of an 'occupational problem'. Dentists complained particularly of musculoskeletal discomfort (Chapter 2) and of stress; surgery assistants complained mainly about allergies and respiratory infections.[6-8] Musculoskeletal problems and fatigue were also fairly common complaints in British dentists, and more frequent than in pharmacists.[9] Stress is more fully discussed later in this chapter, and diseases of specific body systems are outlined in Chapter 2.

Causes of death among dental staff

Dentists' mortality

The first records of mortality among dentists were from the UK in the late 1920s. Various early studies gave equivocal findings as to life expectancy,[10-13] but a series of surveys has since confirmed a lower mortality rate for dentists than for comparable professions (fig. 1.2)[14-17] and lower than for health care workers in social classes II and IV (Table I).

As in non-dental groups in Western countries, the main causes of death among dentists in Britain, USA and other industrialised countries are cardiovascular disease, cancer and suicides.[15,16,18-26] Nevertheless, reports of a significant overall excess of deaths from cardiovascular disease and suicides over others in the same social class have not always been confirmed in recent studies, although there appears to be a risk from cirrhosis[21] and male dentists may be at slightly greater risk of coronary heart disease[27] and of suicide[21,26] than the general population. Reported rates of suicide in any group are probably an underestimate because of the stigma attached to such deaths.

Recent reports of an increased risk of brain tumours (glioblastomas) in dental staff[28] and of nasal cancer[29] have not been confirmed[29a].

The standardised mortality ratio (SMR) is used to assess death rates. This is the ratio of observed deaths in an occupation or from a disease, to the national average death rate for the same age and sex. An SMR of less than 100 indicates a lower death rate; an SMR over 100 indicates a higher rate. The SMR of dentists both in the UK and USA is lower than that of the general population. The most recent studies of dentists' mortality show that male dentists in the UK had

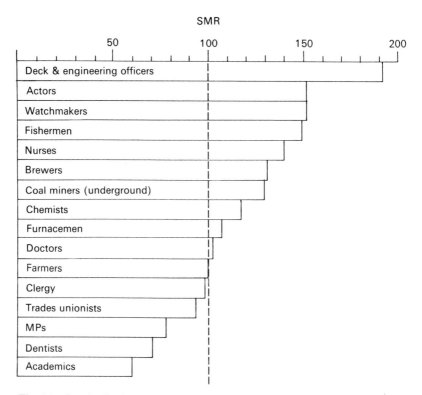

Fig. 1.2   Standardised mortality ratios (SMR) for men aged 15–64 years (social class adjusted); from *Dec Suppl Occup Mort* 1970–72. OPCS, 1978.

an SMR of 59 to 66, which is far better than that for many other professions and others in the same social class, but not as good as University academics who had an SMR of 48.[17,21] This is perhaps a reflection of the latter's relatively leisurely and stress-free life-style— at least until recently. Single women dentists, however, had an SMR of 123, but the reason for this apparently high figure is unclear.[17] Similar findings of lower mortality rates for dentists have been reported from North America and Scandinavia.[30,31] As mentioned earlier, dentists have a higher SMR for suicides and cirrhosis of the liver compared with the overall figures for social class I[21] (Table 1.1), but lower SMR for cancers, ischaemic heart disease, cerebrovascular disease and chronic lung diseases such as bronchitis, emphysema and asthma (Table 1.2).

Table 1.1 Overall mortality of British male dentists compared with other health care workers[a]

Social class	Health care group	Standardised mortality ratio (SMR) from group	SMR for social class
I	Dentists	66	75
	Doctors	69	
	Opticians	72	
	Pharmacists	105	
II	Physiotherapists	79	86
	Radiographers	79	
	Chiropodists	93	
	Nurses	118	
IV	Ambulancemen	109	121
	Porters	151	

[a]After Balarajan R. Br Med J 1989; **299**: 822–825.

In summary therefore, it is reassuring to know that the mortality rate of dentists in Western countries is lower than for others of the same social class. Indeed, it has been estimated that, of the 140 000 dentists practising in the USA, probably 77 die each year from accidents, suicides or murder; this figure far exceeds known mortality from any direct possible occupational risk.[32] Furthermore, it is evident that 73% of dentists now live past retirement age.[33]

Mortality rates among other dental staff

There is little data available on the mortality rates of other dental staff. Medical technicians and dental auxiliaries are grouped together in British government figures, which give an SMR for males of 106 and for single females 55.[17] However, one report found that male American dental laboratory technicians aged 20 to 65 had an incidence of lung cancer 4·05 times higher than that for all other identified occupations.[34] The SMR reported was 405 compared with 70 for dentists, but the effects of cigarette smoking may have been as important as, or more important than any effect from the dusts to which technicians may be exposed (see Chapter 5).

Responses to health education

To what extent dentists' health benefits from their particular education and medical knowledge is unclear. For example, examinations of

OCCUPATIONAL HAZARDS TO DENTAL STAFF

Table 1.2 Mortality of British male dentists from selected major causes compared with other health care workers[a]

Health care group	Suicide	Cirrhosis	All cancers	Cerebrovascular disease	Ischaemic heart disease	Lung cancer	Chronic lung diseases
Dentists	222	165	69	62	60	37	32
Doctors	172	177	66	71	70	33	28
Opticians	83	NR	73	53	78	62	36
Pharmacists	242	254	91	103	109	75	80
Social Class II	82	115	86	87	92	73	61
Social Class IV	116	107	122	122	117	130	144

[a] After Balarajan R. *Br Med J* 1989; **299**: 822–825. (Figures represent SMR.) NR = not recorded

dentists attending the annual meetings of the American Dental Association (presumably a highly motivated group) revealed a significant amount of oral and perioral disease, even malignant neoplasms, in a minority.[35,36]

On the other hand, there is evidence that dentists respond to health education. For example, the percentage of US male dentists who smoked cigarettes fell from 34% in 1967 to 16% in 1982,[37] and there are indications that dentists also now take more physical exercise in order to relieve 'stress' and to lessen any tendency to cardiovascular disease. Nevertheless, dentists tend to be physically unfit and, at least in the USA, there is increasing abuse of alcohol and drugs, as in many other groups.

Stress and mental health among dental staff

Stress and mental ill-health cause up to 40% of all sickness absence from the workplace in the UK, according to the Health and Safety Executive (Mental Health at Work, 1988; ISBN: 0–118839985). Most problems arise from interpersonal relationships, working procedures or the design of the workplace. Factors that give rise to difficulties include resentment at failure to be promoted, promotion beyond ability, too much or too little work, changes in work environment, colleagues, nature or style of work, relocation, role conflicts, irregular or long hours of work, monotony or lack of autonomy, and actual or perceived hazards such as infection or violence. Domestic or personal circumstances can strongly influence the affected person's responses.

Dental students

Dentistry, even for students,[38] appears to be somewhat stressful (fig. 1.3), but perhaps less so than medicine and some other professions.[9,42–51] In some studies, dental students exhibited increasing anxiety and cynicism, and less humanitarianism as they progressed through their education.[39] Anxiety, depression and psychosomatic complaints appeared to become commonplace.[38] However, more recent studies suggest that anxiety and stress in dental students are now, in general, no more than the norm,[41] although, hardly surprisingly, final year students are somewhat more under stress.

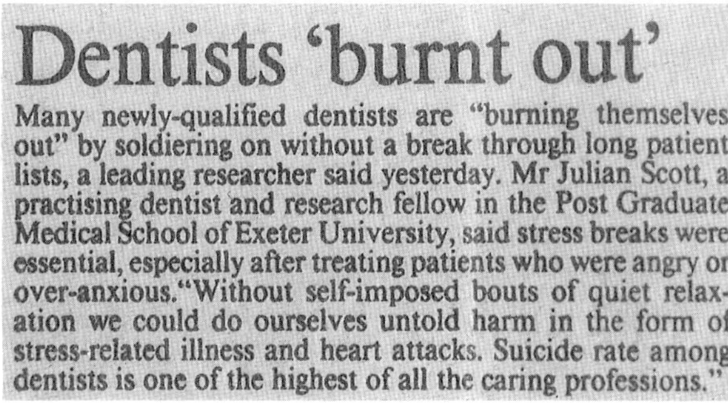

Dentists 'burnt out'

Many newly-qualified dentists are "burning themselves out" by soldiering on without a break through long patient lists, a leading researcher said yesterday. Mr Julian Scott, a practising dentist and research fellow in the Post Graduate Medical School of Exeter University, said stress breaks were essential, especially after treating patients who were angry or over-anxious."Without self-imposed bouts of quiet relaxation we could do ourselves untold harm in the form of stress-related illness and heart attacks. Suicide rate among dentists is one of the highest of all the caring professions."

Fig. 1.3 Newspaper headline on stress among dentists (1989).

General practitioners

Perceived culpable aspects of dental practice relate to piecework remuneration, interpersonal relationships, poor working conditions and a bad public image of dentistry. The disenchantment of dentists has even reached the national press. Many surveys of dentists have shown that they believe themselves to be under stress.[42–51]

Interactions with other staff, colleagues, or patients can be the source of considerable stress, despite the fact that dentists claim that they like human contact. Many factors influence the dentist–patient relationship, not least patients' concepts of a good dentist, and the dentists' expectations of the level of income they should generate. In the constant effort to maintain a high patient flow, the dentist becomes fatigued, irritable and concerned that goals may not be achieved.[47] The patient may not feel that the benefits are commensurate with the cost, time and effort involved in attending for treatment. Complaints may follow and the dentist–patient relationship can easily suffer. Several studies have confirmed that the most common identifiable sources of stress among dentists are from interpersonal relationships and from the conflict of striving to perform good technical dentistry quickly enough to maintain an income at a level regarded as adequate.[42–51]

Other stresses in dentistry, comparable with those in medicine, include those caused by dealing with frightened, difficult or ill patients, especially as, unlike their medical colleagues, they have little or no training in dealing with such problems, and uncertainty about clinical decisions.[52] Interactions with patients are unavoidably emotion-laden since patients' emotional or psychic states can stir up responses, sometimes adverse, in the person caring for them.[53] These can sometimes amount to aversion, guilt, fear, anger or even malice. There are also demands for the dentist to conform to social conventions of behaviour and appearance and these may increase the pressures on the dentist. In contrast, hours of work in practice usually range from 30 to 40 hours a week,[54] which is comparable with many occupations, and dental practitioners can have almost complete control over which patients they will accept for treatment. One study of South African dentists showed a high level of job satisfaction.[55] Interestingly, a recent study also showed that over 75% of US dentists felt they were under less stress than their colleagues.[50] Dentists in practice in the USA also seem to be more content than dental surgery assistants or dental hygienists[56] (see below). However, most practice in South Africa and the USA is private and is not health service-related.

. Nearly one third of British dentists, mostly males over 35 years of age, express job dissatisfaction and male dentists have higher indices of anxiety and Type A (achievement orientated) behaviour than the general population.[44-47] Overall, the evidence from this and other studies suggests that about one in five dentists is dissatisfied, a rate similar to that found in other occupations.[57]

Hospital resident dental staff

Hospital resident medical staff in Britain and many other countries work inordinately long hours and stress is particularly common, especially when there is contact with violent or abusive patients who are, increasingly, dealt with late at night in Accident and Emergency Departments (Chapter 2). Time as a resident house officer can be particularly stressful because of the long hours, the amount of work, repeated calls to the telephone (and irritating telephone calls), ethical dilemmas, exposure to severely ill and sometimes dying patients, and social difficulties.[58] Many of today's hospital patients are more seriously ill, more demanding or more difficult to manage than formerly. There is often little time for the resident to relax or to be with friends or relations. Interpersonal relationships can therefore deteriorate, setting up a vicious circle as personal difficulties start to interfere with work. Residents' messes are also changing as staff often marry younger and live away from the mess. As a result there is less camaraderie and companionship than previously. Depression is common among medical residents; some studies of US first year residents have reported depression in 30% and the situation appears to be worsening.[59–62]

Night work can cause many difficulties. Some resident medical staff have as little as one and a half hours sleep when on duty. The long hours of duty (often over 100 hours per week) and loss of sleep not only contribute to psychological deterioration and mood changes but, worse, impair memory and decision-making,[61–63] almost certainly to the detriment of patient care. An American court ruled that the long working hours of a hospital resident contributed to the death of a patient (the Libby Zion case) and a British judge linked long working hours and medical malpractice claims.[64] Such pressures may also unfortunately produce depression and long-lasting negative attitudes and practices which persist into the later career.[65]

Fortunately, the problem has been recognised in Britain and is less severe in dental residents.[66] Legislation should soon further reduce the hours of work. However, the hours will even then still be about double that expected of most of the population! Dental residents tend to lose less sleep than their medical counterparts and, as a result, are less stressed and, in general, now fairly content, but there are still instances of stress.[66]

Dental hygienists

Dental hygienists appear to have less job satisfaction than dentists, at least in the USA,[56] and more frequently change jobs. There is little recent objective data on stress, although hygienists often leave dentistry entirely.[67–69]

Dental surgery assistants

There seems to be a fair degree of job dissatisfaction, high levels of turnover, and a lack of long-term commitment to dentistry among dental surgery assistants in several countries.[68,70–73] Undue stress is reported by over 50% of assistants,[74–76] and pay is not good.

Dental technicians

No data were found relating to stress in dental technicians.

Reactions of staff to stress

It is only too easy for dentists to become socially involved with dental or medical colleagues and such acquaintances may prevent the dentist from getting any rest from work by constantly 'talking shop'. Non-dental acquaintances may aggravate the dentist with jokes about dentistry or criticisms of his or her financial success. Added to these occupational problems are, of course, domestic and other stresses, particularly among hospital or university dental staff, who find themselves having to move around the country in order to find employment.[58,77]

Most cope with such stresses by adapting their environment and goals, but some react adversely and develop excessive anxiety and depression. The result may be that they leave dentistry, or a vicious circle may develop, in which behaviour becomes increasingly inefficient, worsening the stress, and the physical symptoms of the 'burn-out' syndrome appear (fig. 1.4). Interpersonal relationships may suffer. Depression and indeed suicide are recognised hazards, particularly for hospital residents[60,77,78] and, as discussed above, also for other dentists.

There are many warning signs of the chronic anxiety state that precedes 'burn-out', but they are not always recognised. Anxiety tends to manifest itself as increasing impatience or hostility, suspicion or paranoia, deterioration in appetite, sleep, or bowel habits; dissatisfaction, cynicism or indifference, and multiple minor somatic complaints such as tension headaches, low back pain, dry mouth, cheekbiting or bruxism. Marital problems are commonplace. Dentists seem

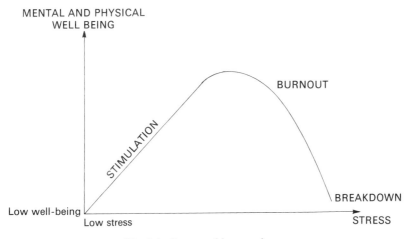

Fig. 1.4   Stress and its sequelae.

to suffer more frequently from low back pain than others (Chapter 3), but there is little evidence for other psychogenic illness.

It has been suggested that dentists undergo five stages leading to burn-out:[79]

(1) The practice honeymoon.
(2) The drill and fill blahs—where the job becomes boring.
(3) The operatory blues—when depression sets in.
(4) The crisis—where agitation and frustration appear and, if no positive behavioural changes are made, finally lead to
(5) The pulp-out, or burn-out.

Although there are no data showing that burn-out is more or less frequent in dentists than in comparable occupations,[57] the cirrhosis, cardiovascular disease and suicide rates discussed above, are cause for some concern.

By the age of 60, one third of American dentists may have suffered stress-related health effects, and 20% have been divorced[80] although, as discussed above, this is no more than in comparable professions. Increased smoking, or abuse of alcohol or drugs may follow (fig. 1.5).

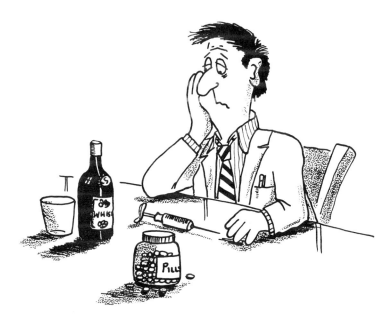

Fig. 1.5 Some of the consequences of excessive stress.

Nevertheless, most dentists are healthy and can cope, and indeed take off about half the time that other workers do.[81]

Drug abuse (see also Chapter 7)

Fortunately, cigarette smoking has been declining among health professionals; for example, 50% or more doctors smoked in 1950, but 25 years later this had dropped to 20%. By 1982, only 16% of American male dentists smoked, compared with 25% of other males.

Drug abuse in dentistry and medicine is, however, increasing. Unfortunately, this is not a new problem, not least because of the ready availability of drugs such as inhalational anaesthetic agents. Freud, who introduced the principle of local anaesthesia (though not a dentist), became a cocaine addict, while Halstead, the pioneer of the inferior dental block, was addicted to both cocaine and morphine. Recent studies have shown alcohol dependence or other drug abuse in over one third of US medical students.[82,83] Dentists are also known to abuse alcohol and drugs of various kinds,[84,85] including nitrous oxide or other inhalational anaesthetics (Chapter 3), but cases of this kind only rarely appear before the General Dental Council in the UK. About 8% of recent US dental graduates resorted to alcohol or drugs in a 1981 survey[86], and another study revealed marijuana abuse in 14%, cocaine abuse in 4%, and nitrous oxide abuse in 4%.[78]

Alcohol is the most widely abused drug. There appears to be a small genetic component to alcoholism, but more important, intolerable stress and easy access increase the likelihood of abuse. The incidence of alcohol abuse by doctors and dentists is probably somewhat higher than comparable groups of the population. Although little is known about the actual level of abuse, it has been estimated that 8% of American dentists are alcoholic.[87] Occasionally, cases come to light as a result, for example of accidents to patients, or police cases where a dentist has been found to be under the influence of alcohol or in illegal possession of drugs. Clearly such cases (as with drug abuse in general) represent only the tip of the iceberg since, as discussed above, cirrhosis and suicides are more prevalent in dentists than others of the same social class.[21]

In short, drug abuse can be both a response to occupational stress and also a threat to the dentist's own health. In addition, there may be medicolegal consequences (Chapter 7).

Management of the sick dentist is also discussed in Chapter 7.

Adapting to stress

If work starts to become too great a burden and a source of undue anxiety, it is important to consider whether the aims or lifestyle should be modified, particularly in view of the fact that at least one half of one's waking hours are usually spent at work (fig. 1.6). It is crucial to avoid drug abuse. Under such circumstances it is important to stop and give serious thought to what one really wants out of life. It seems pointless, for example, to pine for a 140 mile-an-hour Porsche simply for the pleasure of sitting in a 10-mile tail-back on a motorway. It is even less worthwhile to struggle to possess an ocean-going yacht if there is going to be little leisure to use it; a visit to any marina shows innumerable boats floating idle for most of the time.

It is necessary only to strive for a lifestyle that is genuinely desired, but however modest the hoped-for lifestyle may be, it is essential to manage efficiently and not waste time. As many tasks as possible should be delegated without abrogating responsibilities. However, to achieve such aims involves the often difficult task of building up an

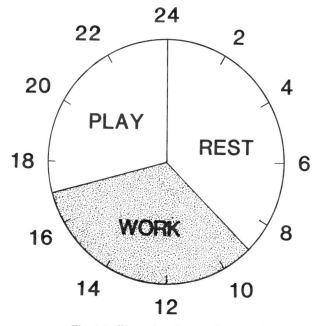

Fig. 1.6 We work to live, not live to work.

efficient team who also feel themselves committed to the success of the practice or laboratory.

Strong family support reduces stress and group practice may also fulfil this role[7]. In single-handed practice there is usually less support from colleagues, and, of course, partnerships themselves can sometimes be the source of anxiety. It *must* be appreciated that, in the long term, it is the health of the dentist that is the hub around which the practice revolves and every effort should be made to keep stress and anxiety under control. These considerations are discussed further elsewhere.[87,88]

The stresses on technical and other dental staff are unclear, but it is important that the staff work at an acceptable pace in a pleasant, comfortable environment, and have adequate rest and relaxation. Above all, *good* dental staff must be encouraged and appropriately rewarded. To be penny-pinching with one's staff can quickly cost considerably more than what little seems to be saved.

Female dental staff and concern about hazards to pregnancy

The possible hazards of exposure to anaesthetic gases, mercury, ionising radiation and infections have caused some concern, quite understandably, particularly among female dental staff. However, although certain points relating to these dangers are discussed in later chapters, most current evidence suggests that there is little if any specific occupational risk in dentistry to the outcome of pregnancy. Indeed, spontaneous abortions are increased in various other occupations, from sales personnel to those in catering; stillbirths are more frequent in, for example, those in agriculture and horticulture, and low birthweight babies are more frequent among those in domestic service and the manufacturing industry.[89]

Reproductive history of dental staff

Female dentists have been reported to suffer less infertility than female hospital doctors, but are reported to have a somewhat greater incidence of spontaneous abortions than controls who do not go to work.[90] In one large study (involving over 30 000 persons) of female dental surgery assistants and the wives of an almost equal number of dentists, there were increased rates of spontaneous abortions[91] as compared to female anaesthetists. Rates of low birthweight babies and foetal malformations were found to be comparable to those in controls. However, female dentists who continued to work during pregnancy seemed to have a tendency to premature deliveries. In contrast, a recent study showed no increase in spontaneous abortions in dental surgery assistants[92] and an enormous prospective study (involving 10 000 women and including 7300 pregnancies) of illness among doctors and a detailed analysis of existing epidemiological studies has revealed no evidence to confirm any relationship between hours worked in a particular specialty, such as anaesthesia, and miscarriage rates.[93]

General anaesthetic agents

In Sweden, there had appeared to be a relationship between the hours worked in the operating theatre and birthweight of babies, but although the birthweight of babies was slightly (though not significantly) less than in controls, this was possibly the result of the slightly higher incidence of twin births in the group studied.[94,95] A Canadian study showed *no* relationship between exposure to anaesthetic agents and either spontaneous abortions or stillbirths.[89]

Mercury

Pregnant female staff may be concerned about possible risks to their foetus from exposure to mercury in the dental surgery (Chapter 3). Provided the guidelines on mercury hygiene are followed, as described in Chapter 3, there appears to be no risk to female clinical or laboratory dental staff. One Polish report did show increased rates of menstrual irregularities, reproductive failures and spina bifida, which appeared to correlate with the mercury content of the females' hair, but the study did not take account of the females' age, despite the fact that spontaneous abortions are strongly age-dependent.[96] In contrast, a recent Swedish study of 8157 infants born of female dental staff showed a lower than normal perinatal death rate and no increase in spina bifida.[97] The study also examined dental staff hospitalised with spontaneous abortions and found no differences from those rates expected in a non-dental population.[97] Furthermore, none of the mothers of 220 infants with neural tube defects born in 1965–1967, was a dentist. This study therefore gives no indication of any significant reproductive hazard in dentistry. Nevertheless, mercury can accumulate in the placenta and foetal membranes[98] and, where work practices are poor, there may be some risk. There are occasional reports suggestive of a foetotoxic effect of mercury where dental surgery mercury vapour levels have been high,[99] but a causal relationship remains to be proven.

Ionising radiation

Pregnant female staff may also be worried about possible risks to their foetus from ionising radiation but, provided the rules of radiation protection are carefully followed (Chapter 4), even female radiography or radiology staff appear to be at no significant risk.[100,101]

Infectious agents

Non-immune, or immunocompromised female staff and their foetuses may be at risk from various infectious agents, notably rubella, cytomegalovirus and other viral infections but preconception immunisation and routine cross-infection control procedures should obviate most of this risk (Chapter 5).

References

1   Foley GPH. A treasury of dentistry: early offices were a dangerous place to practice. *J Am Coll Dent* 1983; **50**: 24–25.
2   Samson E. Dentists still head professional death rate table. *Br Dent J* 1958; **9**: 303–304.
3   Willee AW. How to avoid the occupational hazards of dentistry. *Aust Dent J* 1967; **12**: 348–359.
4   Rimpela AH, Pulkkinen PO, Nurminen MM, Rimpela MK, Valkonen T. Mortality of doctors: do doctors benefit from their medical knowledge? *Lancet* 1987; **1**: 84–86.
5   Harrington JM, Gill S. *Occupational health pocket consultant.* (2nd ed) Oxford: Blackwells, 1987.
6   Briller FE. Occupational hazards in dental practice. *Oral Hyg* 1946; **36**: 1194–1197.
7   Dunlap JE, Stewart JD. Survey suggests less stress in group offices. *Dent Econ* 1982; **72**: 46–56.
8   Murtomaa H. Work-related complaints of dentists and dental assistants. *Int Arch Occup Env Health* 1982; **50**: 231–236.
9   Powell M, Eccles JD. The health and work of two professional groups: dentists and pharmacists. *Dent Pract Dent Rec* 1970; **20**: 373–378.
10 Braun R. Importance of occupational diseases in the dental surgeon. *Rev Franc Odontostomatol* 1962; **9**: 482.
11 Registrar-General Decennial Supplement, England and Wales, 1921 Occupational Mortality. London: HMSO, 1927.
12 Registrar-General Decennial Supplement, England and Wales, 1931 Occupational Mortality. London: HMSO, 1938.
13 Registrar-General Decennial Supplement, England and Wales, 1951 Occupational Mortality. London: HMSO, 1958.

14   Registrar-General Decennial Supplement, England and Wales, 1961 Occupational Mortality. London: HMSO, 1971.
15   Hill GB, Harvey, W. The mortality of dentists. *Br Dent J* 1972; **132**: 179–182.
16   Scarrott DM. Death rates of dentists. *Br Dent J* 1978; **145**: 245–246.
17   Office of Population Censuses and Surveys. Occupational mortality 1979–1980, 1982–1983 Decennial Supplement. London: OPCS, 1986.
18   Bureau of Economic Research and Statistics. Survey of dentists over 60. Illness and injuries. *J Am Dent Assoc* 1963; **67**: 539.
19   Bureau of Economic Research and Statistics. The occupation of dentistry: its relation to illness and death. *J Am Dent Assoc* 1977; **95**; 606–613.
20   Glass RL. Mortality of New England dentists 1921–1960. US Department of Health, Education and Welfare, Public Health Service, Radiology Health Division, Washington DC, 1966.
21   Balarajan R. Inequalities in health within the health sector. *Br Med J* 1989; **299**: 822–825.
22   Blachly PH, Osterud HT, Josslin R. Suicide in professional groups. *New Engl J Med* 1963; **268**: 1278–1282.
23   Orner G, Breslin P. Mortality study of dentists. US Department of Commerce, National Technical Information Service, prepared for National Institute for Occupational Safety and Health, 1976.
24   Dean G. The causes of death of South African doctors and dentists. *South Afr Med J* 1969; 495–500.
25   Rose KD, Rostov, I. Physicians who kill themselves. *Arch Gen Psychiatr* 1973; **29**: 800–806.
26   Simpson R, Jakobsen J, Beck J, Simpson S. Suicide statistics of dentists in Iowa 1968 to 1980. *J Am Dent Assoc* 1983; **107**: 441–443.
27   Russek HI. Emotional stress and coronary heart disease in American physicians, dentists and lawyers, *Am J Med Sci* 1962; **243**: 716–726.
28   Ahlbom A, Norell S, Rodvall Y, Nylander M. Dentists, dental nurses and brain tumours. *Br Med J* 1986; **292**: 662.
29   Glazebrook GA. Occupational nasal carcinogenesis among dentists? *Cancer Detect Prev* 1981; **4**: 31–40.
29a Brownson RC, Reif JS, Chang JC, Davis JR. An analysis of occupational risks for brain cancer. *Am J Publ Health* 1990; **80**: 169–172.
30   Anderson O. Dodelighed og erhverv 1970–1980 (Occupation and mortality) Kovenhavn: Danmarks Statistik, Statiske Undersogelser No 41 (in Danish), 1985.
31   Borgan J-K, Kristofersen LB. Mortality by occupation and socio-economic group in Norway 1970–1980. Oslo: Central Bureau of Statistics of Norway, Statistike analyser 56, 1986.
32   Klein RS, Phelan JA, Freeman K, Friedland GH, Treiger N, Steigbigel NH, Schable C. Dentists and risk of HIV. *New Engl J Med* 1988; **319**: 113–114.
33   Galginaitis C, Gift H. Occupational hazards: is dentistry hazardous to your health? *New Dent* 1980; **10**: 24–27.
34   Mench HR, Henderson BE. Occupational differences in lung cancer. *J Occup Med* 1976; **18**: 797–801.
35   Cutright DE *et al.* Clinical examination of the head and neck. *J Am Dent Assoc* 1977; **94**: 915–917.
36   Goltry RR, Ayer WA. Head, neck, and oral abnormalities in dentists participating in the health assessment program. *J Am Dent Assoc* 1986; **112**: 338–341.
37   CA-A Cancer Journal of Clinicians, 1986.
38   Davis EL, Tedesco LA, Meier ST. Dental student stress, burnout and memory. *J Dent Educ* 1989; **53**: 193–195.

39 Manhold JH, Shatin L, Manhold BS. Comparison of interests, needs and selected personality factors of dental and medical students. *J Am Dent Assoc* 1963; **67**: 601–605.

40 Wexler, M. Mental health and dental education. *J Dent Educ* 1978; **42**: 74–77.

41 Cecchini JG. Differences of anxiety and dental stressors between dental students and dentists. *Int J Psychosom* 1985; **32**: 6–11.

42 Howard JH, Cunningham DA, Rechnitzer, PA, Goode RC. Stress in the job and career of dentists. *J Am Dent Assoc* 1976; **93**: 630.

43 Powers WJ, Brusch WA, Klugman PJ, Mize SA. Stress in dentistry: a survey of military dentists. *Dent Survey* 1980; **56**: 64–68.

44 Cooper CL, Mallinger M, Kahn R. Identifying sources of occupational stress among dentists. *J Occup Psychol* 1978; **51**: 227–234.

45 Cooper CL. Dentists under pressure: a social psychological study. *In* Cooper CL and Marshall J (eds). *White collar and professional stress.* Chichester: Wiley, 1980.

46 Cooper CL, Watts J, Kelly M. Job satisfaction, mental health and job stressors among general dental practitioners in the UK. *Br Dent J* 1987; **162**: 77–81.

47 Cooper CL, Watts J, Baglioni AJ Jr, Kelly M. Occupational stress amongst general practice dentists. *J Occup Psychol* 1988; **61**: 163–174.

48 Furnham A. Social skills and dentistry. *Br Dent J* 1983; **154**: 404–411.

49 Lewis KJ. Stress in dentistry. *In* Davis HC, Forrest JD, Lewis KJ (eds). *Review of dental practice.* Epsom: Morgan, 1982.

50 O'Shea RM, Corah NL, Ayer W. Sources of dentist's stress. *J Am Dent Assoc* 1984; **109**: 48–51.

51 Selor, RJ. Stress: Inherent to dentists or taught to dental students. *Dent Student* 1984; **10**: 14–20.

52 McCue JD. The effects of stress on physicians and their medical practice. *New Engl J Med* 1982; **306**: 458–463.

53 Zinn WM. Doctors have feelings too. *J Am Med Assoc* 1988; **259**: 3296–3298.

54 Deverall A. The health of dentists in South Africa. *J Dent Assoc South Afr* 1969; **24**: 368–371.

55 Coster E, Coetsee L, Van Niekerk A. The quality of working life of a group of dentists. *J Dent Assoc South Afr* 1979; **34**: 563.

56 Chapko MK, Bergner M, Beach B, Green K, Milgram P, Skalabrin N. Development of a measure of job satisfaction for dentists and dental auxiliaries. *Community Dent Oral Epidemiol* 1986; **14**: 76–79.

57 Kent G. Stress amongst dentists. *In* Paynes R, Firth-Cozens J (eds). *Stress in health professionals.* pp 127–149. Chichester: Wiley, 1987.

58 Scully C. Spare a thought for the resident hospital dental surgeon. *Br Dent J* 1989; **166**: 4–5.

59 Walerstein SJ, Rosner F, Wallace EZ. House staff stress. *N Y State J Med* 1989; **89**: 454–457.

60 Smith JW, Denny WF, Wizke DB. Emotional impairment in internal medicine house staff: results of a national survey. *J Am Med Assoc* 1986; **255**: 1155–1158.

61 Friedman RC, Bigger JT, Kornfield, DR. The intern and sleep loss. *New Engl J Med* 1971; **285**: 201–203.

62 Hart RP, Buchsbaum DG, Wade JB. Effect of sleep deprivation on first-year resident's response times, memory and mood. *J Med Educ* 1987; **62**: 940–942.

63 Orton DI, Gruzelier JH. Adverse changes in mood and cognitive performance of house officers after night duty. *Br Med J* 1989; **198**: 21–23.

64 Asch D, Parker R. The Libby Zion case. One step forward or two steps backward? *New Engl J Med* 1988; **318**: 771–775.

65 McCall TB. The impact of long working hours on resident physicians. *New Engl J Med* 1988; **318**: 775–778.

66 Bowden J, Porter SR, Scully C. Resident dental staff (in press).

67 Howell MA, Brumback GB, Newman SH. Dimensions of work satisfaction among federally employed dentists. *J Dent Educ* 1969; **33**: 206–211.

68 Bader JD. Auxiliary turnover in 13 dental offices. *J Am Dent Assoc* 1982; **104**: 307–312.

69 Leatherman GH. Survey of auxiliary dental personnel. *Int Dent J* 1979; **19**: 49–54.

70 Gold IL. The quality of life of the dental assistant. *Int Dent J* 1978; **18**: 289–297.

71 Sapp J. The constant turnover of dental assistants in dental practice. *Dent Assist* 1978; **47**: 36–46.

72 Editorial. Personnel management: keeping the dental team together. *J Am Dent Assoc* 1987; **114**: 772–779.

73 Editorial. The disappearing DSA. *Br Dent J* 1987; **163**: 211.

74 Clark J, Phillips S. Stress and the dental assistant. *Dent Assist* 1981; **50**: 31–33.

75 Willis G, Gruner J. Are you burning out in your career? *Dent Assist* 1983; **52**: 20–23.

76 Locker D, Burman D, Otchere D. Work-related stress and its predictors among Canadian dental assistants. *Community Dent Oral Epidemiol* 1989; **17**: 263–266.

77 Reuben DB. Depressive symptoms in medical house officers: effects of level of training and work rotation. *Arch Int Med* 1985; **145**: 286–288.

78 Clark DC, Slazar-Gruesco E, Grabler P, Fawcett J. Predictions of depression during the first 6 months of internship. *Am J Psychol* 1984; **141**: 1095–1098.

79 Edelwich J, Brodsky A. *Burnout*. New York: Human Sciences Press, 1980.

80 Wilson B. Stress in dentistry: a national survey. *Dent Manag* 1984; July 14–19.

81 Waller TP, Ayer WA. Work loss among practicing dentists. *J Am Dent Assoc* 1984; **108**: 81–83.

82 Clark DC, Eckenfels EJ, Daugherty SR, Fawcett J. Alcohol-use patterns through medical school: A longitudinal study of one class. *J Am Med Assoc* 1987; **257**: 2921–2926.

83 McAuliffe WE, Rohman M, Santagelo S. Psychoactive drug use among practicing physicians and medical students. *New Engl J Med* 1986; **315**: 805–810.

84 Council on dental practice. Chemical dependency and dental practice. *J Am Dent Assoc* 1987; **114**: 509–518.

85 Peterson RL, Avery JK. The alcohol-impaired dentist: an educational challenge. *J Am Dent Assoc* 1988; **117**: 743–748.

86 Godwin WC, Starks DD, Green TG, Koran A. Identification of sources of stress in practice by recent dental graduates. *J Dent Educ* 1981; **45**: 220–221.

87 Bissell L, Haberman PW. *Alcoholism in the professions*. p 26. Oxford: Oxford University Press, 1984.

88 Symposium. Management of stress in the dental practitioners. *Dent Clin North Am* 1986; **30**: No 4 (suppl.).

89 McDonald AD. Work and pregnancy. *Br J Indust Med* 1988; **45**: 577–580.

90 Nixon GS, Helsby CA, Gordon H, Hytten FE, Renson CE. Pregnancy outcome in female patients. *Br Dent J* 1979; **146**: 39–42.

91 Cohen EN, Brown BW, Wu ML, Whitcher CE, Brodsky JB. Occupational disease in dentistry and chronic exposure to trace anesthetic gases. *J Am Dent Assoc* 1980; **101**: 21–31.

92 Heidam LZ. Spontaneous abortions among dental assistants, factory workers, painters and gardening workers: a follow-up study. *J Epidemiol Community Health* 1984; **38**: 149–155.

93 Spence AA. Environmental pollution by inhalation anaesthetics. *Br J Anaesth* 1987; **59**: 96–103.

94 Ericson A, Kallen B. Survey of infants born in 1973 or 1975 to Swedish women

working in operating rooms during their pregnancies. *Anesth Analg* 1979; **58**: 302.

95   Ericson A, Kallen B. Hospitalization for miscarriage and delivery outcome among Swedish nurses working in operating rooms 1973–1978. *Anesth Analg* 1985; **64**: 981.

96   Sikorski R, Juszkiewicz T, Paszkowski T, Szprengier-Juskiewicz T. Women in dental surgeries: reproductive hazards in occupational exposure to metallic mercury. *Int Arch Occup Env Health* 1987; **59**: 551–557.

97   Ericson A, Kallen B. Pregnancy outcome in women working as dentists, dental assistants or dental technicians. *Int Arch Occup Env Health* 1989; **61**: 329–333.

98   Wannag A, Skjaerasen J. Mercury accumulation in placenta and foetal membrane: a study of dental workers and their babies. *Env Physiol Biochem* 1975; **5**: 348–352.

99   Gelbier S, Ingram J. Possible foetotoxic effects of mercury vapour: a case report. *J Public Health* 1989; **103**: 35–40.

100   Langmead, WA. Radiation hazard to female radiographers. *Br J Radiol* 1968; **41**: 75.

101   Wagner LK, Hayman LA. Pregnancy and women radiologists. *Radiology* 1982; **145**: 559–562.

2

Hazards to specific body systems

This chapter discusses specific hazards to the special senses, respiratory system, skin and some other systems. Some of these, and other more general hazards arising from the practice of dentistry, are also discussed in the following chapters.

The eyes

Good eyesight is essential to all aspects of the practice of clinical and laboratory dentistry and every care must be taken to protect the eyes of both staff and patients from damage (fig. 2.1).

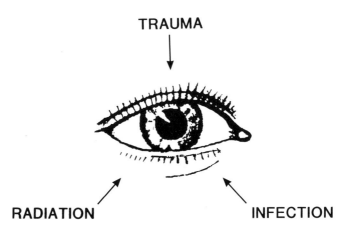

TRAUMA

RADIATION   INFECTION

Fig. 2.1   Hazards to the eyes.

Trauma

With air turbine speeds of 250 000 to 400 000 rpm, small particles can be projected from the bur at velocities of up to 10 m/second.[1] If they hit the eye, they can cause, at the very least, conjunctivitis, or, more important, corneal abrasions or even dangerous penetrating wounds.[2,3] Care should also be taken to protect the eyes from projected particles produced, especially when grinding metals or cutting wire (figs 2.2 and 2.3).

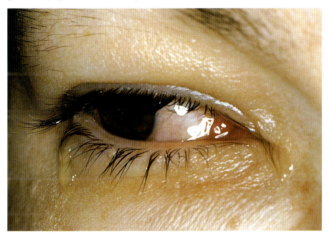

Fig. 2.2   Eye damage caused by a projectile, in a dental technician who was working without protective eyewear.

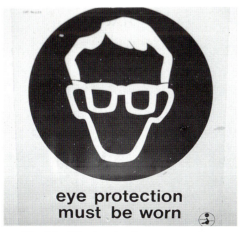

eye protection
must be worn

Fig. 2.3   Warning sign for eye protection.

Penetrating wounds cause deep injuries and can be caused by any sharp instrument such as a dental probe or bur. Particularly dangerous is the use of wires and of bent rotating instruments such as burs. Blunt injury to the eye can cause a subconjunctival haemorrhage; this is usually trivial, but may conceal a deeper injury. Dental staff have been wounded in this way (as have patients), and some have been permanently blinded as a consequence.[4,5] One study showed 18% of dentists to have had eye lesions caused by foreign bodies.[4]

Burns

Chemicals used in clinical dentistry, particularly phosphoric acid, sodium hypochlorite, trichloroacetic and chromic acids can all cause serious chemical burns of the eye (see Chapter 3). Laboratory materials constitute a very significant hazard. Many of the laboratory acids and alkalies can cause serious eye damage. Methyl methacrylate monomer, if splashed into the eye, can cause a painful reaction.[6] Plaster of Paris contains small quantities of lime and quartz that can damage the eye, whilst pumice can abrade it (see also Chapter 3).

Infections

Some 10% of dental practitioners may contract eye infections at some time in their practice.[7] Herpetic keratitis is one of the worst ocular infections that can be contracted by clinical dental staff and endangers sight, but bacterial conjunctivitis caused by Staphylococcus aureus is more common. Other conjunctival pathogens, such as Chlamydia trachomatis, have recently also been reported to have been transmitted in dental practice[8] and some viruses such as hepatitis B virus may, if contaminated fluids splash onto the conjunctiva, cause systemic infection (see Chapter 5).

Radiation damage (see Chapter 4)

Prevention of eye disease

Eyes really *must* be protected from foreign bodies, infected material, chemicals, and the various forms of radiation (Table 2.1). Some 53% of dentists need to wear glasses because of sight defects,[4] but all should wear protective spectacles during work.

Close-viewing distances and treating anterior teeth increase the possibility of exposure to missile damage and injury from blue and

Table 2.1 Eye protection in dentistry

	Use	Comments
Wear protective eyewear and/or a face shield	During active treatment of all patients	Protective eyewear and face shields not only prevent contact with splatter and aerosols, but also prevent missile injury
	During dental laboratory procedures	
	During instrument and surface decontamination procedures and use of acids and alkalies	Some disinfectant/ sterilising solutions/acids, etc, can harm eyes.
	To avoid injury when using ultraviolet or other light sources	

UV-light sources. Exposures to wavelengths shorter than 400–500 nm (this is mainly a UV danger) are cumulative, whilst the shortest wavelengths are most damaging. This will be discussed further in Chapter 4.

The simplest and most effective method of preventing eye injury from missiles is the use of protective spectacles, preferably with plastic lenses and side-shields. Safety spectacles can be obtained from Norville Opticals*, or many opticians (eg Dolland and Aitchison).

As far as possible, direct and prolonged viewing of UV or blue light should be avoided. Ordinary dark glasses do *not* filter the offending wavelengths but, by absorbing visible light, can cause pupil dilatation and therefore aggravate the trouble. Protective glasses should be used to filter out all light under about 500 nm and therefore glasses with red, orange, or yellow coloured lenses of sufficient optical density are indicated when using blue or UV light. A UV400 coating, which is almost colourless, can be applied to ordinary plastic lenses and effectively blocks UV light. Blue-light hazards can be reduced by Guardian protective eye glasses, by Topaz glasses, and by the Premier Cureshield. Laser Bloc spectacles provide total eye protection over the 180 nm to 10 000 nm range and are also virtually unbreakable.

---

*Details can be found at the end of the chapter.

Staff wearing contact lenses should be careful not to get powders or other materials behind the lenses.

Hearing

The *intensity* of sound is measured in decibels (dB), the scale of which runs from 0 to 150 and is logarithmic. Thus, sound of 10 dB is ten times louder than 1 dB, but sound of 20 dB is 100 times louder than 1 dB. Apparently small increases in decibel number in the higher part of the range therefore represent *very* large increases in noise; 100 dB represents a sound which is 10 billion times as intense as 1 dB. A dB level of zero is the threshold of sound. Decibels are often expressed as dB(A); the 'A' indicates a scale which is weighted to represent the human hearing range.

The *frequency* of sound is expressed in hertz (Hz); the lowest frequency detectable to the human ear is about 20 Hz, the highest about 18 kHz. Normal speech has a frequency of about 500 Hz to 2 kHz. With age there is loss of high frequency hearing. The ear tolerates louder sounds better at lower frequencies than at higher ones.

Noise
Loud noise typically produces an initial reduction in hearing sensitivity (a temporary threshold shift) that affects the higher frequencies (3000 to 6000 Hz), but hearing typically recovers after the exposure ceases.

Loud noise (85 dB or more) can, however, irreversibly damage the inner ear hair receptor cells of the organ of Corti in the cochlea. Some of the relevant causes of noise are shown in figures 2.4 and 2.5. This noise-induced damage mainly affects the ability to hear over the range 3–6 kHz and produces a disability ranging from slight loss of hearing for specific frequency ranges, and tinnitus (buzzing or ringing in the ears), to total deafness. Noise of 85 dB or more can also annoy, irritate or fatigue the recipient.[9] Noise of 120 dB or more can irrevocably damage hearing within a very short time; the UK code of practice for reducing the exposure of employed persons to noise (DOE, 1976) recommends a maximum of 30 seconds exposure to a dB level of 120 or more.[10,11]

Vowels are of lower frequency than consonants. Since noise exposure initially damages higher frequency perception, the hearing

	Decibels (dB)	Dental sounds measured at 30 M	Non-dental sounds
Pain	120		Aircraft
			Loud stereo music
	110		Underground train
			Road drill
	100		Motor cycle
	90		
Threshold for damage	80	Aspirator	
		Air turbine	
	70	Ultrasonic scaler	
		Amalgamator	
	60		
	50		Normal conversation
	40		
	30		
	20		Whisper
	10		
	0		Threshold of hearing

Fig. 2.4 Levels of occupational and domestic noise (adapted from Coles and Hoare, 1985[18]).

impairment may thus remain unnoticed for some time. Later, the affected person has difficulty hearing consonants and therefore may be able to hear speech, but be unable fully to understand what is being said. Formal audiometric testing may be needed to reveal the extent of the defect. Unlike age-related hearing loss (presbycusis), noise-induced hearing loss is *not* improved by the use of a hearing aid.[12]

Noise, therefore, is a hazard and the aim should be to maintain all noise levels at work, and elsewhere for that matter, to a minimum. A level of 80–90 dB(A) for 8 hours seems to be the maximum that can be safely tolerated, and the Health and Safety Executive in Britain recommends a maximum of no more than 90 dB(A) or an equivalent

Decibels

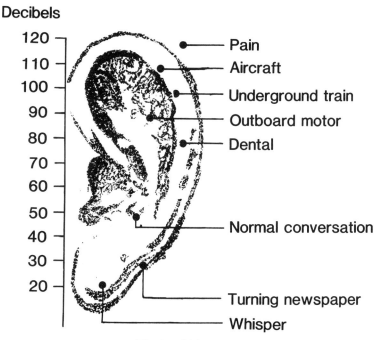

120	● — Pain
110	● — Aircraft
100	● — Underground train
90	● — Outboard motor
80	● — Dental
70	
60	
50	
40	● — Normal conversation
30	
20	● — Turning newspaper
	— Whisper

Fig. 2.5   Noise levels.

continuous noise level (ECNL); however, this level of noise would be unpleasant. Recommended maxima in American hospitals are 45 dB(A) for daytime and 35 dB(A) at night.

Air-rotors

Noise in the dental surgery, especially from high speed dental handpieces has been a source of some concern.[13] Older high speed handpieces, especially those with ball-bearings, produce sufficient noise (about 85 dB) to constitute a very slight hazard to hearing, but modern, well-maintained, ball-bearing or air-bearing handpieces produce no significant hazard (the noise levels are below about 85 dB). The overall evidence from several studies suggests that hearing is not impaired in clinical dental staff compared with age-matched controls, provided modern, well-maintained equipment is used (Table 2.2).[14–32] Surprisingly, the average exposure to drill noise during a day's work seems to be less than 20 minutes,[21,25] although these studies were carried out some years ago. One recent study

Table 2.2 Results of a variety of studies examining the possibility of hearing loss in dentistry

Noise level (dB)	Mean exposure period (years)	Number dental subjects	Hearing loss demonstrated	Reference
80–100	0·5	61	−	Hopp, 1962[14]
72–88	2·0	120	−	Keller et al., 1964[31]
70–100	3·7	40	+	Taylor et al., 1965[30]
70–95	2·9	125	+	Lumio et al., 1965[32]
69–94	2·8	18	−	Arentsschild and Eichner, 1966[22]
?	4·5	31	+	Ward and Holmberg, 1969[23]
?	25	35	−	Cole and Hoare, 1985[18]
?	18	234	−	Rahko et al., 1988[24]

examined the hearing of dentists and dental surgery assistants, most of whom had practised for about 18 years and again no hearing loss was found.[24] However, despite these results some of the older handpieces from the 1950s and 1960s are still in use and these may pose some hazard as may some of the surgical orthopaedic-type bone drills.[33]

Ultrasonic scalers

Ultrasonic scalers may produce slight tinnitus after prolonged use, but this rarely appears to be clinically significant, either to patients or staff.[34–36]

Prevention of hearing loss

Although, as noted above, there is no evidence of hearing damage in most dental staff, noise-induced hearing loss is irreversible and prevention is therefore crucial. All unnecessary noise should be eliminated. Dental high-speed handpieces should be chosen for their quietness (as well as other features) and should be well maintained. Ear protectors could be worn when the air-rotor handpiece or ultrasonic scaler are being used, but these should be amplitude-

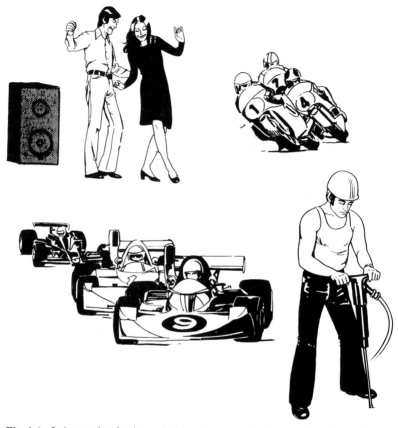

Fig. 2.6   Leisure-related noise and other noises are probably more damaging to dental staff hearing than dental noise.

sensitive in order to exclude high frequency sound, but permit normal speech to be heard (eg Norton Sonic 11 or Gundefenders). Ear plugs are also suitable for this purpose.

Dental staff are much more likely to suffer *leisure-related* hearing loss (from loud stereo music, shooting and so on) or hearing loss from sources other than their occupation (fig. 2.6).[18,23,29] Therefore, should dental staff notice impaired hearing, it is most important that a specialist opinion should be obtained, rather than that the defect be attributed, almost certainly incorrectly, to their occupation.[18]

The respiratory system

Among dental staff the respiratory system can become a site of infection, or can be damaged by various dusts or other materials (fig. 2.7). Apart from accidents, damage to the respiratory system is probably the most important hazard to laboratory dental staff.

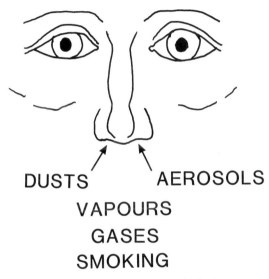

DUSTS   AEROSOLS
VAPOURS
GASES
SMOKING

Fig. 2.7   Respiratory hazards in dentistry.

Dust, splatter and aerosols from dental equipment (see also *Chapter 5*)

Aerosols are suspensions of fine particles of less than 50 µm in size, (most are smaller than 5 µm), which remain airborne for 24 hours or more, are dispersed widely by air currents, and may enter the lungs. These, and larger particles which tend not to pass to the lungs, may also settle on the conjunctiva or nasal mucosa.

Dust can be created by many dental procedures. Air-rotors, ultrasonic scalers, air–water syringes and dental lathes can produce splatter over a distance of 7 feet, as well as an aerosol, containing dental hard tissue material, other hard material, bacteria, fungi and possibly viruses and also oil, persisting 30 minutes or more.[36–43]

Infections

The water supply from dental units should theoretically be sterile, but tends to be contaminated, usually with soil and water saprophytes and oral microorganisms, particularly pseudomonads. Also present are actinomyces species, viridans streptococci and a range of other organisms including, occasionally, pathogens such as *Pseudomonas aeruginosa, Staphylococcus aureus,* and *Legionella pneumophila.*[44-58] Dental handpieces are often contaminated with microorganisms, as are air or air–water syringes, the dental chair and its immediate environment, as well as a large proportion of dental unit water supplies. Indeed, one recent British study showed that all dental unit water supplies in a hospital were contaminated.[45] Such contamination appears to originate from the environment of the dental surgery, and enters the water supply in the unit by back-siphonage, particularly through those dental handpieces which have a suck-back system to prevent the handpiece dripping after use. It is also possible that viruses and other microorganisms may contaminate the unit water supply.

If the drinking water supply can be contaminated by backflow or back-siphonage, a double check valve such as the Conex Saeflo, should be installed.

A variety of infectious agents can also be found in sputum or saliva, particularly if these are contaminated with blood (Chapter 5). Most prevalent are upper respiratory viral infections. There is well documented evidence of transmission to clinical dental staff of a variety of agents, including *Chlamydia trachomatis*[7] and viruses such as adenoviruses,[59] but these incidents are very rare. The agents of most concern are the viruses which cause a high morbidity or mortality, and bacterial infections such as tuberculosis or, possibly, legionellosis (Chapter 5). However, neither HBV nor HIV appear to be transmitted by the airborne route (*see* Chapter 5).

There are few studies of respiratory disease in clinical dental staff, but hygienists appear to be more prone than dental surgery assistants or clerical staff to nasal irritation, breathlessness, chest tightness and sputum production.[60] Technicians may be at risk from infections if work practices are not good (Chapter 5) and there have been *rare* reports of infection (eg mycoplasmal), apparently transmitted from dental appliances brought from the clinic.[61] It must be stressed again that such incidents are extremely rare.

Although there is no reliable direct evidence that transmission of infections from the dental unit water supply is common, there are reports of transmission of *Pseudomonas aeruginosa*[57] and there is at least a possibility of transmission of *Legionella*[62] and possibly other species. Hospital water supplies may be contaminated with *Legionella* and with mycobacteria. Contamination can be reduced by flushing the water line for at least one minute before using the handpiece or by intermittent chlorination with 0·5–1 ppm hypochlorite for 10 minutes daily.[63] In the latter case, there is a possibility of corrosion of aluminium-containing alloys. Povidone–iodine 10% may also reduce contamination.[64]

Microbial contamination of laboratory pumice is discussed in Chapter 5.

Dust injury

Dust can be created during various dental procedures and can constitute a hazard where work practices are poor, especially in the dental laboratory (Table 2.3). There is little evidence of occupational lung disease among clinical dental staff, but the drilling of teeth and old amalgams creates dust if there is inadequate water-cooling, and the mixing of alginates can also create dust (see below).

The possible consequences of inhaling such dust are unclear and a disturbing report of nasal carcinoma in dentists[65] has yet to be confirmed. There are, however, some reports of mild dyspnoea, respiratory infections (for example, mycoplasma causing atypical pneumonia),[61] pneumoconioses,[66,67] and possibly lung cancer[68] in

Table 2.3 Possibly hazardous mineral dusts in dentistry

Mineral	Found in some
Albite	Porcelain veneers
Andalousite	Silicate cement powders
Calcium sulphate	Gypsum products
Chrysolite	Asbestos ring liners
Cristobalite	Casting investments
Diatomite	Alginates (see text)
Labradorite	Porcelain veneers
Metals (various)	See text
Microcline	Porcelain veneers
Orthoclase	Porcelain veneers
Quartz	Casting investments
Sillimanite	Silicate cement powders
Spinelles	Cement powders

dental laboratory technicians. Occupational asthma is rare[69] (see Chapter 3). These hazards and their prevention are discussed below, but dust exposure in the workplace must always be minimised as much as possible.[70,71]

Pneumoconioses
Materials such as silica, beryllium, chromium and cobalt are the best recognised causes of pneumoconioses in technicians.[67,72–84]

One study of 250 dental technicians in Germany revealed pneumoconiosis in 27 and x-ray microanalysis of lung biopsy material has identified deposits of silica, cobalt, chromium, aluminium, iron and molybdenum.[72,73] Other European studies, but not all, have also suggested a risk to technicians of pneumoconiosis and, in a US study, eight out of 178 dental technicians had pneumoconiosis, possibly related to silica or beryllium inhalation.[80] One recent Scandinavian study showed simple pneumoconiosis in 13% and progressive lung fibrosis in 3% of dental technicians.[81]

To date, most reports of pneumoconiosis in dental technicians relate to silica dust inhalation from polishing and sandblasting using outdated equipment which produces considerable amounts of quartz dust. This and beryllium and other dusts are clear hazards.[85–87] Over the past 10–20 years there has been a significant increase in the use of base metal alloys for complex restorations and prostheses. The main alloys contain nickel (Ni), chromium (Cr) and molybdenum (Mo), Ni/Cr and beryllium (Be), or cobalt (Co) and Cr.[88] Often, other elements such as aluminium, boron, carbon, cerium, gallium, iron, manganese, niobium, silicon, titanium and zirconium are included. The risk from these is unclear,[88] but it is clearly wise to minimise inhalation.

However, cigarette smoking is probably a far greater hazard to the respiratory (and other) systems of technicians.

Lung and other cancers and potential carcinogens
Cancer of the lung in dental technicians is well recognised (see below). Mention has been made above and in Chapters 1, 3 and 4 of the oncogenic risks from ionising radiation, and of reports of brain tumours and nasal cancer in clinical dental staff.

A report from the USA revealed a fourfold higher risk of lung cancer in male dental laboratory technicians,[68] based on a survey of cases and deaths over the period 1968–1973. The increased incidence of lung cancer is likely to be related to a high frequency of cigarette smoking, but potential carcinogens and inhaled dusts are other possible causal, potentiating, or predisposing agents. Cigarette smoking also enhances the potential carcinogenicity of many of these inhaled substances as well as being strongly implicated in many different cancers. By contrast, dentists have a reduced SMR from cancers compared with other groups (Chapter 1).

Asbestos is the generic term for various hydrated fibrous silicate minerals which break down to fibres often less than 1 μm wide and 10 μm long. The use of asbestos should be avoided wherever possible because of the dangers, if inhaled or ingested, of asbestosis, carcinomas, or mesothelioma. Asbestos was used in some older periodontal packs, as a liner for casting rings and melting crucibles, and in some fire-resistant gloves. However, although alternatives are available, the aluminium silicate ceramic casting ring liners introduced into dentistry may not be safer than asbestos.[89,90]

Other potentially carcinogenic dusts include nickel, chromium, and beryllium used in some dental alloys.[88] Nickel is a carcinogen which causes nasal and lung cancer in nickel workers. Hexavalent chromium, which is released during welding, can predispose to lung, nasal and antral carcinoma. Beryllium is a suspected carcinogen.[91]

Dusts and smoke increase the risk of respiratory disease, including nasopharyngeal cancer and exposure should therefore be minimised.

Beryllium
Beryllium is possibly still an occupational hazard to technicians. A significant amount of beryllium is released during alloy melting, finishing and polishing unless there is good exhausting. Adverse reactions can range from contact dermatitis to chemical pneumonitis.[88]

Nickel
Nickel is found with chromium (in a ratio of about 8:2) in crown alloys used for porcelain bonding. Overheating or grinding produces nickel vapour and dust. Nickel is a recognised cause of respiratory disease, including carcinoma, in occupations where there is heavy exposure, and it can appear in fairly large amounts in the dust in dental laboratories where ventilation is inadequate. Contact dermatitis to nickel is not uncommon, but is not usually an *occupational* hazard,[88] although there seems to be a slightly increased risk of allergy to nickel in dental professionals.[92]

Cadmium
Acrylic base powders may contain cadmium, which is unlikely to be toxic.[93] However, cadmium in large doses can cause renal damage and hypertension, although this has not been reported in dental technicians.

Cobalt
Cobalt occasionally causes allergic skin reactions.[94]

Asthma
Occupational asthma is rare, but has been precipitated in nurses and dental technicians by methyl methacrylate and cyanoacrylates.[67,95] Formaldehyde, chlorhexidine, glutaraldehyde, cobalt, nickel, beryllium and chromium are other potential causes.[67,69,95–99] Clinical staff have very occasionally developed asthma after exposure to enflurane.[100]

Nasal irritation
Glutaraldehyde may cause nasal and pharyngeal irritation.[98,99]

Alginate inhalation
Alginate impression materials contain alginate salts and calcium sulphate, silica compounds and diatomaceous earth. Many alginates contain fluorine salts, zinc oxide or barium sulphate and various filler particles; a few used to contain lead. These materials may be inhaled, especially during dispensing and mixing, and produce a hazard either because of the lead content or the siliceous fibres, although objective evidence for injury from these is very slender.[101–104] Results of an early study showing high blood lead levels in those using alginates[102] have not been confirmed.[103] However, siliceous particles may be less than 3 μm in diameter and 20 μm long and might constitute a hazard similar to that of asbestos fibres, the carcinogenicity of which is related to particle size, not physicochemical composition.[105] Some impression materials are supposedly dust-free[101] and some, such as 'Dust-free Blueprint', do indeed produce very little dust during mixing. The amount of dust created during the mixing of alginates, however, varies greatly between different persons mixing the material and is probably reduced if sachets and automatic mixers are used.[106,107]

Oil inhalation
It is possible that oil from the lubricants of air turbines may be

inhaled, but what damage this may cause is uncertain.[108] Indeed, the only report on apparent oil-induced lung disease in a dentist proved to be non-occupational, and turned out to be due to siphoning petrol by mouth![109]

Impaired olfactory function

Methacrylate vapours can reversibly impair olfactory function, although there are no reports of this occurring in dental staff.[110]

Prevention of respiratory disease

The most important preventive measures are as follows.
(1) Avoid treating or being in close proximity to persons with acute respiratory infections.
(2) Minimise production of aerosols, splatter, and dusts. In clinical work, use rubber dam and high vacuum aspiration. In the laboratory, use guards and suction.
(3) Avoid inhaling aerosols, dusts, vapours, smoke, or fumes by using masks.
(4) Ventilate the working area adequately.

A simple method of reducing bacterial aerosols from clinical dental procedures is to have the patient rinse pre-operatively with 0·2% aqueous chlorhexidine. Use of high volume aspiration and rubber dam during restorative procedures will significantly reduce the amount of infected aerosol and splatter.

Face masks rarely filter particles smaller than 5 µm in diameter and, as discussed later (Chapter 5), the filtering efficiency of disposable

Table 2.4 Mask use in dentistry

	Use	Comments
Surgical mask	During treatment of each patient, particularly when treatment is likely to involve procedures that produce aerosol, droplets, and splatter	Change mask between patients or when mask is moist
	During any grinding or polishing procedure	May be better to use a system such as Zephyr
		Dispose of used masks in waste receptacle.

face masks varies from 14–99%.[111] Nevertheless, face masks do filter a great deal of debris. They should preferably be changed at least every hour (Table 2.4).

In the laboratory, local lathe ventilation is mandatory and dust extraction is vital. A plexiglass shield will reduce splatter (fig. 2.8). A chamber should be used while grinding and polishing appliances.

Electrostatic or HEPA (High Efficiency Particulate Air) air filters significantly reduce aerosols containing dusts or microorganisms. Face protectors such as the Zephyr have the advantage of giving a flow of filtered cool air to the operator and protecting the eyes and respiratory system simultaneously (fig. 5.21).[112]

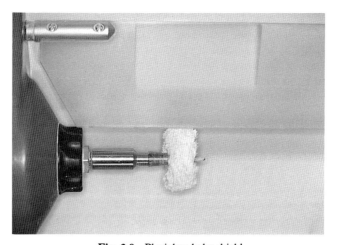

Fig. 2.8   Plexiglass lathe shield.

The skin

Skin complaints make up about half the total number of occupational illnesses in health care workers; in most cases this is direct or contact dermatitis. Occupational skin disease affects about 6 in 10 000 workers. Solvents, resins, plastics, detergents, heat and humidity are common predisposing factors for skin complaints. The health of the skin on the hands is of great importance in dentistry. Dry and cracked skin is difficult to keep clean and skin diseases where the continuity of the integument is impaired can allow access to infections. Patients are justifiably discouraged by a dental surgeon whose hands are not perfectly clean, healthy and well cared for. The main skin problems in dentistry are maceration (water-logging) and dermatitis from repeated hand-washing, occasionally candidosis secondary to maceration, other infections such as herpetic whitlow, and contact dermatitis (fig. 2.9).

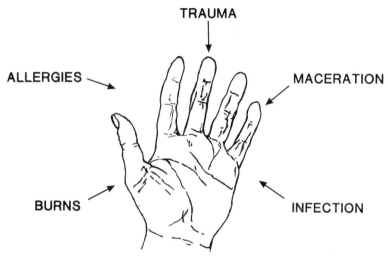

TRAUMA

ALLERGIES

MACERATION

BURNS

INFECTION

Fig. 2.9 Skin problems in dentistry.

Maceration
The use of barrier creams and the wearing of gloves may reduce the maceration which results from repeated hand-washing (see below).

Infections
Up to 98% of clinical dental staff report occasional hand and finger infections resulting from their occupation.[113] Local infections such as herpetic whitlow can be painful and incapacitating. A primary syphilitic chancre on the finger is little more than a theoretical occupational hazard of dental clinical practice (Chapter 5). However, the skin, especially if broken or punctured by a needlestick injury, may be the route for transmission of viral infections such as hepatitis B or HIV (Chapter 5) and for bacterial infections such as local infection of the tendon sheath. Wearing gloves may reduce the rate and risk of infections,[114] but cannot protect against needlestick wounds.

Burns

Obviously, flames can cause burns, but any hot material or instruments, acids or caustics, or very cold material can have the same effect. Staff (or patients) may be wounded and there is a risk of fire, especially in the laboratory (Chapter 3).

Dermatitis

Dermatitis can result from direct chemical irritation of the skin or, in a susceptible individual, from an allergic response (contact allergy) which is a Type 4 (delayed hypersensitivity) reaction. Radiation dermatitis is now virtually unheard of (Chapter 4).[114]

Hand dermatitis in dental staff, however, is most commonly caused by repeated hand washing, with subsequent soreness and chapping, even occasionally to the extent that fungal infections such as candidosis may be induced, particularly around the nails.[114] With the widespread wearing of rubber gloves, this problem should be reduced.

Direct irritation of the skin often produces a reaction almost immediately and the substance responsible is usually well known as an irritant (Table 2.5). Contact allergy is uncommon in dental staff. It typically manifests itself only 24–48 hours after exposure. A patch test, in which the test substance is applied under controlled con-

Table 2.5 Some skin irritants and allergens used in dentistry[a]

Irritants

Soaps and detergents
Abrasives in polishing materials (pumice, silica, calcium carbonate)
Etching compounds (phosphoric acid)
Adhesives (epoxy and cyanoacrylates)
Coumarone-indene resins
Germicidal solutions (glutaraldehyde), benzalkonium chloride)
Resins and catalysts
Essential oils (especially eugenol)
Amalgam
Solvents (alcohol, chloroform, methyl cellusolve)

Recognised allergens

Potassium dichromate
Wood alcohol (medications)
2 Mercaptobenzothiazole (rubber gloves, rubber bands and dams, Band-aids)
Parabens (medications, local anaesthetics, toothpaste)

Neomycin (medications, especially for root canal)
p-Phenylenadiamine (patients' recently dyed hair)

Lanolin (medications)
Epoxy resin (adhesives)
Mercapto products (rubber gloves, rubber bands and dams, Band-aids)
Ethylenediamine dihydrochloride (medications)
p-Chloro-m-xylenol (antiseptics)
Rubber (rubber gloves, rubber bands and Band-aids)
Thiuram products (rubber gloves, rubber bands and dams, Band-aids)
Formaldehyde (germicidal solutions and medications such as Formo-cresol)
Fragrances—various (medications, toothpaste)
Nickel (hand tools)

Table 2.5—*continued*

Recognised allergens—*continued*	Rarely allergenic—*continued*
Resin (colophony), (impression materials and soldering flux)	Glutaraldehyde (disinfectants)
Thiomersal (disinfectants)	Gold (alloys)
	Hexachlorophane (antiseptics)
Rarely allergenic	Hexylresorcinol (medications)
Acrylic monomer	Hydroquinone (inhibitor for acrylic resin systems)
Amethocaine (tetracaine) (topical anaesthetics)	N-Isopropyl-N-phenyl-p-phenylenediamine (IPPD) (rubber)
Balsam of Peru (medications)	MEK peroxide (catalyst for acrylic resin systems)
Beeswax (impression materials)	Menthol (medications)
Benzalkonium chloride (disinfectants)	Mercury
Benzocaine (anaesthetic)	Methyl dichlorobenzene sulphonate (impression materials, Impregum catalyst)
Benzophenone, (light absorber in plastic materials)	Methyl p-toluene sulphonate (Scutan)
Benzoyl peroxide, (catalyst for resins)	Methyl salicylate (toothpastes)
Bronopol (medications)	Nickel
Camphor (plasticiser in acrylics)	Penicillin
Chlorhexidine	Povidone–iodine
Chlorocresol (medications)	Procaine (anaesthetics)
Chlorothymol (medications)	Resorcinol monobenzoate (ultraviolet inhibitor in clear plastics)
Cinnamon oil (medications, toothpaste)	Triethylenetetramine (catalyst for epoxy resins)
Cobalt (alloys)	Zirconium (polishing paste)
Dichlorophene (germicidal agents)	
Eugenol (various dental materials)	

[a]Many of these only *rarely* cause reactions. Check manufacturers' details for contents of particular brands as components have changed.[94]

ditions to an area of skin, is used to determine whether a reaction is due to contact allergy.[115]

Hand dermatitis is frequently seen in dental technicians, where up to one third may suffer;[116] the most common causes are direct irritation and a reaction to acrylic monomer.[116] Clinical dental staff may develop dermatitis from repeated hand washing or chemicals such as glutaraldehyde. Those dentists who develop contact dermatitis most commonly react to eugenol, mercury or chromium.[117] Other causes of contact dermatitis include the following (*see also* Table 2.5).[94]

Certain anaesthetics
Topical anaesthetics, in particular those containing benzocaine or amethocaine, and local anaesthetics containing para-amino benzoic acid esters (procaine) are very rarely used now.

Methyl methacrylate monomer (see also Chapter 3)
Sensitivity is predominantly to the hydroquinone stabiliser in the monomer and has been recorded in surgeons,[118,119] although it is rare in clinical dental staff.

Dental technicians handling acrylic monomer are at risk from dermatitis and it has been estimated that some 10% become hypersensitive;[120] other workers suggest a lower incidence.[116]

Tooth-coloured filling materials[121,122]
Composite resins are based mainly on bisphenol A and acrylates, but can contain several contact allergens, particularly:
(1) chemically reactive pre-polymers, usually acrylated epoxides or acrylated urethanes;
(2) mono- and multi-functional aliphatic acrylates;
(3) initiators (eg benzoyl peroxide);
(4) activators (eg tertiary aromatic amines);
(5) inhibitors (eg hydroquinone).
Most reactions appear to be one or more of the following, although there may also be reactions to impurities, including traces of epoxy resin:[122]
BIS-GMA 2,2-bis[4-(2-methacryloxypropoxy)phenyl]propane
BIS-GA   epoxydiacrylate
MMA   methyl methacrylate
TEGDMA   triethylene glycol dimethacrylate
BIS-EMA 2,2-bis[4-(2-methacryloxyethoxy)phenyl]propane
DEGDA   diethylene glycol dimethacrylate
EGDMA   ethylene glycol dimethacrylate
TEGDA   triethylene glycol diacrylate

Essential oils
Eugenol, cinnamon, peppermint, aniseed, spearmint, eucalyptol, menthol and thymol and related substances such as balsam of Peru, benzoin, rosin, vanilla and perfumes in soaps, cleansers and some dental materials may induce contact dermatitis.[91,114]

Nickel and chromium
Nickel and chromium occur in some alloys and chrome-plated dental instruments as discussed above.[92,94,124]

Mercury (see also Chapter 3)
Very occasionally, clinical dental staff develop clinical contact allergy

to mercury. In view of public anxiety, partly fanned by unscrupulous practitioners, about mercury poisoning or mercury 'allergy', it is important to distinguish the genuine risk of contact sensitivity from more nebulous hazards. The latter include various vague neurological symptoms such as undue fatigue, lassitude or depression and weakness, which are ascribed to 'allergy' to mercury in dental amalgams. There has been no objective evidence of reactions of this type and no relationship has been demonstrated with contact hypersensitivity.

Contact hypersensitivity to mercury consists of an inflammatory and sometimes vesiculating reaction of the skin when exposed to mercury or its salts. However, personal experience has shown that even those patients who can be demonstrated objectively to react to mercury in this way can tolerate amalgams in the mouth provided no mercury comes into contact with their skin. Nevertheless, in patients genuinely sensitive to mercury it is usually simpler to use composite materials.

Contact hypersensitivity to mercury is remarkably rare among clinical dental staff,[125,126] but if it develops, it could be troublesome. The routine use of gloves and coverage of the arms during preparation and insertion of amalgams should obviate such reactions.

Organic chemicals such as in epimines or some impression materials
Methyl dichlorobenzene sulphonate (in Impregum) and methyl p-toluene sulphonate (in Scutan) are examples.[126–130] Chlorhexidine occasionally causes contact dermatitis or even rare severe allergies.[117,131–134] Glutaraldehyde may cause direct or allergic skin irritation[135–137] and has produced contact dermatitis in dental surgery assistants.[135]

Many organic solvents and thinners[94]
Various organic solvents can cause dermatitis.

Latex gloves
Fortunately, allergy to these is very rare! (*see* Chapter 5).

X-ray processing chemicals
Dermatitis can result from contact with various constituents of x-ray processing chemicals (Table 2.6).

Other agents
Very rarely, dentists have reacted to the cosmetics or hair dyes of

Table 2.6 Constituents of some x-ray processing solutions

Fixer	Ammonium thiosulphate
	Acetic acid
	Boric acid
	Sulphuric acid
	Aluminium sulphate
	Acetic acid
	Tartaric acid
Developer	Hydroquinone
	Potassium hydroxide
	Acetic acid
	Ethanediol
	Phenylpyrazolidone
	Glutaraldehyde
	Bisulphite
Starter	Acetic acid
	Inorganic bromide
Screen cleaner	Isopropanol

their patients.[138] Other materials that may produce dermatitis include hexachlorophane, benzalkonium chloride, formaldehyde, alcohols and fibreglass products.[139]

It has been suggested that up to one third of dental staff suffer from contact allergies,[140] but this is not evident in Britain, at least in our experience.

'Dry hand' syndrome

Frequent washing of the hands and handling plaster of Paris may produce dryness and cracking of the skin.[116]

Local neurotoxicity ('white hand' syndrome)

Methyl methacrylate may produce numbness or paraesthesia of the fingers and palms, with pain and whitening in the cold, possibly due to local neurotoxicity as a result of monomer penetrating the skin.[118,141,142]

Prevention of skin disorders

The Health and Safety Executive (HSE) have recently produced a guidance leaflet *'Save your skin'*, available from the Dermatitis

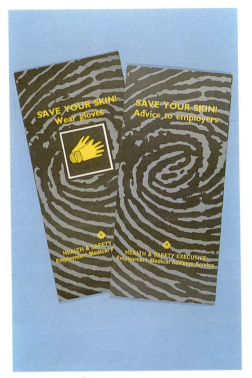

Fig. 2.10　Guide to skin care from the Health and Safety Executive.

Campaign Secretariat, HSE, Room 141, Magdalen House, Trinity Road, Bootle, L20 3QZ (fig. 2.10).

Direct contact with infective material, chemicals and drugs should be minimised and gloves worn wherever possible (*see also* Chapter 5). Disposable latex and vinyl gloves are most commonly used for clinical work, while polymer (especially polyethylene) gloves are needed for some laboratory work. Heavy duty rubber gloves should be worn at other times, except when fire-resistant gloves are more appropriate. Areas of skin which have been exposed to chemicals should be washed liberally in tap water or a suitable neutralising agent (Table 2.7).

Latex gloves protect against many physical, chemical and microbial agents, but they will not, of course, prevent puncture injuries and do not completely prevent penetration of some organic solvents such as methyl methacrylate monomer.[141] It is possible that there is a small amount of monomer penetration of polyethylene gloves during the short period of mixing acrylic[116] and, for clinical work, butyl rubber

46   OCCUPATIONAL HAZARDS TO DENTAL STAFF

Table 2.7 Hand care in dentistry

	Use	Comment
Wash hands thoroughly	At beginning of the day; before gloving for dental treatment; between patients; for breaks; upon return to work; before leaving at the end of the day.	Use an antimicrobial chlorhexidine handwash preparation such as Hibisol or Hibiscrub.
	After touching objects likely to be contaminated with saliva or blood.	Use an antimicrobial handwash preparation as above. Change gloves for next patient.
	After contact with chemicals.	Wash with soap and liberal water.
	When gloves have been torn, punctured or cut.	Remove gloves as soon as possible without compromising patient's or operator's safety. Use an antimicrobial scrub and reglove before proceeding with treatment.
		Dry hands using disposable paper towels and discard after use, or use an electric hand dryer. Cloth towels should be used only once and then discarded into a laundry or disposal bag.
Wear protective latex or vinyl gloves	In all clinical procedures and when touching contaminated instruments or appliances.	*See* Chapter 5
Wear fire-resistant gloves	When handling very hot materials.	

gloves seem less pervious.[143] Other methods used to reduce exposure to monomer in the laboratory also include a protective monoglyceride skin ointment, changing to an injection moulding technique for denture flask packing, or using a no-touch technique.

Gloves must be worn by all staff handling teeth, mucous membranes, saliva, blood and pathology specimens, or instruments or appliances that have been in contact with these (*see* Chapter 5). Gloves vary in the proportion that contain punctures, even when new, and in their durability. Most can be re-used if the external surface is cleaned with an antiseptic such as chlorhexidine or povidone–iodine, which fairly effectively removes microbial contaminants, but fresh gloves should be used for each patient in clinical practice (Chapter 5).

Other systems

Kidneys
In one recent study clinical dental staff were frequently shown to have proteinuria. This may be related to exposure to mercury or other potentially nephrotoxic agents,[144] or to standing posture, but this has yet to be confirmed.

Liver, brain and bone marrow
Liver function may be impaired by alcohol (Chapter 1) or exposure to halothane and other agents; cerebral function can be affected by mercury and inhalational anaesthetic agents, and bone marrow function by nitrous oxide (Chapter 3).

Cardiovascular system
One study of US dentists attending a meeting, showed that 20–30% had blood pressures higher than those of comparable ages in the general population, but it could be argued that the setting in which the measurements were taken was somewhat unusual.[145] As discussed above, although another study showed no increase in cardiovascular disease, this proves to be a major cause of mortality among dentists (Chapter 1).

Gastrointestinal tract
A study of Italian dentists showed that over one third suffered from gastrointestinal complaints (mainly peptic ulcers), and that haemorrhoids were fairly common.[146]

In contrast, a study of American dentists showed no increased incidence of gastrointestinal, rheumatic or cardiovascular disease.[147] As mentioned in Chapter 1, most dental staff in the West suffer less occupational illness than other health care workers, or individuals of similar socioeconomic status.

References

1   Eichner K. Investigation on cutting and grinding procedures on the hard tooth structure and ivory. *Aust Dent J* 1965; **10**: 214–216.
2   Cooley RL, Cottingham AJ Jr, Abrams H *et al*. Ocular injuries sustained in the dental office: Methods of detection, treatment and prevention. *J Am Dent Assoc* 1978; **97**: 985–988.
3   Cooley RL, Barkmeier WW. Prevention of eye injuries in the dental office. *Quintessence Int* 1981; **9**; 953.
4   Gennari U, Galli S. Le malattie professionali dei dentisti. *Rivista Ital Stomatol* 1971; **26**: 747–755.
5   Harley JL. Eye and facial injuries resulting from dental procedures. *Dent Clin North Am* 1978; **22**: 505–515.
6   Spealman CR, Main, RJ, Haag HB, Larson, PS. Monomeric methyl methacrylate—studies on toxicity. *Indust Med* 1945; **14**: 292–298.
7   Fauchard Academy Poll. Nearly a fourth have contracted illness as a result of practicing dentistry. *Dent Survey* 1965; **41**: 29.
8   Midulla M, Sollecito D, Fellepa F, Assensio AM, Ilari S. Infection by airborne *Chlamydia trachomatis* in a dentist cured with rifampicin. *Br Med J* 1987; **294**: 742.
9   Burns W. *Noise and man*. London: John Murray, 1973.
10   Code of Practice: Reducing the exposure of employed persons to noise. Department of the Environment, 1976.
11   International Organisation for Standardisation. Acoustics determination of occupational noise exposure and estimation of noise-induced hearing impairment. ISO/DIS 1999, 1982.
12   Lutman ME, Haggard MP. *Hearing science and hearing disorders*. London: Academic Press, 1983.
13   Zubick HH, Tolentino AT, Boffa J. Hearing loss and the high speed dental handpiece. *Am J Publ Health* 1980; **70**: 633–635.
14   Hopp ES. Acoustic trauma in high-speed dental drills. *Laryngoscope* 1962; **72**: 821–827.
15   Norman DH. A preliminary appraisal of an air-bearing handpiece. *Br Dent J* 1963; **114**: 90–92.
16   Cantwell KR, Tunturi AR, Sorenson FM. Noise levels of a newly designed handpiece. *J Prosthet Dent* 1965; **15**: 356–359.
17   Forman-Franco B, Abramson AL, Stein T. High-speed drill noise and hearing: audiometric survey of 70 dentists. *J Am Dent Assoc* 1978; **97**: 479–482.
18   Coles RRA, Hoare NW. Noise-induced hearing loss and the dentist. *Br Dent J* 1985; **159**: 209–218.
19   Smith AFJ, Coles RRA. Auditory discomfort associated with use of the air turbine dental drill. *J Roy Navy Med Serv* 1970; **15**: 259–260.
20   Taylor W, Pearson J, Mair A. The hearing thresholds of dental practitioners exposed to air turbine drill noise. *Br Dent J* 1965; **118**: 206–210.

21 Schubert ED, Bloomington I, Glorig A. Noise exposure from dental drills. *J Am Dent Assoc* 1963; **66**: 751–757.

22 Arentsschild, O, Eichner K. Untersuchungen zur Frage der Hörschaden bei Verwendung kugel-und luftgelagerter zahnarzlicher Turbinengerät. *Zahnarztl Rdschau* 1966; **6**: 217–223.

23 Ward WD, Holmberg CJ. Effects of high-speed drill noise and gunfire on dentists' hearing. *J Am Dent Assoc* 1969; **79**: 1383–1387.

24 Rahko AA-L, Karma PH, Rahko KT, Kataja MJ. High-frequency hearing of dental personnel. *Community Dent Oral Epidemiol* 1988; **16**: 268–270.

25 Praml GJ, Sonnabend E. Noise-induced hearing loss caused by dental turbines. *Deutsch Zahnarztl* 1980; **35**: 400–406.

26 Man A, Neuman H, Assif D. Effect of turbine dental drill noise on dentists' hearing. *Israeli J Med Sci* 1982; **18**: 475–477.

27 Skurr BA, Bulteau VG. Dentists' hearing: the effect of high speed drill. *Aust Dent J* 1970; **15**: 259–260.

28 Roberts ME. Report of a hearing survey of dentists. *J Canad Dent Assoc* 1976; **44**: 110–113.

29 Weatherton MA, Melton RE, Burns WW. The effects of dental drill noise on the hearing of dentists. *J Tennessee Dent Assoc* 1972; **52**: 305–308.

30 Keller J, Olk E, Opitz J. Untersuchungen über den Einfluss der Turbinengerausche in der zahnarztlichen Praxis auf das Hörvermögen. *Z Laryngol Rhinol* 1964; **43**: 680–690.

31 Lumio JS, Aho J, Lehtinen PV. Ist der durch Zahnturbinenbohrer verursachte Lärm für das Gehör gefährlich? *Monatsschr Ohrenheilkd* 1965; **99**: 192–199.

32 Yrjonheikki E, Anttonen H, Hassi J. Exposure of dental personnel to mercury and noise. *Proc Finn Dent Soc* 1980; **76**: 30–34.

33 Kamal SA. Orthopaedic theatres: a possible noise hazard? *J Laryngol Otol* 1982; **96**: 985–990.

34 Moller P, Grevstad AO, Kristofferson T. Ultrasonic scaling of maxillary teeth causes tinnitus and temporary hearing shifts. *J Clin Periodontol* 1976; **3**: 123–127.

35 Walmsley AD, Hickson FS, Laird WRE, Williams AR. Investigation into patient's hearing following ultrasonic scaling. *Br Dent J* 1987; **162**: 221–225.

36 Grundy JR. Enamel aerosols created during use of the air turbine handpiece. *J Dent Res* 1967; **46**: 409.

37 Travaglini EA, Larato DC, Martin A. Dissemination of organism-bearing droplets by high-speed dental drills. *J Prosthet Dent* 1966; **16**: 132–139.

38 Micik RE, Miller RL, Mazzarella MA. Studies on dental aerobiology. (1) Bacterial aerosols generated during dental procedures. *J Dent Res* 1969; **48**: 49.

39 Madden RM, Hausler W, Leaverton P. Study of some factors contributing to aerosol production by the air turbine handpiece. *J Dent Res* 1969; **48**: 341.

40 Timbrell V, Eccles JD. The respirability of aerosols produced in dentistry. *J Dent* 1973; **12**: 21.

41 Holbrook WP, Muir KF, MacPhee IT, Ross PW. Bacteriological investigation of the aerosol from ultrasonic scalers. *Br Dent J* 1978; **144**: 245.

42 Muir KF, Ross PW, MacPhee IT, Holbrook WP, Kowolik MJ. Reduction of microbial contamination from ultrasonic scalers. *Br Dent J* 1978; **145**: 76.

43 Larato DC, Ruskin PF, Martin A. Effects of a dental air turbine drill on the bacterial counts in air. *J Periodontol* 1967; **38**: 550.

44 McEntegart MC, Clark A. Colonization of dental units by water bacteria. *Br Dent J* 1973; **134**: 140.

45 Fitzgibbon EJ, Bartzokas CA, Martin MV, Gibson MF, Graham R. The source, frequency and extent of bacterial contamination of dental unit water systems. *Br Dent J* 1984; **157**: 98–101.

46   Blake GC. The incidence and control of bacterial infection in dental spray reservoirs. *Br Dent J* 1963; **115**: 413–416.
47   Kellett M, Holbrook WP. Bacterial contamination of dental handpieces. *J Dentistry* 1980; **8**: 249–253.
48   Murray JP, Slack GL. Some sources of bacterial contamination in everyday dental practice. *Br Dent J* 1957; **102**: 172–174.
49   Grun VL, Crott K. Ueber den keingehalt des Türbinen sprays. *Dtsch Zahnarztl* 1969; **24**: 189–193.
50   Neff JH, Rosenthal SL. A possible means of inadvertent transmission of infection to dental patients. *J Dent Res* 1957; **36**: 932–934.
51   Abel LC, Miller RL, Micik RE, Ryge G. Studies on dental aerobiology. IV. Bacterial contamination of water delivered by dental units. *J Dent Res* 1971; **50**: 1567–1569.
52   Clark A. Bacterial colonization of dental units and the nasal flora of dental personnel. *Proc Roy Soc Med* 1974; **67**: 1269–1270.
53   Gross A, Devine MJ, Cutright DE. Microbial contamination of dental units and ultrasonic scalers. *J Periodontol* 1976; **47**: 670–673.
54   Kelstrup J, Funder-Nielsen TD, Theilade J. Microbial aggregate contamination of water lines in dental equipment and its control. *Acta Pathol Microbiol Scand* 1977; Section B **85**: 177–183.
55   Dayoub ME, Rusilko DJ, Gross A. A method of decontamination of ultrasonic scalers and high speed handpieces. *J Periodontol* 1978; **49**: 261–265.
56   Bagga BSR, Murphy RA, Anderson AW, Punwani I. Contamination of dental unit cooling water with oral microorganisms and its prevention. *J Am Dent Assoc* 1984; **109**: 712–716.
57   Martin, MV. The significance of the bacterial contamination of dental water systems. *Br Dent J* 1987; **163**: 152–154.
58   Fiehn N-E. Bacterial contamination of water systems in dental units. *Danish Dent J* 1987; **91**: 755–760.
59   Shreeve WB, Tow HD. Bacteriological and serological surveillance of dentists exposed to dental aerosols. *Bull Tokyo Dent Col* 1981; **22**: 151.
60   Basu MK, Browne RM, Potts AJ. A survey of aerosol-related symptoms in dental hygienists. *J Soc Occup Med* 1988; **38**: 23–25.
61   Sande MA, Gadot F, Wenzel RP. Point source epidemic of *Mycoplasma pneumoniae* infection in a prosthodontics laboratory. *Am Rev Resp Dis* 1975; **112**: 213–217.
62   Reinthaler F, Masher F. *Legionella pneumophila* in dental units. *Zbl Bakt Hyg* B 1986; **183**: 86–88.
63   Fiehn N-E, Henriksen K. Methods of disinfection of the water system of dental units by water chlorination. *J Dent Res* 1988; **67**: 1499–1504.
64   Mills, SE, Lauderdale, PW, Mayhew, RB. Reduction of microbial contamination in dental units with povidone–iodine 10%. *J Am Dent Assoc* 1986; **113**: 280–284.
65   Glazebrook GA. Occupational nasal carcinogenesis among dentists? *Cancer Detect Prev* 1981; **4**: 31–40.
66   Rom WN, Lockey JE, Lee JS, Kimball AC, Bang KM, Leaman H, Johns RE Jr, Perrota D, Gibbons HL. Pneumoconiosis and exposures of dental laboratory technicians. *Am J Publ Health* 1984; **74**: 1252.
67   Leading Article. Lung disease in dental laboratory technicians. *Lancet* 1985; **1**: 1200–1201.
68   Mench HR, Henderson BE. Occupational differences in lung cancer. *J Occup Med* 1976; **18**: 797–801.
69   Lozewicz S, Davison AG, Hopkirk A, Burge PS, Boldy LA, Riordan JF,

McGivern DV, Platts BW, Davies D, Newman Taylor AJ. Occupational asthma due to methyl methacrylate and cyanoacrylates. *Thorax* 1985; **40**: 836.

70 HSE guidance note EH 44. Dust in the workplace: general principles of protection. ISBN: 0–11–883598–X, 1984.

71 Brune D, Belteskrekke. Dust in dental laboratories. Types and levels in specific operations. *J Prosthet Dent* 1980; **43**: 687–692.

72 Kronenberg H, Morgenroth K, Tuengerthal S *et al*. Pneumoconiosis of a dental technician's collective. *Atemwegs und Lungenkrankheiten* 1980; **6**: 279–282.

73 Kronenberger H, Kappos AD, Muller J, Meier-Sydow J. Lung function in dental technicians in comparison to occupationally non-exposed controls. *Am Rev Resp Dis* 1984; **129**: 179.

74 Morgenroth K, Schneider M, Kronenberger H. Histologic features and x-ray microanalysis in pneumoconiosis of dental technicians. *Am Rev Resp Dis* 1981; **123**: 127 (abstract).

75 Lob M, Hugonnaud C. Risks of pneumoconiosis by hard metal and of berylliosis for dental technicians. *Arch Mal Prof* 1977; **38**: 543–549.

76 Huggonaud C, Lob M. Risks encountered by dental technicians during manufacture of metallic prostheses. *Med Soc Prev* 1976; **21**: 139.

77 Carlos P, Fabre J, Pujol M, Duprez A, Bollinelli R. Complex pneumoconioses of dental technicians. *Le Poumon et le Coeur* 1978; **34**: 189–192.

78 Peltier PA, Moulut JC, Demange M. The risk of pneumoconiosis for dental technicians. *Rev Fr Prosthes Dent* 1980; **249**: 60–63.

79 De Vuyst P, Vande Weyer R, De Coster A *et al*. Dental technicians' pneumoconioses: a report of two cases. *Am Rev Resp Dis* 1986; **133**: 316–320.

80 Rom WM, Lockey JE, Lee JS, Kimball, AC, Bang M, Leaman H, Johns RE Jr, Perrota, D, Gibbons HL. Pneumoconiosis and exposures of dental laboratory technicians. *Am J Public Health* 1984; **74**: 1252–1257.

81 Sherson D, Maltbaek N, Olsen O. Small opacities among dental laboratory technicians in Copenhagen. *Br J Industr Med* 1988; **45**: 320–324.

82 Leclerc P, Fiessinger J-N, Capron F, Ameille J, Rochenmaure J. The Erasmus syndrome in a dental technician: value of prevention of occupational diseases. *Ann Med Int* 1983; **134**: 653–655.

83 Hansen HM. A dental technician with silicosis. *Ugeskr Laeger* 1983; **145**: 2378–2379.

84 Briotet A, Magrex LL, Parant C *et al*. The risk of silicosis among dental technicians. *Arch Mal Prof Med Trav Sec Soc* 1979; **40**: 122–123.

85 Brune D, Beltesbrekke H, Melson S. Dust in workroom air of dental laboratories. *Swed Dent J* 1981a; **5**: 247–251.

86 Brune D, Beltesbrekke H. Levels of methylmethacrylate, formaldehyde and asbestos in dental workroom air. *Scand J Dent Res* 1981b; **89**: 113–116.

87 Hinmann RV, Lynde TA, Pelleu CB, Gaugler RW. Factors affecting airborne beryllium concentrations in dental spaces. *J Prosthet Dent* 1975; **33**: 210–215.

88 Council on Dental Materials, Instruments and Equipment. Report on base metal alloys for crown and bridge applications: benefits and risks. *J Am Dent Assoc* 1985; **111**: 479–483.

89 Priest G, Horner JA. Fibrous ceramic aluminium silicate as an alternative to asbestos liners. *J Prosthet Dent* 1980; **44**: 51–56.

90 Davis DR. Potential health hazards of ceramic ring lining material. *J Prosthet Dent* 1987; **57**: 362–369.

91 International Agency for Research on Cancer. IARC Monographs on the evaluation of carcinogenic risk of chemicals to man. *Some Metals and Metallic Compounds* 1980; **23**: 205–323.

92   Franz G. The frequency of allergy to dental materials. *J Dent Assoc South Afr* 1982; **37**: 805.
93   McCabe JF, Wilson SJ, Wilson HJ. Cadmium in denture base materials. *Br Dent J* 1978; **144**: 167.
94   Adams RM. *Occupational skin disease.* New York: Grune and Stratton, 1983.
95   Pickering GA, Bainbridge D, Birtwhistle IH, Griffiths DL. Occupational asthma due to methyl methacrylate in an orthopaedic theatre sister. *Br Med J* 1986; **292**: 1362–1363.
96   Waclawski ER, McAlpine LG, Thomson NC. Occupational asthma in nurses caused by chlorhexidine and alcohol aerosols. *Br Med J* 1989; **298**: 929–930.
97   Benson WG. Exposure to glutaraldehyde. *Soc Occup Med* 1984; **34**: 63–64.
98   Corrado OJ, Osman J, Davies RJ. Asthma and rhinitis after exposure to glutaraldehyde in endoscopy units. *Hum Toxicol* 1986; **5**: 325–327.
99   Burge PS. Occupational risks of glutaraldehyde. *Br Med J* 1989; **299**: 342.
100   Schwettmann RS, Casterline CL. Delayed asthmatic response following occupational exposure to enflurane. *Anesthesiology* 1976; **44**: 166–169.
101   Vrijhoef MMA, Lourens FL, Setcos JC, Phillips RW. Dust formation of alginate impression materials. *Quintessence Int* 1983; **6**: 665–670.
102   Soremark R, Wiktorsson G, Forberg S, Ekenback, J. Bly i Alginat. *Tandlae Kartindingen* 1974; **66**: 241–244.
103   Mjor IA. Blood Pb analysis and alginate impression materials. *Scand J Dent Res* 1974; **82**: 401–402.
104   Mack PJ. Inhalation of alginate powder during spatulation. *Br Dent J* 1979; **146**: 141–143.
105   Stanton MF. Fibre carcinogenesis: is asbestos the only hazard? *J Nat Cancer Inst* 1974; **52**: 633–634.
106   Brune D, Beltesbrekke H. Levels of airborne particles resulting from handling alginate impression materials. *Scand J Dent Res* 1978; **86**: 206–210.
107   Knibbs PJ, Piney MD. An assessment of the relative dustiness of different alginate impression materials under simulated working conditions. *Br Dent J* 1985; **158**: 171.
108   Nixon GS, Tilston DR. Inhalation of oil particles from air turbine handpieces. *Br Dent J* 1965; **119**: 114–117.
109   Fischbein A, Chuang MT, Suzuki Y, Rohl A. Progressive dyspnoea and diffuse pulmonary nodules in a dentist: a diagnostic dilemma. *Mount Sinai J Med* 1978; **45**: 79–795.
110   Schwartz BS, Doty RL, Monroe C, Frye R, Barker S. Olfactory function in chemical workers exposed to acrylate and methacrylate vapours. *Am J Publ Health* 1989; **79**: 613–618.
111   Rogers KB. An investigation into the efficiency of disposable face masks. *J Clin Pathol* 1980; **33**: 1086.
112   Foad T, Sellen P. Keeping one's nose clean. *Dent Tech* 19–20, 1988.
113   Bleicher JN, Blinn DL, Massop D. Hand infections in dental personnel. *Plast Reconstruct Surg* 1987; **80**: 420–422.
114   Zingsheim M. Occupational dermatosis and eczema on the hands of dentists. *Deutsch Zahnarztl Z* 1958; **13**: 241–244.
115   Jobling AP. Contact allergy, the dental surgeon and his patient. *Br Dent J* 1982; **153**: 59–64.
116   Estlander T, Rajaniemi R, Jolanki R. Hand dermatitis in dental technicians. *Contact Derm* 1984; **10**: 201–205.
117   Rudzki E, Rebandel P, Grzywa Z. Patch tests with occupational contactants in nurses, doctors and dentists. *Contact Derm* 1989; **20**: 247–251.
118   Fries IB, Fisher AA, Salvati EA. Contact dermatitis in surgeons from methylmethacrylate bone cement. *J Bone Joint Surg* 1975; **57**: 547–549.

119   Fregert S. Occupational hazards of acrylate bone cement in orthopaedic surgery. *Acta Orthopaed Scand* 1983; **54**: 787–789.
120   Riva F, Pigatto PD, Altomare GF, Riboldi A. Sensitization to dental acrylic compounds. *Contact Derm* 1984; **10**: 245–255.
121   Spiechowicz E. Experimental studies on the effect of acrylic resin on rabbit skin. *Berufsdermatosen* 1971; **19**: 132–144.
122   Kanerva L, Estlander T, Jolanki R. Allergic contact dermatitis from dental composite resins due to aromatic epoxy acrylates and aliphatic acrylates. *Contact Derm* 1989; **20**: 201–211.
123   Nyquist G, Koch G, Magnusson B. Contact allergy to medicaments and materials used in dentistry (III). *Odontol Revy* 1972; **23**: 197–204.
124   Newman SM. The relationship of metals to the general health of the patient, the dentist and office staff. *Int Dent J* 1986; **36**: 35–40.
125   White RR, Brandt RL. Development of mercury hypersensitivity among dental students. *J Am Dent Assoc* 1976; **92**: 1204–1207.
126   Frykholm KO. On mercury from dental amalgam. Its toxic and allergic effects and some comments on occupational hygiene. *Acta Odontol Scand* 1957; **15**: 22.
127   Nally FF, Storrs J. Hypersensitivity to a dental impression material: A case report. *Br Dent J* 1973; **134**: 244–246.
128   Duxbury AJ, Turner EP, Watts DC. Hypersensitivity to epimine containing materials. *Br Dent J* 1979; **147**: 331–333.
129   Lui JL. Hypersensitivity to a temporary crown and bridge material. *J Dent* 1979; **7**: 22–24.
130   Kulenkamp D, Hausen BM, Schultz KH. Kontaktallergie durch neuartige, zahnarztlich verwendete Abdruck-materialen. *Hautarzt* 1977; **28**: 353–358.
131   Osmundsen PE. Contact dermatitis to chlorhexidine. *Contact Derm* 1982; **8**: 81–83.
132   Ljunnggren B, Moller H. Eczematous contact allergy to chlorhexidine. *Acta Dermatol Venereol* 1972; **52**: 308–310.
133   Cheung J. O'Leary JJ. Allergic reaction to chlorhexidine in an anaesthetised patient. *Anaesth Intensive Care* 1985; **13**: 429–430.
134   Bergqvist-Karlsson A. Delayed and immediate-type hypersensitivity to chlorhexidine. *Contact Derm* 1988; **18**: 84–88.
135   Nethercott JR, Holness DL, Page E. Occupational contact dermatitis due to glutaraldehyde in health care workers. *Contact Derm* 1988; **18**: 193–196.
136   Norback D. Skin and respiratory symptoms from exposure to alkaline glutaraldehyde in medical services. *Scand J Work Env Health* 1988; **14**: 366–371.
137   Jackuck SJ, Bound CL, Steel J, Blain PG. Occupational hazard in hospital staff exposed to 2% glutaraldehyde in an endoscopy unit. *J Soc Occup Med* 1989; **39**: 69–71.
138   Hindson C. O Nitro-paraphenylene diamine in hair dye: an unusual dental hazard. *Contact Derm* 1975; **1**: 333.
139   Fisher AA. Contact dermatitis in medical and surgical personnel. *In* Maibach, HI, Gellin GA (eds). *Occupational and industrial dermatology*. pp 219–228. London: Year Book Publishers, 1982.
140   Djerassi E, Berowa N. Contact allergy in stomatology as an occupational problem. *Berufsdermatosen* 1966; **14**: 225.
141   Seppalainen AM, Rajaniemi R. Local neurotoxicity of methyl methacrylate among dental technicians. *Am J Industrial Med* 1984; **5**: 471–477.
142   Pegum JS, Medhurst FA. Contact dermatitis from penetration of rubber gloves by acrylic monomer. *Br Med J* 1971; **2**: 141–143.
143   Darre E, Vedel P. Surgical rubber gloves impervious to methyl methacrylate monomer. *Acta Orthopaed Scand* 1984, **55**: 254–255.
144   Verschoor MA, Herver RFM, Zielhuis RL. Urinary mercury levels and early

changes in kidney function in dentists and dental assistants. *Community Dent Oral Epidemiol* 1988; **16**: 148–152.
145 Cutright D, Carpenter W, Tsaknis P, Lyon T. Survey of blood pressure of 856 dentists. *J Am Dent Assoc* 1977; **94**: 918–919.
146 Gennari U, Galli S. Le malattie professionali dei dentisti. *Rivista Ital Stomatol* 1971; **26**: 821–840.
147 Austin LJ, Kruger GO. Common ailments of dentists. A statistical study. *J Am Dent Assoc* 1947; **35**: 797–805.

Norville Opticals: Magdala Road, Gloucester GL1 4DG.
Jencons Ltd: Cherrycourt Way Industrial Estate, Leighton Buzzard LU2 8UA.
Iles Optical Ltd: Walmgate Road, Perivale, Greenford, Middlesex UB6 7LG.
Coltene (UK) Ltd: Teknol House, Victoria Road, Burgess Hill, West Sussex.
BLC blue-light coating: Stiltint Ltd.
Guardian protective eye glasses: Laclede Professional Products, California, USA.
Topaz glasses: Davis, Schottlander and Davis, City Road, London EC1V 7LU.
Premier Cureshield: Austenal Dental, Harrow, Middlesex HA1 2HG.
Laser Bloc spectacles: Jencons, Cherrycourt Way Industrial Estate, Stanbridge Road, Leighton Buzzard LUZ 8UA.
Norton Sonic 11 ear protectors: Siebe Norton Inc., 16624 Edwards Road, Cerritos, California 90701, USA.
Gundefender: The Game Conservancy, Fordingbridge, Hants.
Ear plugs: EAR division, Cabot Safety Ltd, First Avenue Pynton, Stockport, Cheshire SK12 1YJ.
Conex Saeflo: Whitehall Road, Tipton, West Midlands DY4 7JU.
Zephyr face protector: Racal Ltd, Beresford Avenue, Wembley, Middlesex HA0 1QJ.

3

Physical and chemical dangers in dentistry

Some of the more common hazards in dentistry result from the use of sharp, rotating or hot instruments, exposure to various dusts, aerosols, chemicals and drugs, and poor posture. Serious injuries and accidents are, fortunately, uncommon. Needlestick injuries, with the possibility of serious infection, and eye injuries, with the possibility of damage to sight, are among the main dangers (fig. 3.1; *see* Chapters 2 and 5). Musculoskeletal complaints are not infrequent. Drug abuse is discussed in Chapters 1 and 7.

Fig. 3.1   Hazard warning signs relevant to dentistry.

Physical dangers and their avoidance

Accidents
British data on workplace accidents show that there were 1·6 reported fatal injuries at work per 100 000 employees in 1987–1988. There are

at least 95 reported serious injuries at work per 100 000 employees per year in the UK.[1] Non-fatal accidents are commonplace, but probably under-reported by a factor of about five. The highest injury rate is in the construction industry.

Accidents are common in dental premises, but many can be prevented by care and common sense (Table 3.1). A little thought about the design and furnishing of premises, especially flooring (Table 3.2), and thoughtful behaviour at work (such as not running), can prevent many accidents (*see below*, under Accident Notification). Non-slip flooring is needed, but carpeting should be avoided because of possible contamination with mercury and microorganisms. Much of the equipment used in dentistry constitutes some hazard to staff and sometimes to the patient. There are then also the risks of

Table 3.1 Twenty precautions to minimise accidents in the surgery and laboratory

(1) No unnecessary rushing about or horseplay.
(2) Safe paths and doors that are unobstructed by trailing wires or any other hazard.
(3) Well-lit, firm, secure and unobstructed passageways, steps and stairs that are cleaned daily.
(4) Clean, non-slip, secure floor surfaces with a minimum of joins.
(5) Furniture that is strong, safe and secured where necessary; staff should use appropriate steps or stepladders when reaching high objects.
(6) Fires, heaters, Bunsen burners, etc, must be guarded.
(7) Safe storage and correct labelling of flammables, explosives and toxic materials, including domestic bleach.
(8) Regular maintenance of all equipment, but especially autoclaves and compressors, because of the explosion hazard.
(9) Heat treatment and casting equipment should be housed adequately and tongs used for handling heated casting rings.
(10) Acid baths must be properly housed and protected.
(11) All electrical equipment must be installed, earthed, fused, and connected and maintained properly.
(12) Cables and tubing from electrical and other equipment must not trail on floor.
(13) All gas appliances should be installed, connected and maintained properly.
(14) Electrical, radiographic, general anaesthetic and gas appliances must be turned off out of working hours.
(15) Staff and others should avoid sharps injuries by using appropriate waste disposal.
(16) Staff should wear protective attire as appropriate.
(17) Staff must adhere to the safety policy.
(18) Staff must not smoke, eat or drink except in safe designated areas.
(19) Staff should know the hazards of, and preferably stop, smoking.
(20) Safety training and refresher courses should be taken by all appropriate staff.

Table 3.2 Characteristics of some non-carpet flooring materials

Type	Comment
Concrete	Dense and smooth. Very hard-wearing. Slip resistance improved if carborundum incorporated. Unaesthetic but can be tinted.
Concrete tiles	Similar to above but may be more attractive.
Terrazzo	Attractive, hard-wearing, easily cleaned but very slippery if wet or contaminated with soap or wax.
Ceramic	Attractive and hard-wearing but very slippery if wet. Ribbed or studded surfaces prevent slipping but make cleaning more difficult.
Epoxy resin	Not very hard-wearing unless additives included (eg bauxite). Addition of sand decreases slip. Not resistant to strong acids or solvents or heat.
PVC (thermoplastic or vinyl)	Water may seep through joins. Liable to scorch or show burn marks from hot substances. Grease and oil affect some types. Slippery when wet.
Cork	Attractive but damaged by high point loads such as chairs, high-heeled shoes. Porous unless sealed. Liable to damage from acids.
Wood	Requires regular maintenance and can easily be made slippery. Unsuitable where there is frequent wetting.
Linoleum	Best for places not liable to contamination with chemicals, oil or grease. Liable to curl at edges and to wear.
Rubber	Silent, warm, attractive surface but not suitable where there is underfloor heating or exposure to sunlight. Slippery when wet. Some types are attacked by solvents, oil or grease.
Granwood	Characteristics similar to wood. Attractive. May be damaged by acids, alkalis, oils or grease.
Megesite	Needs sealing. Not suitable where there is frequent wetting. Attractive surface finish like smooth concrete. *Not* affected by oils or grease, but damaged by acids or alkalis.

litigation (*see* Chapters 6 and 7). All equipment must therefore be carefully and regularly maintained.

Obvious dangers, apart from slipping, or tripping over objects such as carpet edges, wires and so on (figs 3.2 and 3.3), and the annoyance of hitting the head or face on the dental light (fig. 3.4), include trapping fingers or limbs when moving the dental chair, and damage from the drill or hot or sharp instruments (fig. 3.5). Injuries to the fingers or hands can be most incapacitating (fig. 3.6). The hands and eyes are especially vulnerable when needles, scalpels, wires or hot or rotating instruments are used. Discs should always be used with guards. Resheathing needles is particularly dangerous, and if a safe system cannot be used, they should be discarded into a special sharps container (*see* Chapter 5). The ends of wires should be held in mosquito forceps to avoid eye injuries, and wires should always be cut between forceps, lest the cut end shoots off and causes damage (fig. 3.7).

Eye injuries are potentially very disabling and, for this reason, staff and patients should always be protected with glasses or other eye

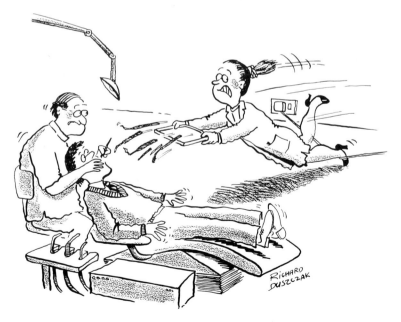

Fig. 3.2   Simple slips, trips and falls are the main physical dangers in dentistry.

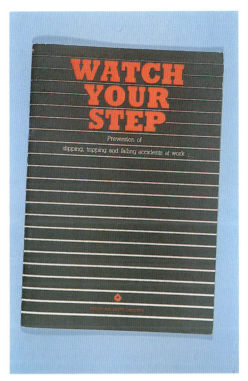

Fig. 3.3 Health and Safety Executive brochure on prevention of accidents at work.

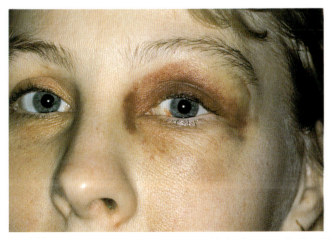

Fig. 3.4 A black eye in a dental surgery assistant hit by the arm of a dental light.

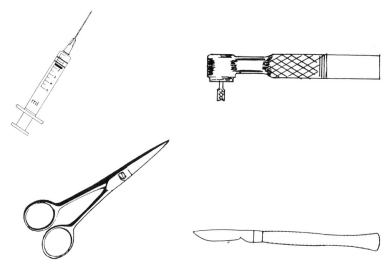

Fig. 3.5   Sharps hazards.

protection when procedures involve dental drills, grinding, polishing, or cutting wires (fig. 3.8 and Chapter 2). Projectiles can leave the mouth at speeds of over 10 metres per second when using drills at 250 000 rpm.[2] Half-glasses are not adequate protection. Patients, of course, should have adequate eye protection—particularly if treated in the supine position and for procedures under general anaesthesia (*see also* Chapter 2).

Accidents are more likely to happen when personnel are not concentrating on what they are doing or are distracted. A novel problem is that of radio headsets and overloud music, which isolate the wearer from the surrounding environment and have resulted in a number of accidents. Several health and safety organisations now recommend that radio headsets should not be worn in the workplace.[3]

Assaults

Occasionally dental staff, especially resident hospital staff, are the victims of assault, especially by psychiatrically disturbed patients or drug abusers. Many patients attending accident and emergency departments and dental casualty units have drunk too much alcohol.[4-6] Obviously, potentially dangerous incidents should be defused where possible, but this may be more easily said than done.

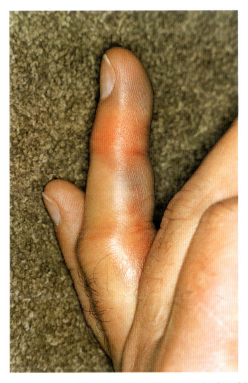

Fig. 3.6 Trauma to the fingers of dental staff can be incapacitating. Most is due to simple accidents but this was non-occupational—one of the authors went skiing (more hazardous than dentistry!).

Musculoskeletal complaints

Particularly in the past, dentists tended to develop musculoskeletal complaints,[7-9] probably as a result of poor working positions and possibly stress (Chapter 1). Only about 20% take regular exercise.[8] Between 30% and 88% of dentists complain of back pain[7-11] and this complaint is made by a similar proportion of hygienists.[11] Seated dentistry may have reduced this problem, since standing dentists adopted awkward postures for nearly 40% of the day, but many still adopt bad postures.[12] Dentistry is now one of the most sedentary occupations and many dentists and hygienists work in a somewhat hunched position. Although there appear to be few reliable objective studies of postural and skeletal problems in dental staff, one radio-

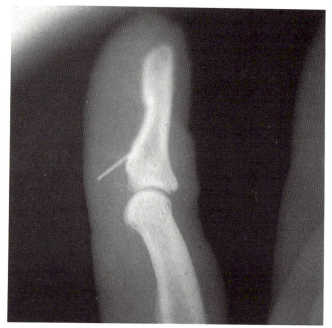

Fig. 3.7   Piece of wire in the finger of a consultant orthodontist. (Courtesy of Professor C. D. Stephens, N. Killingback, and the *British Journal of Orthodontics*.)

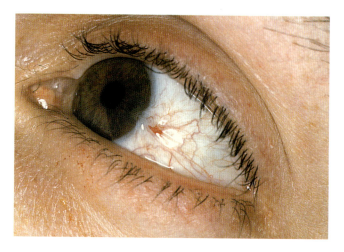

Fig. 3.8   Eye damage is a serious occupational hazard to all dental staff. Protective eyewear should be worn routinely (*see* Chapter 2).

graphic survey carried out in Finland showed cervical spondylosis in about 50% of dentists compared with about 20% of farmers of the same age. Dentists also had somewhat more radiographic changes in the shoulder joint, but less lumbar spondylosis.[13] Despite this, few dental staff need to take time off because of back or musculoskeletal pain[11] and back pain is not uncommon in non-dentists.

Guidelines for good seated posture during clinical dentistry include the following:[14]

(1) The feet should be flat on the floor.

(2) The angle between calf and thigh should be more than 90°, usually 90°–115°.

(3) The torso should be vertical.

(4) The patient's head should normally be at the operator's mid-chest height.

(5) Dentists should move about, and arch and straighten their backs from time to time.

(6) Awkward movements such as twisting should be avoided. Surgery layout is important.

It is highly advisable, therefore, to use comfortable and supportive seating and to take up physical leisure activities (unfortunately, golf is also a potential source of back injuries) and, at work, to take every opportunity to change posture and move about. Heavy equipment or material should be lifted correctly by all dental personnel.

Activities involving repetitive wrist and hand movements, especially in women, may result in oedema beneath the transverse carpal ligaments at the wrist. This can lead to compression of the median nerve and subsequent pain (especially at night), paraesthesia, hyperaesthesia and weakness in the wrist and hand (carpal tunnel syndrome). Although this is a not uncommon consequence of a variety of activities such as knitting or playing musical instruments, and is predisposed to by, for example, pregnancy and hypothyroidism, carpal tunnel syndrome has been reported in hygienists and endodontists especially.[15–17] Typists may also suffer from this condition. Interestingly, mechanical typewriters appear to cause fewer problems than electronic keyboards.

Symptoms and signs consistent with partial carpal tunnel syndrome have been noted in one quarter or more of hygienists in some surveys, but the diagnosis is made in only 1–6% of cases.[15–17] Complaints are more common, the more work that is done manually and the longer the hygienist has been in practice.

Rest and analgesics usually provide adequate relief but, occasion-ally, splinting or corticosteroid injections are required. Surgical decompression may be indicated for recalcitrant cases.

Fires and explosions (see also Chapter 6)

Official regulations govern fire precautions, but common sense, particularly in avoiding the use of naked flames and care in the use and storage of combustible materials, will prevent many fires. Human error is responsible for most fires and explosions (fig. 3.9). The main causes of fire in a practice or similar place are electrical faults (23%), cigarettes and matches (21%), incorrect use of flammable anaesthetic gases and vapour, oxygen and flammable fluids (Table 3.3) (19%), and non-electrical heating (11%)[18]. However, there are many other causes, including some lasers (Chapter 4). Asphyxia by smoke and

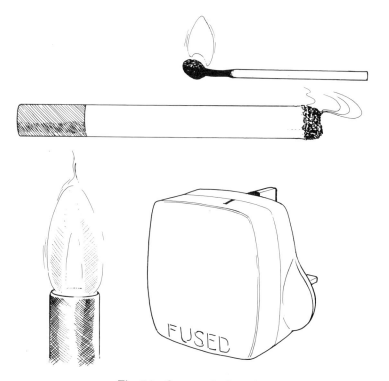

Fig. 3.9 Common fire hazards.

Table 3.3 Especially hazardous fluids that may be used in dentistry

Flammable
Acetone
Alcohols
   Ethyl alcohol
   Methyl alcohol
   Isopropyl alcohol
Benzene[a]
Butane
Ethers
Ethylene oxide[a]
Methyl methacrylate monomer
Propane
Toluene
Vapour sterilisers containing:
   Alcohols
   Acetone
   Methyl ethyl ketone

Acids	**Alkalis**
Chromic	Ammonium hydroxide
Hydrochloric	Sodium hydroxide
Hydrofluoric	Sodium hypochlorite
Nitric	
Phosphoric	
Sulphuric	
Trichloroacetic	

Other dangerous fluids
Carbon tetrachloride[a]
Chloroform[a]
Methylene chloride

[a]Possible carcinogens.

fumes, and poisoning by toxic gases such as cyanide from plastic foam upholstery account for most subsequent morbidity and mortality.[18]

All pressure vessels, including autoclaves, must be regularly maintained. Gas cylinders should be securely stored so that they cannot fall, in a room separate from any flammable materials (*see* below and Chapter 6).

For this, and other health reasons, smoking should, if possible, be forbidden in all parts of the practice and laboratory.

Autoclaves can be an explosive risk if the door is not secured or maintained properly. The Dentists Provident Society (*see* p. 98) can arrange regular autoclave examinations through Ajax Engineering Policies at Lloyds. Laboratory and surgery compressors can be similarly covered. Compressors should be serviced regularly and must be checked every 26 months (*see* p 249).

Electrical accidents

The Electricity at Work Regulations (1989) cover supply and use of electricity (*see* Chapter 6). Electrical equipment must be safely installed and maintained. Equipment must be switched off before repairs are carried out, and at night.

Measures needed to reduce electrical accidents are the same as those used in the home. These are (1) instruction of personnel in the correct use of equipment; (2) frequent periodic maintenance of apparatus and wiring; (3) earthing of all apparatus; (4) the separation of mains circuits; (5) the use of earth leakage circuit breakers; and (6) not touching electrical equipment with wet hands.

A far more trivial but probably more frequent cause of electrical shocks is the large static charge generated when personnel wear non-conductive footwear and/or nylon overalls in a dry atmosphere. This can lead to arcing, which may startle the person and cause, in turn, another, unrelated, accident. Furthermore, static discharges in areas where there are flammable vapours such as operating theatres have caused serious explosions and deaths. To prevent this, both the flooring and footwear should be conductive. Where this is difficult, floors should be of wood, footwear of antistatic rubber, and clothing of cotton, polyester or polyamide materials.

Heat burns

In dentistry, obvious but avoidable causes of heat burns are instruments just removed from the autoclave or hot air oven. This is often the result of difficulty in gauging their temperature through the rubber gloves that all staff should wear in the clinic. Extraction forceps, elevators and metal mouth gags, in particular, retain heat for many minutes and have caused burns to staff and severe orofacial burns to patients.

High-speed handpieces, if the water-cooling is working efficiently, cannot cause burns but, if not cooled, they can overheat and burn the patient's mouth. Hot wax knives and Bunsen burners are often causes of burns, and long hair and gloves or clothing can catch light in a Bunsen flame. Hot air blowers can obviate this danger, although they take somewhat longer to heat objects (fig. 3.10). One versatile type of flameless wax knife/hot air blower is the Portasol Professional, which

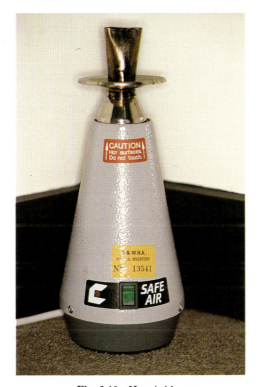

Fig. 3.10 Hot air blower.

runs off a standard gas lighter butane refill. Burns from the melting and casting of alloys can be quite severe.

Other possible causes of thermal burns include hot gutta-percha, hot dental composition, hot wax, boiling water, steam, naked flames, flammable or explosive fluids, lasers or diathermy and even operating lights.[19] Fluid heated in a microwave oven may be hotter than it appears as the container remains cooler.[20] Lasers are rarely used in routine dental practice, but are considered in Chapter 4.

Diathermy is a form of high frequency electrical energy used either for local tissue warming or cutting. The principle of diathermy is that agitation of molecules by passing radio-frequency electrical current through tissue causes heating. The current density determines whether the heating is gentle and non-destructive (used, for example, in short-wave diathermy for physiotherapy), or so great that cell contents boil and explode with complete denaturation of the protein along the line of contact with the electrode. Short-wave diathermy has also occasionally been used for temporomandibular joint pain and to accelerate healing after oral surgery. For this purpose, relatively low-powered diathermy is used. This is restricted to the industrial, scientific and medical (ISM) frequency (27·12 MHz) to avoid interference with short-wave radio reception. Short-wave diathermy is safe provided that the power levels are restricted to avoid excessive temperature rises.

In dentistry, cutting diathermy units are available to provide about 70 watts of energy at 0·2–3·0 MHz for electrosurgery. The fine needle electrodes produce a high current density over a minute area, resulting in destruction of tissue. These electrodes are often unipolar. In this case the current path is completed by capacitative coupling between the diathermy unit and the patient. However, accidents have resulted from metallic parts of the dental chair becoming involved in the current path. The localised increase in current density can then cause superficial burns to the skin. Some serious accidents of this nature have also resulted from the use of diathermy units in operating theatres, where higher powers are used and the current path is normally completed by a large area electrode placed under the patient, to reduce the current density. The risk from such diathermy is that of superficial burning, should the current be misdirected, but any part of the body can be involved if the current density is high enough.

There is no evidence that exposure to electromagnetic radiation at these radio frequencies and power levels poses any other health hazard to normal persons, but some individuals fitted with cardiac pacemakers could be at risk (Chapter 4).

Cold burns

Cold burns are rare in dentistry, but spillage of liquid nitrogen is a problem attendant on the use of cryosurgical equipment.

Radiation burns

Radiation burns in association with diagnostic radiation are now unheard of, but burns may be caused by laser treatment. These hazards and those of ultraviolet and blue lights are discussed in Chapter 4.

Vibration injury

A case has been reported of sensory loss over the web between thumb and forefinger, presumably induced by the vibration from a dental air-rotor affecting the sensory nerves, in a dentist,[21] but this is a rare complication.

Chemical and other hazards

The Control of Substances Hazardous to Health (COSHH) Regulations (1988 SI No 1657) place specific obligations on employers and the self-employed, to control hazardous substances (figs 3.11 and 3.12; *see* Chapter 6). Such substances include 'any natural or artificial substance, whether it is in solid or liquid form or in the form of a gas or vapour (including microorganisms), which can constitute a

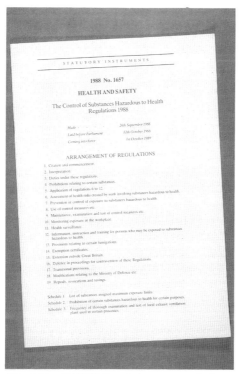

Fig. 3.11 COSHH Regulations are now in force.

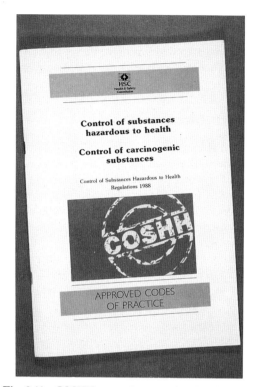

Fig. 3.12 COSHH notes of approved codes of practice.

hazard'. The Health and Safety Executive have produced a guide to COSHH (ISBN 011 885470 4) to complement the one brought out by the Health and Safety Commission (ISBN 011 885468 2).

In summary, employers must fulfil the following requirements and keep written records of their measures to:

(1) Assess health risks created by work involving substances hazardous to health. Assessment consists of gathering relevant information and drawing up an inventory of all hazardous substances on the premises and must take account of planned and unplanned (eg accidents) events. If the assessment shows no risk, the process is complete.

(2) Prevent or control exposure to substances hazardous to health.

(3) Provide and use control measures, personal protective equipment, etc, and take all reasonable steps to ensure that these are properly used or applied.

(4) Maintain control measures in an efficient state, in good working order and repair.

(5) Monitor exposure to substances hazardous to health.

(6) Provide suitable health surveillance where appropriate for the protection of all employees exposed to substances hazardous to health.

All employees, and so far as is reasonably possible, persons on the premises where the work is being carried out who may be exposed to substances hazardous to health, must be protected and properly informed, instructed and trained. Employees must take steps to protect themselves and others, must make full use of control measures and should immediately report any defects.

COSHH is enforced in the same way as the Health and Safety at Work etc Act or any other Regulations made under it (Chapter 6).

Product labels should be checked for details of hazards. Part IA1 of the Approved List for the Classification, Packaging and Labelling of Dangerous Substances Regulations (1984) (ISBN 011 8839012) lists very toxic, corrosive, harmful or irritant substances hazardous to health. All these come under COSHH.

Where work practices are poor, staff can be exposed to a wide range of noxious substances in the dental environment, including gases, vapours, liquids, fumes, dusts and solids (Tables 2.6, 3.4 and 3.5). Occupational exposure should be minimised wherever possible. Recommended limits for various hazardous substances used in the UK are laid down in Health and Safety Executive (HSE) guidance note EH 40/87 (1987), but it should be a fundamental principle to reduce exposure as much as possible by safe work practices (Table 3.6). In particular, this means storing materials in correctly labelled, appropriate, preferably unbreakable, containers, avoiding spills and splatter, avoiding contacts with eyes and skin, and washing away spilt material with running tap water.[22] Consideration should be given as to whether a hazardous substance can be substituted with an innocuous one.

Non-anaesthetic agents
Chemical burns
Chemical burns are all too common. Acids such as phosphoric acid, chromic acid and trichloroacetic acid, and corrosives such as paramonochlorphenol and sometimes even glutaraldehyde can cause burns to clinical dental staff. These chemicals have sometimes also been spilt

Table 3.4 Other dental chemicals that can pose a hazard

Substance	Contained in some	Substance	Contained in some
Acetic acid	Photographic solutions	Iodine	Iodophor
Acetone	Solvents		disinfectants,
Aluminium oxide	Polishing disks		dressings, hand cleansers
Asbestos	Casting ring liners	Isopropyl alcohol	Solvents, wiping agents
Benzoyl peroxide	Denture resins		
Beryllium	Casting alloys	Lead/inorganic lead compounds	Impression materials (polysulphides)
Calcium carbonate	Polishing agents		
		Mercury	Amalgam
Carbon tetrachloride	Solvents	Mercury, organic	Topical antiseptics
Chloroform	Solvents	Methyl acetate	Solvents
Chromic acid	Caustics	Methyl alcohol	Solvents
Chromium	Casting alloys	Methyl methacrylate	Denture base resins
Cobalt	Casting alloys		
Copper	Amalgam, casting alloys	Methylene chloride	Solvents
Cresol	Endodontic materials	Molybdenum	Casting alloys
Cyanide	Electroplating		
		Nickel	Casting alloys, stainless steel, orthodontic appliances
Dibutylphthalate	Impression materials Denture resins	Nitric acid	Pickling solutions, bleaching solutions
Ethyl acetate	Solvents		
Ethyl acrylate	Resins	Oils	Lubricants
Ethyl alcohol	Solvents		
Ethyl chloride	Solvents, topical refrigerants	Phenol	Disinfectants
Ethyl silicate	Silicate investments, impression materials (silicone)	Phosphoric acid	Etching agents, phosphate cements
		Phthalic anhydride	Resins
Ethylene oxide	Sterilising agents	Picric acid	Pickling agents
		Platinum	Impression materials (silicones), alloys
Fluoride	Composites, various fluorides		
Formaldehyde	Disinfectants	Rouge	Polishing agents
Glutaraldehyde	Disinfectants	Silica	Composites, impression materials
Hydrochloric acid	Pickling solutions, bleaching agents	Silicon carbide	Polishing disks, cutting wheels
Hydrofluoric acid	Etching agents for porcelain	Silver	Amalgam, endodontic points, casting alloys, photographic solutions
Hydroquinone	Denture base resins, photographic and x-ray solutions		

Table 3.4—*continued*

Substance	Contained in some	Substance	Contained in some
Sulphuric acid	Etchant for alloys, copper plating solutions	Uranium	Porcelain
		Vinyl chloride	Maxillofacial plastics
Talc	Gloves	X-ray processing chemicals	*See* Table 2.6
Tantalum	Casting alloys		
Tin	Amalgam, polishing pastes	Xylene	Solvents
Titanium dioxide	Porcelain, impression materials	Zirconium	Porcelain, polishing paste
Toluene	Solvents		
Trichloroethane	Solvents		

Table 3.5 Examples of possible levels of risk from dental substances[a]

Level of risk	More common examples	Comments in relation to COSHH
High	Virus-infected body fluids or tissues Laboratory acids (eg hydrofluoric, nitric, sulphuric and hydrochloric) Cyanide Disinfectants such as glutaraldehyde	This group includes substances with defined maximum exposure limits and others with an intrinsically high risk. Careful control measures are essential. Written assessment and staff instruction required
Lower	Inhalational anaesthetic agents Mercury Cleaning solutions (ultrasonic, etc) Radiographic solutions Acid-containing solutions (phosphoric, sulphuric, hydrochloric)	Less stringent control measures are required; written assessment, and staff instruction required
Virtually none	Most restorative dental materials Impression materials. Mouth rinses	Written assessment not required

[a] Relevant to COSHH regulations.

Table 3.6 Minimisation of risks from toxic materials

---

(1) Handle in accordance with manufacturer's instructions.[a]
(2) Avoid skin contact (consider wearing gloves).
(3) Where appropriate, wear protective eyewear and masks.
(4) Avoid spills and splatter. Ensure adequate ventilation of working area.
(5) Store material in sealed, correctly labelled containers. Do not leave bottles open.
(6) Do not eat, drink, or smoke in an area where a toxic material is used.
(7) Wash spills off skin with running water and wipe up other spills.
(8) Dispose carefully all toxic materials into the appropriate place.
(9) Ensure safety policy is in effect.
(10) Train staff in the risks and precautions to take.

---

[a]Suppliers are now obliged by law to provide information for safe use.

in patients' mouths, on their skin or eyes or, worse, have been accidentally injected. Many other, stronger acids and corrosives are used in dental practice, particularly in the laboratory. Hydrofluoric, sulphuric and nitric acids, and caustic soda are especially dangerous.[23] Such acids and pickling solutions should be stored safely in appropriate and clearly labelled containers, and with proper safety precautions (see below).

Flammable or explosive agents
Volatile, highly flammable liquids such as methyl methacrylate monomer, and gases such as oxygen are commonly used in dentistry. If they are not stored properly in a strong, correctly labelled container and are used near flames, a fire or explosion could result (see Health and Safety at Work etc Act, and Factories Act, Chapter 6). Some of the flammable liquids used in dentistry include those shown in Table 3.3. Fatal accidents have resulted from the misuse of these liquids in dentistry.

Chemical sterilisers
Although rarely used in British dental practice, chemical vapour and ethylene oxide sterilisers are also potential hazards. Chemical vapour sterilisers may use various alcohols, acetone and methyl ethyl ketone, which is a flammable mixture, particularly in vapour form. Flames or lighted cigarettes should therefore be kept well away from these sterilisers.

Ethylene oxide sterilisation is mainly used in hospital practice, to sterilise articles that must not be exposed to heat. This is a highly toxic, explosive and flammable gas and appropriate exhausting to the exterior is therefore needed; protective gloves and forceps should be used to handle sterilised equipment, since traces of ethylene oxide remain on material sterilised in this way. Ethylene oxide is highly dangerous, on either skin or eye contact or inhalation. Ethylene oxide may be neurotoxic and carcinogenic and there is therefore great interest in replacing it with alternative sterilising procedures, such as propyl oxide or gamma radiation.

Disinfectants
Glutaraldehyde and chlorhexidine are discussed in Chapter 2 and, with hypochlorite, in Chapter 5.

Solvents
Many alcohols, acetone, solvents and thinners are toxic and may be flammable. They can cause dermatitis, many are irritant to the eyes and respiratory tract and some are suspected carcinogens (Table 3.3 and 2.4). Chronic exposure to high levels of solvents may cause renal or liver damage and some, such as toluene, are teratogenic.[18]

Acrylic monomer is the most common organic solution used in dentistry. The main component of acrylic monomer is methyl methacrylate, but it may also contain other monomers such as N-butyl-methacrylate, isobutyl methacrylate, lauryl methacrylate, 1,4-butanediol dimethacrylate or ethylene glycol dimethacrylate. Polymerisation inhibitors such as hydroquinone, p-methoxyphenol or butylated cresols, plasticisers such as dibutyl phthalate, ultraviolet light absorbers such as benzophenone, and activators such as dimethyl-p-toluidine may also be found in some monomers.[24]

Methyl methacrylate and cyanoacrylate may be used for solvent abuse, but, in the absence of abuse, there is little evidence of a serious hazard if reasonable care is taken. Chemical hepatitis due to overexposure to methyl methacrylate monomer has been reported in one dentist.[25] Rarely, methyl methacrylate monomer and cyanoacrylate have induced occupational asthma or dermatitis.[26–28] Technicians using methyl methacrylate may notice symptoms and the monomer is absorbed through skin to some extent, even where 'protective' creams are used. Urine analysis shows low methacrylate levels in the morning, but clear evidence of absorption throughout the working day.[29–31] Methyl methacrylate is embryotoxic and foetotoxic to rats (as is toluene).[32,33] Therefore, although there is no evidence of such a danger to humans from methyl methacrylate, this should be borne in mind as a hazard, even if no more than a theoretical one, in the case of female dental technicians. There is no evidence of any permanent toxic or carcinogenic effects from methyl methacrylate monomer under conditions of normal use. It may cause transient nausea if inhaled in large quantities,[34] possibly by central depression of gastric motor function and, *rarely*, dyspnoea and hypertension.[35] It may also soften soft contact lenses.

Handling of methyl methacrylate may occasionally cause transient finger and palmar paraesthesia, pain and whitening of the fingers in the cold and local neurotoxicity and an eczema-like reaction.[36–38] Contact dermatitis as a result of handling methyl methacrylate monomer is also a possibility, but is surprisingly uncommon (Chapter 2). Unfortunately, many gloves are permeable to monomer, and barrier creams may impede the setting of acrylic (*see also* Chapters 2 and 5).

Methyl methacrylate monomer has a very low flash point (11°C) and this has resulted in at least one dental technician dying in an explosion. Exposure to acrylic monomer rarely presents serious hazards if used with reasonable care, but, nevertheless, it should be kept to a minimum by safe work practice. Acrylic should be mixed under a glass screen, with extraction (fig. 3.13) (eg Mix-Kit II or CMW mixing cabinet) and skin contact avoided or minimised.

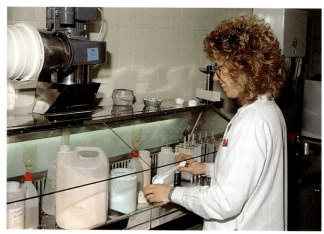

Fig. 3.13   Methyl methacrylate should be mixed under a glass plate with extraction.

Poisons

Many noxious substances are used in the clinic and laboratory (Tables 3.3 and 3.4). Cyanide in plating baths is probably the most lethal, but in the case of all poisons, great care should be taken to avoid inhalation, or contact with eyes or skin. All should be stored in appropriate and correctly labelled containers and kept safe from children (figs 3.14 and 3.15). Under the Medicines Act (1968), drugs must be kept in a locked receptacle.

X-ray processing chemicals

Developers for radiographs contain hydroquinone; fixatives contain acetic acid and sodium thiosulphate. These solutions should be handled carefully and with rubber gloves, avoiding contact with the eyes (it is best to wear protective eyewear) and avoiding excessive inhalation, since they can cause dermatitis, conjunctivitis or bronchitis (Tables 2.6, 3.5, 3.6).

Skin should never come into contact with processing fluids, and any spillages should be washed off immediately in running water. Spilt chemicals should be mopped up straight away.

Formaldehyde

Formaldehyde is used as a fixative for biopsy or surgical specimens, and has been used for disinfection and in some endodontic materials.

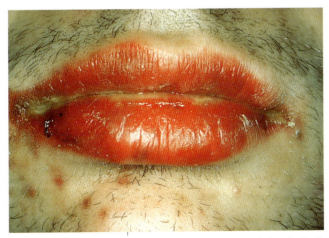

Fig. 3.14   A severe oral burn caused by drinking from a lemonade bottle that had been filled with a caustic.

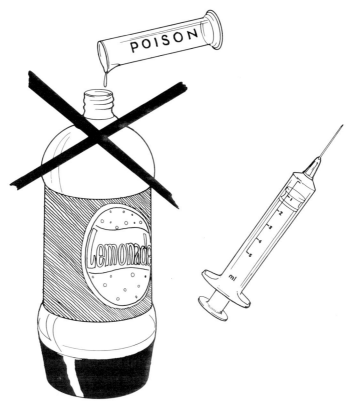

Fig. 3.15 Never fill the wrong or unlabelled bottles or syringes with poisons or corrosives.

Traces are found in some composite dental restorative materials. There are also non-medical sources such as in cigarette smoke, chipboard, plywood, carpet glues, and in foams such as urea-formaldehyde foams used for building insulation.

Formaldehyde is absorbed mainly through the respiratory and digestive systems and can cause ocular and respiratory irritation and dermatitis. Formaldehyde has been implicated as a carcinogen in rodents, but the evidence in humans is controversial. One study, of 26 561 workers, found little evidence of a cancer risk from formaldehyde, and no dose-response effect.[39] However, some other studies have suggested that formaldehyde, especially where there is also airborne particulate matter, may be carcinogenic and may induce nasal, oropharyngeal, CNS or lymphoreticular neoplasms.[40] In the

United States, despite the limited and controversial evidence of a risk in humans, the Environmental Protection Agency and Occupational Safety and Health Administration have decided to regard formaldehyde as a potential carcinogen and propose to regulate it accordingly. In 1984, these bodies estimated the level of risk of health care and other workers potentially exposed to formaldehyde. They suggested that the excess, lifetime risk of cancer per 100 000 ranged from over 1000 in the case of pathologists and nearly 2000 in the case of funeral service workers to less than 1·0 in the case of dentists and most other health service workers. It seems reasonable to conclude, therefore, that the carcinogenicity of formaldehyde in humans is not completely proven but, even if the risk does exist, it is of a very low order indeed for dental staff.[40] Nevertheless, exposure should be minimised.

Reducing exposure to toxic agents

All toxic agents and poisons should be stored in appropriate leak-proof, preferably unbreakable containers, with correct labelling stating:
(1) the identity of the substance;
(2) appropriate hazard warnings;
(3) information on how to handle accidental exposure to the substance.
Any material safety data sheets should be retained for information about the agent, and good work practices followed, as set out in Table 3.5.

It is important to dispose of any unmarked material safely. Never relabel bottles incorrectly, and *do not use domestic bottles or containers to hold toxic materials.* Spills should be quickly cleaned up, using, for example, a Baker spill clean-up kit.

Inhalational anaesthetic agents (see also *Chapter 1*)
Dental clinical personnel may be chronically exposed to anaesthetic gases and vapours, especially if the anaesthetic equipment is faulty, poorly maintained or used without an effective scavenging system,[41] or if the agents are abused. Nitrous oxide and halothane have known adverse effects, but there is as yet little data on the possible adverse occupational effects of isoflurane, enflurane or other agents, apart from occasional asthma (*see* Chapter 2). However, such pollutants are

inhaled and absorbed and appear in the blood and in secretions such as breast milk.

Mental and neurological performance are not significantly affected by exposure to inhalational anaesthetic agents under normal working conditions,[42] but are, not surprisingly, impaired after exposure to excessive amounts of inhalational anaesthetics (to a greater degree by nitrous oxide than by halothane). Headache is common, especially where halothane is used, and there are rare confirmed cases of occupationally acquired halothane hepatitis.[43,44] However, occupational exposure does not appear to give rise to neuropsychiatric disorders.

Abuse of nitrous oxide is a well-recognised hazard in medicine and dentistry[45–49] (Chapter 7) and can produce neurological damage, a myeloneuropathy similar to that of subacute combined degeneration of the spinal cord. This causes early sensory impairment, Lhermitte's sign (shooting pains when the neck is flexed), leg weakness, ataxia, impotence and loss of sphincter control. The myeloneuropathy is caused by nitrous oxide interfering with vitamin B12 metabolism and subsequent DNA production. Nitrous oxide impairs the enzyme methionine synthetase which normally catalyses the conversion of homocysteine to methionine. Fortunately, the myeloneuropathy improves once exposure to the gas is stopped, although some damage remains, especially in the central nervous system.[50]

Interference with vitamin B12 metabolism probably also underlies the bone marrow damage leading to megaloblastosis seen in bone marrow biopsies of dentists chronically over-exposed to nitrous oxide, but, surprisingly, macrocytic anaemia does not seem to result.[51] There is also an increase in neurological symptoms in dentists chronically over-exposed to other inhalational agents, as mentioned earlier, although less than 2% of the 30 000 dentists that were surveyed had such symptoms.[49]

Chronic occupational exposure to traces of inhalational anaesthetics in anaesthetists and operating room nurses has been reported to produce increased rates of various other disorders; such reports have produced considerable anxiety in those occupationally exposed to these agents (see also Chapter 1). Probably some 20% of general dental practitioners and surgery assistants, and 75% of oral surgeons are exposed to inhalational anaesthetic agents regularly for more than 3 hours each week.[52] Various studies of non-dental anaesthetic personnel have revealed increased rates of spontaneous abortions in female anaesthetists and in the wives of male anaesthetists, a higher rate of congenital abnormalities in children born to female anaesthetists who worked during pregnancy and to wives of male anaesthetists, a greater incidence of cancer in children of female anaesthetists (claimed but not substantiated), and an increased risk of cancer, hepatic and renal diseases in female anaesthetists (controversial). An increased risk of hepatic and renal diseases has been reported in male anaesthetists. However, many of these studies have been biased or subject to severe criticism, and it cannot reliably be confirmed that these phenomena are caused by anaesthetic gases and vapours rather than other, associated factors. Overall, the evidence indicates that these risks are those of medical personnel in general, not of anaesthetists in particular[53,54] (Chapter 1).

Dental personnel may be occupationally exposed to higher concentrations of inhalational anaesthetics than are hospital operating room personnel, particularly if the room is small and poorly ventilated and no scavenging system is used. In contrast to anaesthetic personnel, exposure of dental staff to inhalational anaesthetic agents is usually for short periods, except where relative analgesia is frequently used. Nitrous oxide appears to be the agent most frequently responsible for occupational anaesthetic exposure. Dentists have been exposed to levels of about 900 ppm or even up to 6700 ppm nitrous oxide.[41,55–63] American regulations indicate that 25 ppm nitrous oxide and 2 ppm halothane (0·5 ppm in combination with nitrous oxide) are 'safe' levels of exposure.[64] Although these regulations have little scientific basis and have not been updated since 1977, levels of 30–5380 ppm nitrous oxide and 0·1–115 ppm halothane have been recorded in operating theatres, including one dental hospital operating theatre in Britain[65–68] (fig. 3.16), the higher values being peak levels.

Scavenging systems reduce air pollution by inhalational anaesthetic agents,[65] but even when used, nitrous oxide levels in dental surgeries using relative analgesia can still exceed 150 ppm. Many studies have confirmed how difficult it is to reduce nitrous oxide levels,[69–74] although levels approaching 100 ppm are attainable in practice.[67,73] In the zone in which the dentist is working, the level may still be 139–239 ppm, depending on the system used.

It has been suggested that dental personnel exposed to inhalational anaesthetics may be predisposed to disorders of health and reproduction but, as discussed earlier, the evidence is not unequivocal. Male dentists have been reported to have more liver, kidney and neurologi-

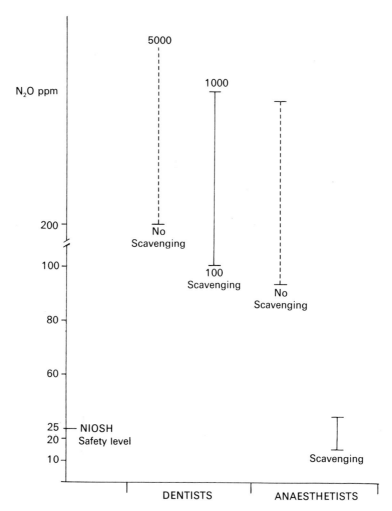

Fig. 3.16 Nitrous oxide levels (ppm) in the atmosphere in dental surgeries and operating theatres. NIOSH, National Institute for Occupational Safety and Health (USA).

cal disorders than controls, while their wives have been reported to have an increased rate of spontaneous abortions. Female dentists exposed to inhalational anaesthetics have been reported to have an increased risk of spontaneous abortion, congenital abnormalities in children and higher rates of cancer, renal and hepatic diseases. Dental surgery assistants chronically exposed to anaesthetic agents may suffer from similar problems and (it has been suggested) may have an increased incidence of cancer of the cervix.

A recent critical review of the available evidence has indicated that none of the criteria for the demonstration of toxicity by trace concentrations of anaesthetic agents have been adequately fulfilled, and that anxieties over occupational exposure may have been unjustifiably exaggerated.[54] Nevertheless, ill-health retirements and deaths in post are more common in anaesthetists than other consultants.[76] This may be *unrelated* to exposure to anaesthetic agents since surgeons, who are also exposed, appear not to suffer similar ill-health.[76]

An illustration of how difficult it is to assess the toxic effects of general anaesthetic agents is that of the extensively studied problem of halothane. Although halothane has recognised hepatotoxic properties, the incidence of abnormal liver function tests *pre-operatively* is actually appreciably higher than the incidence of hepatotoxic reactions *after* exposure to halothane.

Cryosurgery
Nitrous oxide is used in some cryosurgery instruments. Good ventilation and scavenging systems should be used, as high surgery air levels of nitrous oxide may result.[77] There is also a danger of cold burns.

Reducing exposure to inhalational anaesthetic agents

However small the real risks may be, exposure to inhalational anaesthetics should clearly be minimised. The necessary precautions are summarised in Table 3.7, but, in essence, pollution can be reduced by up to 95% by careful use of well-maintained equipment, adequate room ventilation, high volume vacuum ejectors, and effective scavenging systems.[59] New systems are becoming available for scavenging nitrous oxide and other inhalational anaesthetics from both the nose mask and gases escaping from the mouth (for example, the Anevac-D).[78]

Leaks around the nosepiece or face masks and mouth breathing should be avoided. Air extraction and good surgery ventilation are essential. Passive scavenging systems, venting gases from the expiratory valve of the anaesthetic apparatus to the exterior are useful and

Table 3.7 Minimisation of risks from inhalational anaesthetics

---

(1) Advise dental staff about undesirable effects of exposure.
(2) Make medical advice available to all exposed staff.
(3) Check anaesthetic machine, tubing and masks for leaks, and service equipment regularly.
(4) Use an effective scavenging system, exhausted to the exterior.
(5) Monitor anaesthetic waste regularly (eg with Miral 1-A infra red spectrophotometer or Perkin-Elmer diffusive sampler).
(6) Ensure good air ventilation in surgery; use a non-recirculating system.

(Based on National Institute for Occupational Safety and Health. Criteria for a Recommended standard: occupational exposure to waste anaesthetic gases and vapours US Dept. of Health. Education and Welfare 1977; ADA Council on Dental Material, Instruments and Equipment. Nitrous oxide scavenging equipment and nitrous oxide trace gas monitoring equipment (*J Am Dent Assoc* 1977; **95**: 791–797); and Department of Health Circular HC (76) 38 on Pollution of Operating Departments, etc, by Anaesthetic Gases. HMSO, 1976).

inexpensive. However, active systems which draw gases away are more reliable. Regular monitoring using, for example, diffusive samplers (Perkin-Elmer) is indicated.[66]

Mercury

Mercury exists as an element (liquid mercury and vapour), inorganic (mercurous and mercuric salts) and organic (organomercurials such as ethyl- and methyl-mercury) forms. The most volatile form is metallic mercury, which can form one of the most obvious occupational hazards in dentistry. Inorganic and organic forms of mercury can be environmental hazards.[79]

Mercury is highly lipid-soluble, is absorbed through the skin and lungs, rapidly penetrates the blood–brain barrier and infiltrates neurones, and also accumulates in liver, kidneys, spleen, muscle and glands such as the thyroid gland, salivary glands and testes. The average half-life for clearance from the body is 58 days. Mercury is found in trace amounts in the air, water and food, and levels of 30–40 ng/ml in blood and up to 20 μg/litre in urine have been found in non-dental individuals.[79]

Elemental mercury vapour can be readily absorbed (about 75%) through the respiratory tract, and mercury can be absorbed through the skin. *Organic* mercury is highly absorbed from the gut. Mercury is released into the environment from industrial uses, especially as a catalyst in the production of vinyl chloride and acetaldehyde and in the manufacture of electrical apparatus.

Mercury is therefore a constituent of the normal environment and its level is increased especially by air pollution from fossil fuels; it is found in some food additives and contaminants, in a few largely obsolete pharmaceuticals (a diuretic and some preservatives), in cosmetics (bleaching ointment), and in fungicides (for example phenyl mercuric acetate) in some countries. Mercury enters rivers, lakes and seas via waste disposal and is methylated by microorganisms to methyl mercury, which is taken up by plankton and then, in turn, by fish. The highest levels are found in tuna, swordfish and shark. In Britain, skate and dogfish are probably the main sources.[80]

Environmental poisoning from methyl mercury was widespread in Minimata Bay and Nigata, Japan between 1953 and 1960, when numerous persons were poisoned, some died, and there was, subsequently, a high incidence of cerebral palsy in newborn children. In both outbreaks the ingestion of fish contaminated by mercury from industrial discharge was clearly incriminated. Similar poisoning has followed the inadvertent ingestion of seed grain contaminated with mercurial fungicides, in Iraq, Ghana, Guatemala and Pakistan.[81]

Mercury can also cause poisoning if there is exposure to some face creams containing calomel (mercurous chloride), or antiseptics such as merbromin, tincture of mercresin, and merthiolate.

Occupational exposure to mercury can, in rare cases, produce contact dermatitis and the frequency of positive patch tests to mercuric salts increases as dental students progress through their course. Nevertheless, such hypersensitivity (allergy) gives rise to clinical problems surprisingly rarely.

The health hazards of mercury have been a source of concern in dentistry for more than a century and a half, and have recently been reviewed[82] (fig. 3.17). Some 2 to 3 lb of mercury are used by each dental practitioner every year. Several surveys have shown mercury vapour in the surgery atmosphere,[83-89] and in dental hospitals,[90,91] and levels of mercury in the blood, hair, nails and urine in dentists at levels which are often above control levels.[92-100] Mercury levels in urine and hair tend to be higher in dentists than dental surgery assistants. Scalp hair mercury levels are higher than body hair mercury levels because of surface contamination, and it is important to bear this in mind if assays are carried out.[98]

Mercury hygiene can reduce the hazard.[101] Although a decade ago about 10% of American dental practices had higher levels of mercury than recommended by the National Institute for Occupational Safety

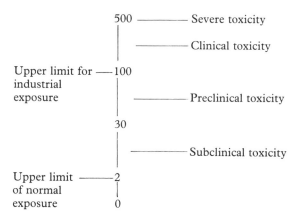

Fig. 3.17   Urinary mercury levels showing levels (μg/l) at which toxicity is seen.

and Health, this does not now appear to be so great a problem and the same is true in Britain.[102] Indeed, no dental staff in one recent study had blood levels of mercury over the recognised 'safe' limit of 35 μg/l. In fact, levels were highest in eaters of fish and this indicates that at least part of the mercury burden is from non-dental sources.[99] In another study, farmers (who are exposed to the fungicide phenyl mercuric acetate) had hair mercury levels comparable with dentists.[100] Furthermore, some studies of dentists and dental surgery assistants have not shown greatly increased urinary levels of mercury where work practice is good and have shown lower urinary mercury levels in dentists in 1986 than in 1983,[103] as a result of improved mercury hygiene.

In the past, a few dentists and dental surgery assistants have suffered from chronic mercury toxicity with tremor, incoordination, polyneuropathies, and accelerated senility. Rarely, deaths have been reported after prolonged heavy exposure[104–109] such as follows mer-cury spills. In the past, objective investigations of nerve function in those chronically exposed to mercury over several years has shown evidence of a subclinical polyneuropathy in dentists with high tissue mercury levels, but this was not obvious clinically, was only detect-able by appropriate testing,[101] and was not correlated with the level of exposure. Autopsies have also shown mercury deposits, particularly in the pituitary glands.[110,111] Mercury poisoning falls under RIDDOR (*see* p 90). The possibility of foetotoxicity is discussed in Chapter 1.

Reducing exposure to mercury

The most recent recommendations on dental mercury hygiene are summarised in Table 3.8 based on the Fédération Dentaire Internationale Report.[112] The Health and Safety Executive (HSE) have recommended that mercury vapour air concentrations should be less than $0.05 \, mg/m^3$. Good work practices can keep mercury levels in dental practice within these limits.[112-117]

The greatest hazard from mercury comes from spillage of free mercury and inhalation of the vapour, or when mercury comes into contact with the skin such as can happen during hand trituration, which greatly increases mercury absorption. The use of mercury should be confined to areas that have impervious surfaces and are suitably lipped to confine and facilitate recovery of spilt mercury— stainless steel trays are ideal. Contaminated instruments should be cleaned before autoclaving as heat will vaporise the mercury. Mercury spilt near hot areas (such as sterilisers) or accumulating in surgery floor coverings and other nooks and crannies, gives rise to mercury vapour, as do other sources (Table 3.8). The type of floor covering, perhaps surprisingly, has minimal effect on mercury contamination, but it is best to avoid carpet and to cover any gaps and holes.[82] Continuous seamless floor covering, such as non-porous sheet polyvinyl chloride is preferable. Waste amalgam should be stored in sealed containers under a sulphur-containing solution such as radiographic fixative.

Removal of old amalgams from teeth with an air-rotor produces a small but not significant amount of mercury vapour if adequate water-cooling and aspiration are used. However, a mask and protective eyewear should be worn.

Apart from avoiding sources of mercury contamination, the most effective methods of reducing levels of mercury vapour in the surgery include adequate room ventilation (iodised charcoal filters help to remove mercury) and the use of pre-portioned mercury capsules. Mercury levels can be monitored using room sniffing devices, palladium chloride impregnated discs (Williams Detectors), various badge monitors, or by analyses of urine excretion or by mercury levels in blood, nails or hair.[82] Thomson Laboratories, or Dr P J Warren, Department of Biochemistry, Queen Mary and Westfield College, Mile End Road, London E1 4NS, or Health Options Ltd (*see* p 98) can undertake urinalysis for mercury and provide further advice.

Table 3.8 Minimisation of risks from mercury

(1) Alert staff to the potential hazard and need for good mercury hygiene practices.
(2) A no-touch technique should be adopted with mercury and amalgam at all times. Skin contaminated by mercury should be washed immediately. It is wise to wear gloves, as always.
(3) Work in well-ventilated spaces. Air conditioning filters may act as mercury reservoirs and should be periodically replaced. Mercury vapour decontamination filter units are available.
(4) Check surgery atmosphere periodically for mercury vapour.
(5) Continuous seamless sheet flooring carried up the walls for at least 10 cm is preferable.
(6) Store mercury in unbreakable, tightly sealed containers, away from heat.
(7) Use mercury and amalgam equipment only on impervious surfaces (eg formica) with suitable lipping and sealed joins so that spills are confined and recovery facilitated. Surfaces should be cleaned weekly with 1% calcium oxide/flowers of sulphur. Mercury vapour/spill control cabinets are available.
(8) Use pre-proportioned single-use capsules if possible.
(9) Use only capsules that remain sealed during amalgamation. The seal of new or used capsules can be checked by wrapping adhesive tape around the capsules. A leak will be shown up by the presence of small drops of mercury on the tape after vibration in a mechanical amalgamator.
(10) Select an appropriate alloy : mercury ratio to avoid the need to remove excess mercury before packing.
(11) Use an amalgamator with completely enclosed arms and place in a tray to catch any spills.
(12) Immerse single-use capsules in radiographic fixer solution or in a screw-top container until disposal, as in (21) below.
(13) Handle mercury dispensers with care and periodically check for leakage.
(14) Examine the mercury dispenser orifice after use. Any remaining mercury droplets should be disposed of, as in (16) below.
(15) Salvage and store scrap amalgam in a tightly closed container under radiographic fixer solution, or under glycerine or potassium permanganate.
(16) Immediately clean up spilt mercury. Pick up drops either with a plastic pipette, or with narrow-bore tubing connected (via a wash-bottle trap) to a low volume aspirator or a wide-bore needle attached to a hypodermic syringe. Do not use a vacuum cleaner. Strips of adhesive or the lead from x-ray packets may be used to clean up small spills.[a] Droplets that cannot be reached can be dusted with sulphur powder or a paste of sulphur and lime can be spread to produce a protective coating effective while the mercury droplets remain undisturbed. Amalgam alloy powder or fragments can be used.
(17) Do not use ultrasonic amalgam condensers.
(18) Use water spray and high-volume suction when removing old or finishing new dental amalgam restorations. The exhaust should go outside the surgery.
(19) Wear a mask to prevent inhalation of amalgam dust.
(20) Do not heat mercury, amalgam or any equipment used with amalgam. Clean instruments before heat sterilisation.
(21) Place any disposable materials contaminated with mercury or amalgam in a polyethylene bag and seal.
(22) Waste systems into which amalgam scrap may enter, (eg cuspidors, sinks and suction systems) should be provided with plastic traps from which amalgam scrap can be recovered, and stored as described in recommendation (15) above.

(23) Do not eat, drink or smoke in the surgery.
(24) Have periodic mercury urinalysis carried out if mercury hygiene is suspect.
(25) Avoid wearing jewellery since mercury combines with silver and gold.

Adapted from FDI technical report No 7.
Int Dent J 1988; **38**: 191–192 and *NY State Dent J* 1986; **52**: 21–25.
*a*Mercury spillage kits are available from Techmate Ltd, Luton and Linton Products; Mercury 'sponges' from May & Baker Ltd.

Mercury is a potent neurotoxin and spilt mercury an undoubted hazard to those in the environment. Mercury spills should be recovered with a syringe or aspirator (*not* a vacuum cleaner since these vent mercury vapour into the atmosphere) and the area decontaminated by absorbing the mercury onto adhesive tape, tin foil, lead foil or amalgam powder or waste. Flowers of sulphur appears to be of little value. A bulb aspirator is available from Jencons Ltd (see p 98). Mercury spillage cleanup kits and a mercury cleanup sponge are also available from Linton Products, Health Options Ltd, and Techmate (see p 98). The effects of mercury poisoning have been effectively reduced using N-acetyl-D,L-penicillamine, which should be used only by a physician.[113]

There is ample evidence then, that provided care is taken, there need be little mercury contamination in dental practices, and no hazard to personnel.[115-117]

'Sick building syndrome'

It has recently been recognised that some office workers develop vague symptoms during the working week, that abate at weekends and vacations. If this has an organic basis, there appear to be several possible variants of this 'sick building syndrome'.

(1) Least common is *hypersensitivity* pneumonitis caused by various microorganisms that breed in ventilation systems.

(2) Most serious is Legionnaires' disease. The causative organisms (primarily *Legionella pneumophila*) colonise cooling systems, humidifiers and elsewhere (*see* Chapters 2 and 5).

(3) Skin or mucosal irritation may be caused by exposure to fibres such as glass fibre or mineral wool from insulation.

(4) Allergy to antigens such as those of mites and moulds in carpeting, etc, and cleaning agents, aerosols or volatile agents such as typewriter correcting fluid.

(5) Mass hysteria caused by strange smells or fear of spread of disease within the building.
(6) An annoyance/irritation syndrome that might possibly be related to an excess of positive ions in the air.
(7) Extensive use of fluorescent lighting, perhaps incorrectly sited, which may, by a flicker effect, give rise to visual problems and headaches.

This 'syndrome' has yet to be reported from a dental surgery or laboratory, although *Legionella* infection is perhaps more than a theoretical hazard (*see* Chapters 2 and 5).

Minerals
A range of minerals can be encountered in dental clinical and especially laboratory practice; possible hazards are discussed in Chapter 2.

Accident notification

Regulations came into force in the UK in 1981 and were updated in 1985, on the notification of accidents and dangerous events at work (*see also* Chapter 6). These regulations apply to all places of work, including dental premises. Serious accidents to members of the public resulting from attending the surgery or laboratories are also now notifiable. However, the regulations exclude accidents to 'patients when undergoing treatment in a hospital or surgery of a doctor or dentist'. The exclusion only applies to patients when undergoing treatment; the new notification rules *do* have to be followed if, for example, a patient breaks a leg on the surgery doorstep.

· Briefly, the Notification of Accidents and Dangerous Occurrences Regulations (1980) and the Reporting of Injuries, Diseases and Dangerous Occurrences Regulations (RIDDOR: SI 2023: HMSO ISBN 0-110-580230 1985: *see* HSE booklet HSE 18) require employers to notify the Health and Safety Executive of accidents causing death or 'major injury' to any person, or 'dangerous occurrences' even if there has been no death or injury. Such accidents and incidents must be notified with minimum delay, by telephone if possible, so that any necessary investigation can begin promptly. The employer must also confirm the information in writing within 7 days on form F2508, which is available from HMSO (reference ISBN 0

11883367 7). Planning procedures for dealing with occupational risks should include, initially, reference to 'Reporting an Injury or Dangerous Occurrence – RIDDOR', (HSE 11 (Rev) and HSE 18) and 'Reporting a case of disease – RIDDOR', (HSE 17) both of which may be obtained from the Health and Safety Executive (fig. 3.18).

'Major' injuries, as defined in the Regulations, include fractures of the skull, spine or pelvis, fractures of any bone in the arm or leg (except in the wrist, hand, ankle or foot), amputation of a hand or foot, loss of sight of an eye, or any other injury which results in the person injured being admitted to hospital as an in-patient for more than 24 hours, unless detained only for observation.

Notifiable 'dangerous occurrences' are also defined in the Regulations (schedule 1) and include the following:

(a) Explosion, collapse or bursting of any closed vessel, including a

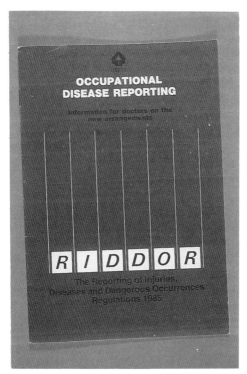

Fig. 3.18 Health and Safety Executive pamphlet HSE 18 on Reporting an Injury or Dangerous Occurrence (RIDDOR).

boiler or a boiler tube, in which there was any gas (including air) or vapour at a pressure greater than atmospheric and which might have been liable to cause major injury to any person or which resulted in significant damage to the plant.

(b) Electrical short circuit or overload attended by fire or explosion which resulted in the stoppage of the plant involved for more than 24 hours and which, taking into account the circumstances of the occurrence, might have been liable to cause major injury to any person.

(c) An explosion or fire in any plant or place, resulting in the stoppage of that plant or suspension of normal work in that place for more than 24 hours and where such explosion or fire was due to the ignition of process materials, their by-products (including waste) or finished products.

(d) The uncontrolled release or escape of any substance or agent in circumstances which might be liable to cause damage to the health of, or major injury to, any person.

(e) Any incident in which any person is affected by the inhalation, ingestion or other absorption of any substance, or by lack of oxygen to such an extent as to cause ill-health requiring medical treatment.

(f) Any case of acute ill-health where there is reason to believe that this resulted from occupational exposure to particular pathogens or infected material.

(g) Any ignition or explosion of explosives, where the ignition or explosion was not intentional.

Compressor or autoclave explosions could therefore be notifiable, as could a mercury spillage or a case of viral hepatitis. In case of doubt, the advice of the local Health and Safety Executive (HSE) office should be sought. The regulations also require employers to keep a record of all notifiable accidents and dangerous events and make it available to the HSE or to a safety representative. HMSO publish an Accident Book which is suitable. The use of this particular record system is not compulsory, but for those who wish to purchase it, the reference for the HMSO Accident Book is form F250 9, (ISBN 0 118 8336 8 5). In the case of less serious accidents, where injuries are not 'major', there is no requirement to notify the HSE, but employers may have to provide details of the accident to the Department of Health (DH) in due course, to support any claims for Industrial Injury Benefit. The local DH office will send a Form Bl 76 for this purpose, for use when employees are absent from work for more than 3 days as a result of any injury at work.

The Regulations also require notification of poisonings (eg mercury), lung diseases (eg pneumoconiosis) and infections (eg viral hepatitis or tuberculosis) that are relevant to dentistry. The Employment Medical Advisory Service can advise (*see* Chapter 6: Appendix).

References

1 Webb T, Schilling R, Jacobson B, Babb P. Health at Work? A report on health promotion in the workplace. Health Education Council Research Report No 22, 1988.
2 Eichner K. Investigation on cutting and grinding procedures on the hard tooth structure and ivory. *Aust Dent J* 1965; **10**: 214–216.
3 Spencer GT. Radio headsets in the workplace. Hamilton, Ontario: Canadian Centre for Occupational Health and Safety, 1989.
4 Rund DA, Summers WK, Levin M. Alcohol use and psychiatric illness in emergency patients. *J Am Med Assoc* 1981; **245**: 1240–1241.
5 Walsh ME, Macleod DAD. Breath alcohol analysis in the accident and emergency department. *Injury* 1983; **15**: 62–66.
6 Shepherd JP, Irish M, Scully C, Leslie I. Alcohol intoxication and severity of injury in victims of assault. *Br Med J* 1988; **296**: 1299.
7 Willee AW. How to avoid the occupational hazards of dentistry. *Aust Dent J* 1967; **34**: 348–359.
8 Fauchard Academy. One of every three practitioners affected with back trouble. *Dent Survey* 1965; **41**: 69–70.
9 Diakow PR, Cassicy JD. Back pain in dentists. *J Manipul Physiol Ther* 1984; 7: 85–88.
10 Powell M, Eccles JD. The health and work of two professional groups: dentists and pharmacists. *Dent Pract Dent Rec* 1970; **20**: 373–378.
11 Bassett S. Back problems among dentists. *J Canad Dent Assoc* 1983; **4**: 251–256.
12 Hope-Ross A, Corcoran D. A survey of dentists working posture. *J Irish Dent Assoc* 1985; **32**: 13–20.
13 Katevuo K, Aitasalo K, Lehtinen R, Pietala J. Skeletal changes in dentists and farmers in Finland. *Community Dent Oral Epidemiol* 1985; **13**: 23–25.
14 Ellis PJ. Are you sitting comfortably. *Dent Update* 1981; **8**: 559–566.
15 Bauer ME. Carpal tunnel syndrome: an occupational risk to the dental hygienists. *Dent Hygiene* 1985; **59**: 218–221.
16 Macdonald G, Erikson JA, Robertson MM. The incidence of carpal tunnel syndrome among Californian dental hygienists. *J Dent Res* 1986; **65**: 320.
17 Boyer EM, Elton J, Preston C. Precautionary procedures. Use in dental hygiene practice. *Dent Hygiene* 1986; **60**: 516–523.
18 Gestal JJ. Occupational hazards in hospitals: accidents, radiation, exposure to noxious chemicals, drug addiction and psychic problems, and assault. *Br J Indust Med* 1987; **44**: 510–520.
19 Eisenbaum SL. Facial burns as a complication of office surgery lighting. *Plast Reconstr Surg* 1989; **83**: 155–159.
20 James MI. Burns from fluid heated in a microwave oven. *Br Med J* 1989; **298**: 1452.

21   Srinivas CR, Balachandran C, Bhat KS, Mgtwani BK, Rao SN, Subramanya R. Air rotor and clinical micromotor induced sensory loss. *Int J Leprosy* 1987; **55**: 559–560.
22   Scully C. Substances of hazard in the dental surgery, 1989. *In* Derrick D (ed). *Dental annual, 1990*. Guildford: Butterworths (in press).
23   Rosenstiel E. Hydrofluoric acid in dental laboratories. *Br Dent J* 1974; **136**: 413.
24   Ruyter IE, Sjovik IJ. Composition of dental resin and composite materials. *Acta Odontol Scand* 1981; **39**: 133–146.
25   Bardis RS. Hazards of organic materials. *J Am Dent Assoc* 1983; **106**: 444.
26   Losewicz S, Davison AG, Hopkirk A. Occupational asthma due to methyl methacrylate and cyanoacrylates. *Thorax* 1984; **39**: 712–713.
27   Nyquist G, Koch G, Magnusson B. Contact allergy to medicaments and materials used in dentistry. *Odontol Revy* 1972; **23**: 197–204.
28   Estlander T, Rajaniemi R, Jolanki R. Hand dermatitis in dental technicians. *Contact Derm* 1984; **10**: 201–205.
29   Rajaniemi R. Clinical evaluation of occupational toxicity of methylmethacrylate monomer to dental technicians. *J Soc Occup Med* 1986; **36**: 56–59.
30   Rajaniemi R, Tola S. Subjective symptoms among dental technicians exposed to the monomer methyl methacrylate. *Scand J Work Env Health* 1985; **11**: 281–286.
31   Rajaniemi R, Pfaffli P, Savolainen H. Percutaneous absorption of methyl methacrylate by dental technicians. *Br J Indust Med* 1989; **46**: 356–357.
32   Singh AR, Lawrence WH, Autian J. Embryonic–fetal toxicity and teratogenic effects of a group of methacrylate esters in rats. *J Dent Res* 1972; **51**: 1632–1638.
33   Nicholas CA, Lawrence WH, Autian J. Embryotoxicity and fetotoxicity from maternal inhalation of methyl methacrylate monomer in rats. *Toxicol Appl Pharmacol* 1979; **50**: 451–458.
34   Tansey MF, Benhayem S, Probst S, Jordan JS. The effects of methyl methacrylate vapor on gastric motor function. *J Am Dent Assoc* 1974; **89**: 372–376.
35   Scolnick B, Collins J. Systemic reaction to methylmethacrylate in an operating room nurse. *J Occup Med* 1986; **28**: 196–198.
36   Seppalainen AM, Rajaniemi R. Local neurotoxicity of methyl methacrylate among dental technicians. *Am J Indust Med* 1984; **5**: 471–477.
37   Rajaniemi R. Clinical evaluation of occupational toxicity of methylmethacrylate monomer to dental technicians. *J Soc Occup Med* 1986; **36**: 56–59.
38   Rajaniemi R, Tola S. Subjective symptoms among dental technicians exposed to the monomer methylmethacrylate. *Scand J Work Env Health* 1985; **11**: 281.
39   Blair A, Stewart P, O'Berg M *et al*. Mortality among workers exposed to formaldehyde. *J Nat Cancer Inst* 1986; **76**: 1071–1084.
40   Council on Scientific Affairs. Formaldehyde. *J Am Med Assoc* 1989; **261**: 1183–1187.
41   Ship JA. A survey of nitrous oxide levels in dental offices. *Arch Env Health* 1987; **42**: 310–314.
42   Smith G, Shirley AW. Failure to demonstrate effect of trace concentrations of nitrous oxide and halothane on psychomotor performance. *Br J Anaesthesia* 1977; **49**: 65–70.
43   Belfrage S, Ahlgren I, Axelson S. Halothane hepatitis in an anaesthetist. *Lancet* 1966; **2**: 1466–1467.
44   Klatskin G, Kimberg DV. Recurrent hepatitis attributable to halothane sensitisation in an anaesthetist. *New Engl J Med* 1969; **280**: 515–522.
45   Paulson GW. Recreational misuse of nitrous oxide. *J Am Dent Assoc* 1979; **98**: 410–444.
46   Gutmann L *et al*. Nitrous oxide-induced myelopathy-neuropathy: potential for chronic misuse by dentists. *J Am Dent Assoc* 1979; **98**: 58–59.

47 Layzer RB, Fishman RA, Schaffer JA. Neuropathy following abuse of nitrous oxide. *Neurology* 1978; **28**: 504–506
48 Gutman L, Johnsen D. Nitrous oxide-induced myeloneuropathy: report of cases. *J Am Dent Assoc* 1981; **103**: 239–241.
49 Brodsky JB, Cohen EN, Brown BW, Wu ML, Whitcher CE. Exposure to nitrous oxide and neurologic disease among dental professionals. *Anesth Analg* 1981; **60**: 297–301.
50 Layzer RB. Myeloneuropathy after prolonged exposure to nitrous oxide. *Lancet* 1978; **2**: 1227–1230.
51 Sweeney B, Bingham RM, Amos RJ, Petty AC, Cole PV. Toxicity of bone marrow in dentists exposed to nitrous oxide. *Br Med J* 1985; **291**: 567–568.
52 Cohen EN, Brown BW, Bruce DL, Cascorbi HF, Corbett TH, Jones TW, Whitcher CE. A survey of anaesthetic health hazards among dentists. *J Am Dent Assoc* 1975; **90**: 1291–1296.
53 Eckenhoff JE. *Controversy in anesthesiology*. Philadelphia: WB Saunders, 1979.
54 Spence AA. Environmental pollution by inhalation anaesthetics. *Br J Anaesth* 1987; **59**: 96–103.
55 Millard RI, Corbett TH. Nitrous oxide concentrations in the dental operatory. *J Oral Surg* 1974; **32**: 593–594.
56 Scaramella J, Allen GD, Adams D, Randall F. Nitrous oxide pollution levels in oral surgery offices. *J Oral Surg* 1978; **36**: 441–443.
57 Vean AH, King KJ. Measuring N$_2$O levels in the dental operatory. *J Dent Child* 1979; **46**: 22–27.
58 Whitcher C, Zimmerman DC, Tonn EM, Piziali RL. Control of occupational exposure to nitrous oxide in the dental operatory. *J Am Dent Assoc* 1977; **95**: 763–776.
59 Whitcher C, Zimmerman DC, Piziali RL. Control of occupational exposure to nitrous oxide in the oral surgery office. *J Oral Surg* 1978; **36**: 431–446.
60 Swenson RD. Scavenging of dental anesthetic gases. *J Oral Surg* 1976; **34**: 207–214.
61 Parbrook DG, Davis PD. Anaesthetic pollution in the dental out-patient surgery. *Anaesthesia* 1979; **34**: 47–52.
62 Campbell RL, Hannifan MA, Reist PC, Gregg JM. Exposure to anesthetic waste gas in oral surgery. *J Oral Surg* 1977; **35**: 625–630.
63 Middendorf PJ, Jacobs DE, Smith KA, Mastro DM. Occupational exposure to nitrous oxide in dental operatories. *Anaesth Prog* 1986; **33**: 91–97.
64 National Institute for Occupational Safety and Health. Occupational exposure to waste anesthetic gases and vapors. Criteria for a recommended standard. Washington: US Government Printing Office, 1977. Publication No NIOSH 77–140.
65 Davenport HT, Halsey MJ, Wardley-Smith B, Bateman PE. Occupational exposure to anaesthetics in 20 hospitals. *Anaesthesia* 1980; **35**: 354–259.
66 Gray WM. Occupational exposure to nitrous oxide in four hospitals. *Anaesthesia* 1989; **44**: 511–514.
67 Thompson JM, Barratt RS, Hutton P, Robinson JS, Belcher R, Stephen WI. Ambient air contamination in a dental outpatient theatre. *Br J Anaesth* 1979; **51**: 845–855.
68 Harrington JM. The health of anaesthetists. *Anaesthesia* 1987; **42**: 131–132.
69 Allen WA. Nitrous oxide in the surgery: pollution and scavenging. *Br Dent J* 1985; **159**: 222–230.
70 Hillman KM, Saloojee Y, Brett II, Cole PV. Nitrous oxide concentrations in the dental surgery: atmospheric and blood concentrations of personnel. *Anaesthesia* 1981; **36**: 257.
71 Sher AM, Mallet J, Braude BM, Moyes DG, Cleaton-Jones, PE. A comparison

of the Cyprane and Samson nasal mask scavengers during relative analgesia. *Br Dent J* 1987; **163**: 111–115.

72 Brown JP, Bell S. Efficiency of three nitrous oxide relative analgesia scavenging systems. *Dent Anaesth Sedation* 1984; **13**: 5–7.

73 Christensen JR, Vann WF Jr, Linville DR. Measurement of scavenged nitrous oxide in the dental operatory. *Pediatr Dent* 1985; 7: 192–197.

74 Ross AS, Riekman GA, Carley BL. Waste nitrous oxide exposure. *J Canad Dent Assoc* 1984; **50**: 561–563.

75 Davenport HT, Wright BM. Measurement and reduction of occupational exposure to inhaled anaesthetics. *Br Med J* 1976; **2**: 1219.

76 McNamee R, Keen RI, Corkill CM. Morbidity and early retirement among anaesthetists and other specialists. *Anaesthesia* 1987; **42**: 133–140.

77 Shepherd JP, Jones DC. Nitrous oxide contamination during out-patient cryo-surgery. *Int J Oral Maxillofac Surg* 1988; **17**: 4–5.

78 Andersson-Wenckert I, Haggmark S, Johansson G, Lindkvist R, Reiz S. Anevac-D, a new system for close scavenging of anaesthetic gases in dental practice. *Scand J Dent Res* 1989; **97**: 456–464.

79 Clarkson TW. Mercury. *Ann Rev Publ Health* 1983; **4**: 375–380.

80 Anonymous. Mercury in fish. *Bull World Health Org* 1986; **64**: 634.

81 Elhassani SB. The many faces of methylmercury poisoning. *J Toxicol Clin Toxicol* 1982; **19**: 875–906.

82 Langan DC, Fan PL, Hoos AA. The use of mercury in dentistry: a critical review of the recent literature. *J Am Dent Assoc* 1987; **115**: 867–879.

83 Ochoa R, Miller RW. Report on independent survey taken of Austin dental offices for mercury contamination. *Texas Dent J* 1983; **100**: 6–9.

84 Kantor L, Woodcock C. Mercury vapor in the dental office—does carpeting make a difference? *J Am Dent Assoc* 1981; **103**: 402–407.

85 Skuba A. Survey for mercury vapour in Manitoba dental offices. *J Canad Dent Assoc* 1984; **50**: 517–522.

86 Chopp GF, Kaufman EG. Mercury vapor related to manipulation of amalgam and to floor surface. *Oper Dent* 1983; **8**: 23–27.

87 Schulein TM, Reinhardt JW, Chan KC. Survey of Des Moines area dental offices for mercury vapor. *Iowa Dent J* 1984; **70**: 35–36.

88 Jones DW, Sutow EJ, Milne EL. Survey of mercury vapour in dental offices in Atlantic Canada. *Canad Dent Assoc J* 1983; **49**: 378–395.

89 Joselow MM, Goldwater LJ, Alvarez A, Herndon J. Absorption and excretion of mercury in man. XV Occupational exposure among dentists. *Arch Environ Health* 1968; **17**: 39–43.

90 McGinnis JP, Mincer HH, Hembree JH. Mercury vapour exposure in a dental school environment. *J Am Dent Assoc* 1974; **88**: 785–788.

91 Wilson SJ, Wilson HJ. Mercury vapour levels in a dental hospital environment. *Br Dent J* 1985; **159**: 233–234.

92 Pritchard JG, McMullin JF, Sikondari AH. The prevalence of high levels of mercury in dentists' hair. *Br Dent J* 1982; **153**: 333–336.

93 Carell R *et al.* Trace metals in dental practitioners: a three-year study. *ASDC J Dent Child* 1981; **48**: 205–207.

94 Francis PC *et al.* Mercury content of human hair: a survey of dental personnel. *J Toxicol Env Health* 1982; **10**: 667–672.

95 Naleway C *et al.* Urinary mercury levels in US dentists 1975–1983: review of health assessment program. *J Am Dent Assoc* 1985; **111**: 37–42.

96 Bang MS. Mercury levels in the blood of dentists. *Taehan Chikkwa Visa Hypohoe Chi* 1985; **23**: 161–164.

97   Iyer K, Goodgold J, Eberstein A, Berg P. Mercury poisoning in a dentist. *Arch Neurol* 1976; **33**: 788–790.
98   Nilsson B, Nilsson B. Mercury in the dental practice. I. The working environment of dental personnel and their exposure to mercury vapor. *Swed Dent J* 1986; **10**: 1–14.
99   Moller-Madsen B, Hansen JC, Kragstrup J. Mercury concentrations in blood from Danish dentists. *Scand J Dent Res* 1988; **96**: 56–59.
100 Yamanaka S, Tanaka H, Nishimura M. Exposure of Japanese dental workers to mercury. *Bull Tokyo Dent Coll* 1982; **23**: 15–24.
101 Wilson J. Reduction of mercury vapour in a dental surgery. *Lancet* 1978; **1**: 200–201.
102 Warren PJ, Das AK. Mercury excretion in dental personnel—a comparative study. *Dent Update* 1973; **7**: 73–79.
103 Herber RFM, de Gee AJ, Wibowo AAE. Exposure of dentists and assistants to mercury: mercury levels in urine and hair related to conditions of practice. *Community Dent Oral Epidemiol* 1988; **16**: 153–158.
104 Cook TA, Yates PO. Fatal mercury intoxication in a dental surgery assistant. *Br Dent J* 1969; **127**: 553.
105 Iyer K, Goodgold, J, Eberstein A, Berg P. Mercury poisoning in a dentist. *Arch Neurol* 1976; **33**: 788.
106 Merfield DP, Taylor, A, Gemmell DM, Parrish JA. Mercury intoxication in a dental surgery following unreported spillage. *Br Dent J* 1976; **141**: 179.
107 McCord CP. Mercury poisoning in dentists. *Indust Med Surg* 1961; **30**: 554.
108 Symington IS, Cross JD, Dale IM, Lenihan JMA. Mercury poisoning in dentists. *J Soc Occup Med* 1980; **30**: 37–39.
109 Shapiro IM, Cornblath DR, Sumner AJ, Uzzell B, Spitz LK, Ship II, Bloch P. Neurophysiological and neuropsychological function in mercury-exposed dentists. *Lancet* 1982; **1**: 1147–1150.
110 Nylander M. Mercury in pituitary glands of dentists. *Lancet* 1986; **1**: 442.
111 Nylander, M, Weiner J. Relation between mercury and selenium in pituitary glands of dental staff. *Br J Indust Med* 1989; **46**: 751–752.
112 Beech DR *et al*. Recommendations on dental mercury hygiene: revision of FDI Technical Report No 7. *Int Dent J* 1988; **38**: 191–192.
113 Hryhorczuk DO, Meyers L, Chen G. Treatment of mercury intoxication in a dentist with N-acetyl-D,L-penicillamine. *J Toxicol* 1982; **19**: 401–408.
114 Wirz, J, Catagnola L. Mercury vapors in dental practice. *Schweiz Monatsschr Zahnheilkd* 1977; **87**: 570–577.
115 Kelman GR. Urinary mercury excretion in dental personnel. *Br J Indust Med* 1978; **35**: 262–265.
116 Warren PJ. The excretion of urinary mercury from dental personnel. *Rev Env Health* 1986; **6**: 297–309.
117 Mann J, Eisman Y, Ernest M. Mercury: health hazards in dentistry. *N Y State Dent J* 1986; **52**: 21–25.

Portasol Professional wax knife/hot air blower: Quayle Dental, Dominion Way, Worthing, West Sussex BN14 8QN.
Mix-Kit II: Howmedica UK Ltd, 622 Western Avenue, London W3 0TF.
CMW mixing cabinet: CMW Laboratories, Falcon Road, Cauton Estate, Exeter EX2 7NA.
Baker spill clean-up kit: Linton Products, Hysol, Harlow, Essex CM18 6QZ.
Anevac-D: Norslands Gas AB, Sweden.

Diffusive samples: Perkin-Elmer,Maxwell Road, Beaconsfield, Bucks HP9 1QA.
Williams Detectors: Williams Gold Refining Co. Inc, Buffalo, USA.
Thomson Laboratories: The Stocks, Cosgrove, Milton Keynes.
Mercury screening: Dr P. J. Warren, Department of Biochemistry, Queen Mary and Westfield College, Mile End Road, London E1 4NS
Bulb aspirator: Jencons Ltd, Cherrycourt Way Industrial Estate, Stanbridge Road, Leighton Buzzard, Bedfordshire.
Mercury cleanup kit and cleanup sponge: Linton Products, Hysol, Harlow, Essex CM18 6QZ, and Techmate, 10 Bridgeturn Avenue, Wolverton, Milton Keynes.
Dentists Provident Society: 9 Gayfere Street,London SW1 3NH.
Met-Scan mercury screening: Health Options Ltd, Technology Drive, Beeston, Nottingham NG9 2ND.

4

Radiation Hazards and Protection

Radiation hazards in dental practice are mainly from ionising radiation, as in x-rays, but there may also be hazards from the light sources used mainly for curing composite materials and, occasionally, other sources such as lasers. Ionising radiation is radiation with a wavelength shorter than 10 nm and may be artificial (such as x-rays) or can come from natural sources.

Ionising radiation

Radiographs are taken so frequently in dentistry that the attitude towards radiation hazards may readily become disastrously casual and the risks ignored. The system of payment for each film taken, and possibly anxiety to avoid medicolegal complications, has stimulated the taking of unnecessary films, often of poor quality. The increasing public concern about such hazards has already reached the national press. However, it is not merely the patient who is at risk; clinical dental staff are also exposed to radiation from x-ray apparatus.

Radiation injury
Acute high level over-exposure may cause radiation sickness, gastrointestinal and haematological damage, but most occupational exposure is at a lower level and is prolonged; radiosensitive, rapidly dividing cells (such as in skin or bone marrow) are then at risk from neoplastic change. Even now the possibility of an increased risk from leukaemia among diagnostic radiologists cannot be entirely dismissed, but rates of leukaemia do not appear to be higher in dentists than the normal population.[1]

Ionising radiations, particularly x-rays, are the main hazard, especially to the foetus or young child, or where cells are proliferating rapidly, as in the gonads and bone marrow. Because of the capacity of ionising radiation to induce genetic mutations in the germinal tissues (teratogenic effect), or to induce malignant tumours in other tissues (oncogenic effect), exposure to ionising radiation must be kept to the absolute minimum. Since there is no known threshold dose (stochastic effects), even normal dosage may ultimately contribute to neoplastic change and radiographs should therefore be taken only when absolutely essential. Ionising radiation can also produce threshold effects such as dermatitis and cataracts, whose severity increases with dose of radiation (non-stochastic effects).

Hazards from dental radiography

Intra-oral and panoramic radiography are widely used but relatively safe, while cephalometry is more hazardous. There has been a dramatic increase in the use of dental radiography over recent years, much in excess of any increase in medical radiography, where there is likely to be a greater element of defensive investigation. The necessity of some dental radiography has therefore been seriously questioned in an editorial in the *Lancet* entitled 'Dental x-rays, for caries or cash?'.[2] Between 1957 and 1977 in the UK there was an almost 6-fold increase in the number of dental radiographs, but only a 0·5-fold increase in medical radiography. Subsequently, there has been a continued increase particularly in dental panoramic radiography.[3,4] Even larger numbers of dental radiographs per head of population are taken in some other countries, such as the USA.[5] The American Dental Association has now produced guidelines to the prescribing of dental radiographs,[6] shown in Table 4.1, which may help rationalise this type of investigation.

There is little doubt that ionising radiation has been an occupational hazard to clinical dental staff since its introduction nearly a century ago.[7-11] Only 30 or so years ago it was reported that 55 dentists developed radiation-induced dermatitis of their hands, resulting from holding x-ray films in the patients' mouths during radiography.[8] Of these 55, 17 developed malignant changes, and similar results were reported in a later study from another centre.[9] At least one stomatologist has died as a result of such exposure; others have lost digits.[10] The question of possible foetal damage is discussed in Chapter 1.

There have been great improvements in technology, technique and ionising radiation safety since the early days of dental radiography.[12]

Table 4.1 Guidelines for prescribing dental radiographs[a]

	Child			Adult	
	Before eruption of first permanent tooth	Later	Before eruption of third molar	Dentate	Edentulous
New patient	BW	BW ± PA or ± panoramic	BW ± PA	BW ± PA	Panoramic
Recall patient High risk caries	BW 6 monthly	BW 6 monthly	BW at 6–12 monthly	BW at 12–18 monthly	
Low risk caries	BW annually	BW annually	BW at 18–36 months	BW at 2–3 years	
High risk periodontal disease	Selected PA or BW	Selected PA or BW	Selected PA or BW	Selected PA or BW	

PA = periapical; BW = bitewing
[a]For caries and periodontal disease. Adapted from ADA guidelines (*J Am Dent Assoc* 1989; **118**; 115–117)

In Britain, following the Radiological Protection Act 1970, the National Radiological Protection Board (NRPB)* was created as the authority primarily concerned with the safety of ionising radiation. Dentists are now more likely to use lead rubber apron protection for patients[13] and few, although still too many, dentists hold the x-ray film in the patient's mouth.[14] Most use film at least as fast as Kodak Ultraspeed and staff usually leave the room where the radiograph is being taken; some dentists wear film monitors.[13,14] Nevertheless, very recent studies have shown that there is great scope for improvements in equipment;[15,16] too many operators still stand closer than the recommended 2 metres from the x-ray source[14] and radiation safety in dental practice is still well recognised as sometimes being wanting.[1,7–17] One example is that of a dentist and his dental surgery assistant who were recently judged to have been exposed to radiation for as long as 1·5 hours because of faulty x-ray equipment. Some 25%

*Details can be found at the end of the chapter.

of x-ray sets in UK dental practices were over 15 years old in 1987/88, over 40% operated at less than the recommended minimum 50 kilovolts (kV), and 40% of intra-oral and 70% of panoramic assessments gave an unnecessarily high dose.[16] A report from 1972 showed that 39% of British dentists still held x-ray films in patients' mouths.[7] Having one's hand in the x-ray beam gives about 4000 times the exposure compared with that received 2 metres away (the recommended 'safe' distance).

Radiation accidents and natural radiation
Additional and possibly more important radiation hazards are those from accidents (eg Chernobyl), nuclear explosions and from domestic radon exposure in dental surgeries situated over uranium-bearing strata, in such areas as parts of Cornwall, Devon, Somerset, and Aberdeen, but also in some areas of Cumbria, Staffordshire, the West Midlands, Mid-Glamorgan and elsewhere. Although this radon hazard has only lately received serious attention, it has recently been suggested that it may account for 5000 to 20 000 excess deaths per year in the United States alone.[18] More than 75% of the annual exposure of the UK population to ionising radiation is from natural sources. Radon is now recognised as a hazard which might equal in magnitude that from cigarette smoking and from toxic waste. The chief danger is from inhalation of radon (an alpha-emitting gas), which can induce lung cancer and this risk is greatly potentiated by smoking. It must be presumed that radon exposure would have a cumulative effect with diagnostic radiation.

Radiation precautions in practice
Despite the higher risks from environmental and nuclear explosion radiation, there are moral and legal needs to reduce exposure to diagnostic radiation (Tables 4.1 and 4.2), not least the Ionising Radiation (Protection of Persons Undergoing Medical Examination or Treatment) Regulations 1988 (figs 4.1, 4.2 and 4.3). The NRPB provide a Dental Monitoring Service (*see* p 140) (fig. 4.4). The NRPB Dental Monitoring Service can provide practitioners with the information needed to meet the statutory requirements, with data on radiation dose rates, and with advice as to the necessity of appointing a Radiation Protection Adviser (page 111). The Standing Dental Advisory Committee (SDAC) has recently produced useful guidelines on 'Radiation Protection in Dental Practice' (1988) which

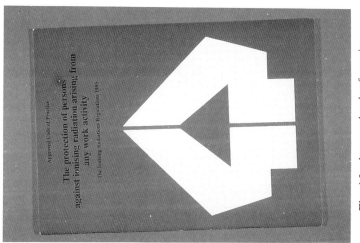

Fig. 4.2 Approved code of practice.

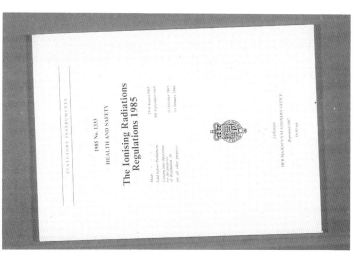

Fig. 4.1 Ionising Radiations Regulations.

Table 4.2 Minimisation of risks from dental radiology

---

(1) Only x-ray a patient if clinically necessary and use the minimum number of films and the fastest film available consistent with good film quality. Intensifying screens must be used for extra-oral and vertex occlusal views.
(2) Only allow a trained and competent operator to use the x-ray equipment.
(3) Ensure that the equipment is of adequate tube rating (preferably about 70 kV). Elderly equipment may emit soft quality x-rays.
(4) Ensure correct beam filtration and diameter.
(5) Ensure that the equipment is regularly properly checked and maintained. Checks are now required at 3-year intervals.
(6) Never hold the film, the patient or the tube housing during exposure and exclude from the x-ray room persons whose presence is unnecessary for the examination.
(7) The operator must stand at least 2·0 m from the tube and the patient, and outside the primary beam.
(8) Ensure that the exposure is correctly set, a minimum exposure time used and that the exposure is completely terminated. Disconnect the x-ray unit from the mains supply after use in order to eliminate the possibility of an inadvertent exposure.
(9) Monitor staff if their individual workload exceeds 150 intra-oral or 50 panoral films per week. Consider wearing a lead protective apron.
(10) All films should be correctly processed and routine checks should be made to detect any deterioration in the quality of radiographs.

Based on: Radiation Protection in Dental Practice. SDAC, 1988.

should be consulted (fig. 4.5). The Department of Health and the British Postgraduate Medical Federation have also issued a teaching videotape 'ALARA!* Radiation protection in dentistry' (fig. 4.6). The following is a synopsis of the SDAC guidelines, but the essence is to (a) reduce time of exposure, (b) increase distance from the x-ray source and (c) use shielding.

(1) Minimise radiographs taken
Legislation lays down controls for radiation safety (*see* Chapter 6) but the best way to reduce exposure is to take radiographs only when and where they are absolutely essential for diagnosis or treatment. The risk/benefit ratio should always be considered on each occasion. Radiographs may also need to be taken to avoid medicolegal difficulties. For example, if there is post-extraction pain but no dry socket apparent, it is prudent to take a film to exclude particularly a fracture of the jaw.

---

*As Low As Reasonably Achievable.

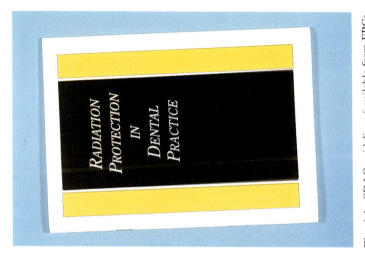

Fig. 4.4 SDAC guidelines (available from FPCs or Health Authorities or Health Boards).

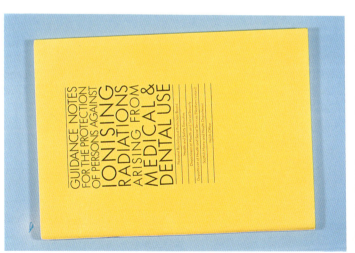

Fig. 4.3 Guidelines to radiation protection.

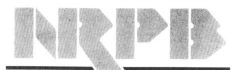

▶RADIATION PROTECTION
IN DENTISTRY

THE
DENTAL
MONITORING
SERVICE

▶a comprehensive service for
the Dental Profession

THE IONISING RADIATIONS REGULATIONS, 1985
THE IONISING RADIATION (PROTECTION OF
PERSONS UNDERGOING MEDICAL EXAMINATION
OR TREATMENT) REGULATIONS, 1988

Fig. 4.5   NRPB Dental Monitoring Service.

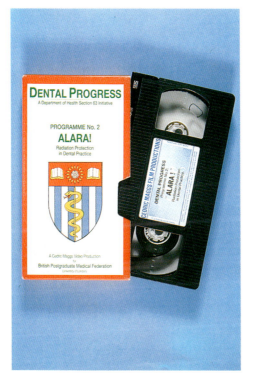

Fig. 4.6 'ALARA' video on radiation safety in dentistry.

(2) Take and develop films correctly
Films should be taken and developed correctly. Each film should yield the maximum amount of diagnostic information possible. To achieve this, the following are required:
(a) Correct alignment and collimation of the x-ray beam;
(b) Correct placing of the film and patient and correct exposure time;
(c) Choice of the fastest film *compatible with image quality*;
(d) Choice of the most effective intensifying screens *compatible with image quality*;
(e) Correct processing of the film to give optimum image quality.

The need for correct x-ray beam alignment is obvious, but collimation is important to reduce unnecessary exposure,[19] and is especially important in cephalometry.[20] The use of film holders and rectangular collimation for intra-oral films eliminates exposure of the patient's fingers and further reduced exposure.

It cannot be emphasised too strongly, therefore, that it is well worthwhile, in the interests of both safety and economy, to make sure that radiographic apparatus and techniques are up to the highest possible standards. An added incentive to the latter is the recent recommendation in the UK that the Dental Estimates Board (Dental Practice Board) may not reimburse practitioners for diagnostically useless radiographs. Processing solutions should be used at the recommended temperature and changed regularly, as advised by the manufacturer. The developer should be changed at least once a month but preferably fortnightly (*see also* Chapter 3). Processing must be carried out in a light-proof environment, either an automatic film processor or a dark room. Panoramic films are particularly light-sensitive and a special filter is required for the dark-room safelight if they are used. Films, once processed, should be washed for 20 minutes to remove chemicals and then dried in a dust-free atmosphere before viewing. They should be filed carefully in the patient's records afterwards.

(3) Maintain radiation equipment carefully

All x-ray equipment leaks radiation. Modern and well-maintained apparatus must therefore be used to keep this leakage to a minimum (see later). Collimating diaphragms must be used to restrict the useful x-ray beam to the area under study and aluminium filters to reduce skin absorption must be installed. It is also important to check that the duration of x-ray emission corresponds exactly with what is indicated on the timer switch.

(4) Keep well away from the x-ray source

The x-ray film should not be held by the operator during exposure and only the patient and operators should be in the room during the exposure. Distance is important since trebling the distance from an x-ray source reduces the radiation dose to about one-ninth (the inverse square law).

The exposure switch should be arranged such that it cannot be operated accidentally and that the operator can stand at least 2 metres away from the x-ray tube, out of line of the direct beam. Failing that, or if the x-ray workload exceeds 150 mA minutes per week for panoramic tomography and 30 mA minutes for other procedures (50 panoramic or 300 intra-oral films per week), a protective lead barrier equivalent to 0·5 mm lead must be provided for the operator. Persons in adjoining rooms should be protected by brick or concrete walls, or lead shielding. Partition walls are insufficient protection, unless specifically prepared to attenuate ionising radiation, for example by thin lead sheet or barium plaster.

(5) Use shielding
Plastic or rubber aprons incorporating lead salts are available and should be used for protecting patients, especially their radiosensitive tissues (gonads, bone marrow, thymus, thyroid, and any foetus) from radiation.[21]

An apron of lead-equivalent of at least 0·25 mm thickness (BS5783) is adequate for routine dental use and reduces exposure by 95%.[22] For panoramic radiation and cephalometry a double apron that covers the patient's back and front as well as sides, should be used. The use of lead aprons by staff would also reduce their occupational exposure.[22] Aprons should not be folded (they may crack) and should be examined annually to ensure that they still afford adequate protection.

(6) Use fast films
The fastest x-ray film consistent with adequate image quality (at least of ISO speed group D or faster) should be used, as this reduces radiation exposure. The fastest films currently available are the group E films, Kodak Ektaspeed and AGFA DM4, which reduce patient dose by 50% compared with D group Kodak ultraspeed films.[19,24,25] Ektaspeed and AGFA DM2 are available for periapical, bitewing, and occlusal films. Many now believe that E-speed films should be used almost exclusively.[14]

(7) Use of cassettes, intensifying screens and panoramic radiography
X-ray tubes produce x-rays that span a range of energies, including some above and some below those for which the x-ray film is most sensitive. Therefore, both high and low energy x-rays are produced which are not merely of no value, but also contribute to the radiation dose to patient and any exposed staff. The higher energies are limited by the kilovolt (peak) of the x-ray generator; the lower energies are limited by aluminium filtration, by the voltage wave form of voltage applied to the tube and by the kV(p) setting. Filters can reduce the dose of radiation (see below), but there is always some unnecessary radiation and efforts should be made to minimise this.

Extra-oral radiography uses cassettes containing intensifying screens. Cassettes are light-tight containers for light-sensitive film and contain sheets of card covered with calcium tungstate or other crystals which emit light when struck by x-radiation and thereby expose the film. Such cassettes reduce the radiation to about one tenth of that necessary to produce an image of the same density on wrapped packet film, but the detail is not as good as with intra-oral film. This results from the very poor edge definition produced by the crystals' diffuse light emission. The larger the crystals the poorer the definition, but the shorter the exposure. Rare earth screens (eg Kodak Lanex or 3M Trimax or Fuji RX ranges) not only further reduce the exposure, but the x-ray tube also lasts longer because of the reduced load.[26] However, for ordinary dental use there is little if any advantage because of the relatively low kilovoltage used in dental sets and for oblique lateral films the exposure may be made unmanageably short.

Panoramic films *may* also reduce exposure to radiation if used appropriately. A panoramic film gives about the same radiation dose as three bitewings or five periapicals and may be preferred when a whole mouth survey is indicated (Table 4.3). A panoramic film may also reveal unsuspected disease in the jaws or elsewhere. However, the limitations of panoramic films, especially in the anterior region, and the lesser quality of detail of the periodontal and periapical tissues, must be borne in mind. The reduction in exposure using rare earth screens for panoramic work is a major advantage and in the case of the Siemens rare earth screen there is also a significant improvement in overall definition. Unfortunately, these rare earth screens are expensive.

(8) Follow radiation protection regulations
Guidance notes for the protection of persons against ionising radiation arising from medical and dental use have been introduced in the UK.[27–31] These and the SDAC guidelines should be consulted, but

Table 4.3 Radiation doses from various examinations

Radiographic examination	Mean dose equivalent (μSv)*
1 intra-oral film	10
1 extra-oral film	15
1 panoramic tomograph	80

* See p 117.

the essential points in the regulations are outlined below and in Table 4.4 and in Chapter 6. Relevant signs are shown in figure 4.7.

Radiation Protection Adviser (RPA). The NRPB can suggest how to avoid the need to appoint an RPA who is otherwise needed to advise on observance of the Regulations and other health and safety matters connected with ionising radiation. An RPA is not needed in the general dental practice if:

(a) only the person undergoing a medical exposure enters a Controlled Area (1·5 m around the dental x-ray set when it is in use);

(b) no employee is exposed to an instantaneous dose rate exceeding 7·5 μSv h^{-1} (microsieverts per hour). If a distance of at least 2 m from the x-ray tube can be achieved, this exposure is unlikely to be exceeded.

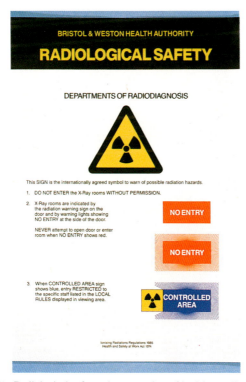

Fig. 4.7   Radiological safety; signs warning of ionising radiation hazard.

Table 4.4 Radiation rules

Check-list of essential actions to meet legislative requirements:

(1) *Notify the Health and Safety Executive* (HSE) of the use of x-rays in the practice.

Date of notification . . . .

(2) Decide whether or not there is a need to appoint a *Radiation Protection Adviser (RPA)* (see note 7).

(3) Appoint a suitably qualified and trained person within the practice as a *Radiation Protection Supervisor* (RPS).

Name of RPS . . . .

(4) Ensure equipment meets all *appropriate standards* in respect of radiation safety and is *regularly checked and maintained.*

Date of last equipment check . . . .

(5) *Provide Local Rules* which must include the name of the RPS(s), description of Controlled Area(s) and any special provisions of a local nature.

Date Local Rules provided . . . .

(6) *Provide adequate information, instruction* and *training* for all staff.

(7) *Ensure that staff cannot be exposed to an instantaneous dose rate exceeding 7·5 μSv per hour*, to avoid the need to appoint a Radiation Protection Adviser.

(8) *Provide a contingency plan* to specify actions to be followed in the event of an equipment malfunction.

(c) the limitations and conditions of use in Part I, paragraph 60 of the Approved Code of Practice are complied with;

(d) the x-ray equipment is properly maintained.

However, exemption only covers the operation of standard dental x-ray units when taking intra-oral and oblique jaw views and of panoramic units using intra-oral and extra-oral sources. It is, however, questionable whether intra-oral panoramic units should ever be used, because of high mucosal exposure.

Cephalometry should not be undertaken without the advice of a RPA, and the latter is also needed where there is the simultaneous use of more than one x-ray set in a room.

A dental practitioner will need to appoint an RPA if any persons other than those undergoing a medical exposure enter a controlled area, or employees are exposed to an instantaneous dose rate exceeding $7.5\,\mu Sv\,h^{-1}$. Advice regarding the implications of this can be obtained from the NRPB, who can also appoint an RPA if needed. An RPA is normally a medical physicist.

Radiation Protection Supervisor (RPS). The employer must appoint a suitably qualified and trained person from within the practice as RPS, to play a supervisory role in assisting the employer to comply with the requirements of the Regulations. The person appointed should be directly involved with the work with ionising radiations and preferably in a position to be able to exercise close supervision and ensure that the work is done in accordance with the Local Rules. Although the RPS need not be present at all times, adequate supervision must be maintained in their absence. No person should be appointed as a RPS unless that person:
(1) knows and understands the requirements of the Regulations and Local Rules as they affect the work that has to be supervised;
(2) commands sufficient respect from the people doing the work to allow the exercise of the necessary supervision for radiation protection;
(3) understands the necessary precautions to be taken in the work which is being done and the extent to which these precautions will restrict exposure.

The RPS should normally be a dentally qualified member of the practice. In a single-handed practice the RPS would normally be the dentist. The employer carries the ultimate responsibility for compliance with the Regulations. This cannot be delegated to an RPS.

Local Rules. Every employer who undertakes work with ionising radiation must devise and set down in writing the Local Rules, for the purpose of enabling the work with ionising radiation to be carried out in compliance with the Regulations, and shall ensure that such of those rules as are relevant are brought to the attention of employees and other persons who may be affected by them (Table 4.5).

X-ray tube voltage, beam size and filtration, and distance control. Dental x-ray equipment should be designed, constructed and installed in compliance with British Standards (eg BS 5724) and maintained in accordance with the recommendations of its manufacturer or the manufacturer's authorised representative.

Table 4.5 Example of Local Radiation Rules

(1) The Local Rules for the use of diagnostic x-rays and the Bristol Dental Hospital Supplementary Local Rules are based on current British legislation. The Bristol and Weston Area Health Authority Rules are available for inspection in the radiography department.
All these rules must be known and observed.

(2) All diagnostic views taken must be recorded, with the date, in the patient's notes.

(3) Radiographs may only be taken on the written prescription of a member of the professional staff.

(4) The patient must wear a lead apron which extends from the shoulders to the thighs for all radiographic procedures using dental x-ray machines.

(5) All extra-oral radiography in the Bristol Dental Hospital must only be performed by the radiography staff.

(6) Radiography rooms must not be entered when the red '*no entry*' warning sign is illuminated. The doors of radiography rooms must be closed when an exposure is made.

(7) Staff and students must be behind the protective screens whilst an exposure is being made. Extraneous people, such as the patient's relatives, must be outside the radiography room or area. Very young children or disabled patients may only be radiographed when being assisted by a parent or relative with the prior approval of the Radiation Protection Adviser who will prescribe the necessary protection required, which shall include the use of protective gloves.

(8) Spacers, filters and diaphragms must never be removed from dental x-ray machines.

(9) Any incident involving possible damage to an x-ray machine must be reported to the Radiation Protection Supervisor or his deputy immediately. The affected machine must not be used again until declared safe by the radiation physics department. This regulation particularly applies to accidental dropping or other damage to the exposure timers.

(10) No dental student shall take radiographs until in possession of a certificate of training, issued by the Clinical Dean's Office after successful completion of the prescribed course of instruction.

(11) Dental x-ray units situated in departments other than the department of dental radiography must not be used for routine examinations. These units must be used only for patients undergoing treatment which makes it impractical for the examination to be carried out in the radiography department of the dental hospital (eg patients undergoing endodontic treatment).

(12) All notices, rules, labels, safety instructions and exposure charts must be maintained in a legible condition and remain close to the exposure control behind the protective screens.

(13) Women who are, or who are likely to be, pregnant must not be radiographed unless special clinical needs make this absolutely essential. Any such prescription must be signed by a consultant and be further approved, finally, by the Radiation Protection Supervisor who will ensure maximal safeguards are afforded to both patient and foetus during exposure.

(14) In the event of an emergency involving exposure of persons to ionising radiation, the Radiation Protection Supervisor, or his deputy, must be informed immediately.

    (A)   Radiation Protection Adviser

    Name and Address

    (B)   Radiation Protection Supervisor

    Name and Address

The x-ray tube voltage should not be lower than 50 kilovolts (kV) and for intra-oral radiography should be preferably 70 kV, since lower kV values necessitate higher localised patient exposure.

Every x-ray source assembly (comprising an x-ray tube, an x-ray tube housing and a beam limiting device) should be constructed so that, at every rating specified by the manufacturer for the x-ray source assembly, the air kerma from the leakage radiation, at a distance from the focal spot of 1 m averaged over an area not exceeding 100 cm², does not exceed 1 mGy* in one hour. In practice, for equipment intended for dental radiography with an intra-oral film, radiation leakage should not exceed 0·25 mGy in one hour.

The total filtration of the beam (made up of the inherent filtration and any added filtration) should be equivalent to not less than the following:
(1) 1·5 mm aluminium for x-ray tube voltages up to and including 70 kV;
(2) 2·5 mm aluminium of which 1·5 mm should be permanent for x-ray tube voltages above 70 kV.

Equipment for radiography using an intra-oral film should be provided with a field-defining spacer-cone which will ensure a minimum focal-spot to skin distance of not less than 20 cm for equipment operating above 60 kV and not less than 10 cm for equipment operating at lower voltages. The correct setting of the equipment is particularly important where two or more interchangeable cones for different radiological techniques are available. The field diameter at the patient's end of the cone should not exceed 6 cm.

For panoramic tomography the beam size at the cassette holder should not exceed 10 mm × 150 mm. The total beam area should not exceed the area of the receiving slit of the cassette holder by more than 20%.

Exposure control (timer). Timers must operate accurately and reproducibly, and repeat exposures must not be possible without first fully releasing the exposure switch. Older timers are likely to need replacing. The calibration and correct exposure times need to be checked, since the characteristics of electronic timers differ markedly from the old mechanical types.

Exposure switches on all dental x-ray equipment should be so arranged that exposure continues only while continuous pressure is

---

*Gy = Gray = 100 Rads.

maintained on the switch and terminates immediately the pressure is released. To guard against automatic timing failure, an additional means of termination should be provided and must be independent of the normal means. Release of the exposure switch may be regarded as the additional means when this action overrides the timer.

Exposure switches should be designed to prevent inadvertent production of x-rays. If resetting is automatic, it should be ensured that pressure on the switch has to be released completely before the next exposure can be made.

All dental equipment control panels should be fitted with a light which gives a clearly visible indication (and preferably also an audible warning) to the operator, that an exposure is taking place. The light should be triggered by the flow of current directly responsible for the start and termination of the emission of radiation. For equipment fitted with an audible warning, the warning should be triggered by the same conditions. The exposure should be terminated automatically when a predetermined condition, such as a pre-set time, has been attained.

Monitoring is discussed below (*see* p 120).

Radiography room. Dental radiography should be carried out in a room (the x-ray room) from which all persons whose presence is unnecessary are excluded while x-rays are being produced. This room, which may be a dental surgery or a separate examination room, should not be used for other work or as a passageway whilst radiography is in progress. It should be large enough to provide safe accommodation for those persons who have to be in the room during x-ray examinations.

It is unlikely that the workload in most dental surgeries would exceed 300 intra-oral films or 50 panoramic examinations each week. Protective panels having a protective equivalent of not less than 0·5 mm of lead should be provided if the workload is likely to exceed this; that is:

(1) 150 mA minutes per week for panoramic tomography; or
(2) 30 mA minutes per week for other procedures.

Persons in all occupied areas immediately outside the x-ray room should be adequately protected. The x-ray room should be arranged so that:

(1) the radiation beam is directed away from those areas;
(2) use is made of the natural shielding of the walls, floor, and ceiling

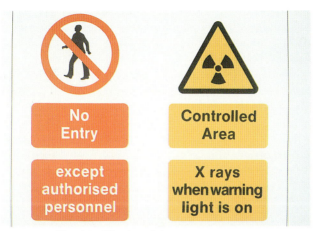

Fig. 4.8   Warning of Controlled Area.

of the x-ray room where these are relatively thick or dense, for example of brick or concrete;

(3) advantage is taken of the reduction in radiation level by distance.

If the normal structural materials do not afford sufficient shielding (for instance, a light-weight partition wall may sometimes be in the radiation beam), protective material such as lead ply should be attached to the wall concerned. The equipment must be installed so that the useful beam is directed away from any door or window, if the space immediately beyond is occupied. Adjacent areas, for example those used as waiting rooms, should not be controlled or supervised areas.

There should be a radiation warning sign, together with appropriate words on any x-ray room door that opens directly into an area where the instantaneous dose rate is greater than $7.5\,\mu\text{Sv}$* per hour (fig. 4.8). When the Controlled Area extends to any entrance of the x-ray room, an automatic warning signal should be given at that entrance while radiation is emitted.

If more than one x-ray unit is sited in any room, for instance in open plan accommodation, then arrangements should be made, in consultation with the Radiation Protection Adviser (RPA), to ensure that patients and staff are adequately protected.

---

* Sv = Sievert (the SI unit of radiation absorbed dose producing the same biological effect, in a specified tissue, as 1 Gray of high energy x-rays = 100 rem).

Since the beam is not always fully absorbed by the patient, it should be considered to extend beyond the patient until it has been attenuated by distance or intercepted by a primary protective shielding such as a brick wall.

If it is necessary to support a handicapped patient or child, this should only be done in accordance with the Local Rules drawn up with the advice of the RPA.

The tube housing should never be held by hand during an exposure. The operator must stand at least 2 m away, making use of the full length of cable to the exposure switch. A protective panel should, if possible, be provided and the operator should stand behind it. If the advice on avoidance of the beam and the protection afforded by distance is followed for ordinary dental radiography and for panoramic tomography, the operator should be outside the Controlled Area and should not therefore need to be designated as a classified person.

Any staff who enter a Controlled Area should either be classified persons or do so under a written system of work, which may include the need to wear a personal dosimeter (fig. 4.9). Operators who undertake significant numbers of radiographs (more than 150 intra-oral or 50 panoramic films per week) should wear a personal dosimeter; the period of issue may be up to 3 months (*see* p 120).

As mentioned earlier, the operator should check that the equipment

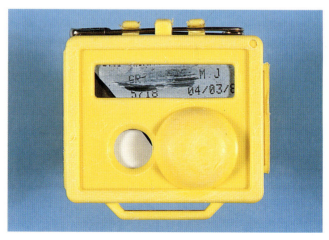

Fig. 4.9 Personal radiation dosimeter.

warning light and, where provided, any audible warning signal operates at each exposure and ceases at the end of the intended exposure time. If the warning does not operate or there is reason to think that the timer is defective or that there may be some other fault (for example, signs of damage, or excessive x-ray tube temperature), the equipment should be disconnected from the supply and not used again until it has been checked and, if necessary, repaired (see below)

Intra-oral radiography. A field-defining spacer tube or cylinder with an open end should be used. When alternative spacers are available or interchangeable spacers are provided, the one most suited to the technique to be employed should be fitted. The open end must be placed as close as possible to the patient's head to minimise the size of the incident beam: beam diameters should not exceed 6 cm and preferably should be collimated to a rectangular field. If a larger focal-spot to skin distance is required, a longer spacer should be employed. Cones should not be used since the field is not defined and the material of the cone in the x-ray beam gives secondary radiation. Cracks or chips on the cone lead to artefacts on the films.

The beam should not be directed towards the gonads. If the patient is a woman who is, or who may be, pregnant, care should be taken that the foetus is not irradiated inadvertently. Where x-rays are essential and such a beam direction cannot be avoided, the body should be covered by a protective apron with a protective equivalent of not less than 0·25 mm lead.

The dental film should be held by the patient only when it cannot otherwise be kept in position. It should virtually never be hand-held by anyone else. Exceptionally it may be held by someone other than the patient using a pair of forceps to avoid direct irradiation of the fingers, for example, when a child or a handicapped person cannot hold it themselves. In such cases, protective gloves and aprons should be worn, in accordance with advice obtained from the RPA.

The exposure factors should be checked by the operator on each occasion before an examination is made. This is particularly important when a short spacer is used after a long one and when there is more than one beam size setting. The larger apertures may be quite unsuitable for use with intra-oral films.

Intensifying screens should be used with all extra-oral films and for vertex occlusal views, and a lead apron should also be provided for the patient.

Panoramic tomography. If the rotational movement fails to start, or stops before the full arc is covered, the switch should be released immediately to avoid high localised exposure of the patient.

Panoramic radiography with an intra-oral x-ray tube. Beam applicators should be used to protect tissues such as the tongue, which do not have to be irradiated for the production of a satisfactory radiograph. Care should be taken in positioning the x-ray tube in order to get satisfactory and consistent results. Because of the unnecessary exposure of tissues not being examined, intra-oral panoramic units still in use should be phased out as soon as practicable.

Monitoring. If any individual's workload exceeds 150 intra-oral radiographs (or 50 panoramic films) per week, that person should be provided with a dosimeter (fig. 4.9). A 3-month wearing period is suitable. The recorded doses should be reviewed by the RPS on receipt, and action taken if any dose exceeds that expected; for example, 150 exposures per week should result in a dose no greater than 0·25 mSv.

When personal dosimeters are not in use they should be stored outside the radiography room, in a dry place away from heat. The NRPB provides an advice and monitoring service (figs 4.5 and 4.10) (The Dental Monitoring Service) and personal dosimeters can be

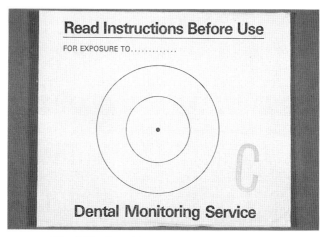

Read Instructions Before Use

FOR EXPOSURE TO............

Dental Monitoring Service

Fig. 4.10 Dental Radiation Monitoring Service.

obtained from the NRPB (*see* p 140). At least two companies offer electronic personal devices that give an audible and visual alarm of acute and chronic over-exposure (X-Alert: GXR1 alarm).

Accidents. If the exposure warning light remains on after the set time has elapsed, or any other fault is apparent or suspected, the x-ray unit should be immediately isolated from the mains supply. It should not be used again until an investigation has resulted in a satisfactory explanation and remedial action has been carried out by service agents. A contingency plan should be prepared and available, to specify the actions to be followed.

If, as a result of malfunction of an x-ray unit, a patient may have been exposed to considerably more ionising radiation than intended, the incident must be investigated immediately. If the investigation shows beyond reasonable doubt that such an incident has happened, the Health and Safety Executive must be notified and arrangements made for a detailed investigation of the circumstances of the exposure and an assessment of the dose received. A copy of the report of any such investigation is supposed to be kept for *at least 50 years* from the date on which it was made!

Maintenance. Equipment should be checked and maintained in accordance with the manufacturer's directions. A record of maintenance, including any defects found and their repair, should be kept for each item of x-ray equipment. X-ray developer should be changed at least monthly, but preferably fortnightly.

Radiation survey. A thorough radiation safety assessment of all x-ray equipment, including measurements of radiation dose, must be carried out by a competent authority *at intervals not exceeding 3 years.* Any recommendations made as a result of this assessment should be implemented within 3 months. The NRPB can provide such a service.

Cross infection control. This is discussed in Chapter 5, but barrier envelopes for intra-oral films are now available (fig. 4.11).

Dose reduction in dental radiography. This is discussed in detail by Horner and Hirschmann (*J Dent* 1990; **18**: 171–184).

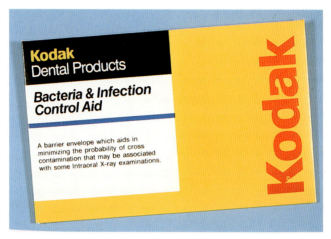

Fig. 4.11   Barrier envelope for intra-oral x-ray film.

Non-ionising radiation (fig. 4.12)

Electromagnetic radiation

Electromagnetic radiation is emitted by a variety of sources, ranging from transmitter towers to electric power lines, computer terminals, electric clocks, microwave ovens and electric blankets. The public has become concerned about possible adverse effects from electromagnetic fields emanating from power transmission lines, but the evidence indicates that, although under special circumstances weak low frequency electromagnetic fields can produce changes at the cellular level *in vitro*, there is little, if any, reliable evidence for a health risk and, in any event, there is more exposure to electromagnetic radiation from household appliances and wiring than from power lines. Moreover, *natural* electromagnetic radiation is at least 100 times as intense as that induced by power lines.[32-34] Nevertheless, electromagnetic radiation can sometimes interfere with pacemakers (page 137). Recently there has been an unconfirmed report of a higher incidence of male breast cancer in workers exposed to high electromagnetic fields.

Ultraviolet light

The most obvious source of ultraviolet light is exposure to the sun. The universally recognised consequence is sunburn, but less obvious are hazards to the eyes and predisposition to melanoma and squamous

Wave lengths or frequencies

nM

10^{-4}	Cosmic rays	100	Extreme Ultraviolet UVC
	Gamma rays	280	UVB (Sunburn range)
	X-rays (medical x rays: TV:VDU)		
10	Ultra-violet light (Sun, UV curing, VDU)	315	UVA (Pigment darkening)
400	Visible light		
700	Infra red Light (Sun, VDU)	400	Violet Indigo Blue 'Blue light'
10^6	Microwaves and UHF (Radar, microwaves, VDU)		Green Yellow Orange Red
80–100 Hz	VHF		
4–12 MHz	Short-wave bands (Radio: VDU: TV)		
500–1500 KHz	Medium-wave band		
150–250 KHz	Long-waves		
10–100 KHz	Very low frequencies (High voltage lines: VDU)		

VDU = Visual display units

Fig. 4.12   The electromagnetic spectrum.

or basal cell carcinoma of the skin. These dangers are all too real, as shown by the rapidly increasing incidence of malignant melanoma. Ultraviolet C consists of wavelengths below 286 nm and these are effectively filtered out by the ozone layer surrounding the earth. The amount of absorption varies and is less near to the equator and at high altitudes owing to the reduced atmospheric thickness. UVB consists of wavelengths between 286 nm and 320 nm; these are responsible for sunburn and snow blindness (actinic retinitis). The amount of such ultraviolet light received is substantially increased by reflection from surfaces such as snow, sand and water. UVA (wavelengths between 320 nm and 400 nm) is possibly the most dangerous and causes chronic damage to the eyes, especially if there is low dose exposure over a long period of time. UVA light can induce cataracts, but the longer wavelength components can also damage the retina.[35-39] UVA light sources in dentistry include UV sources for the curing of restorative resins and fissure sealants and UV plaque lights (320 nm to 365 nm) but these have largely been replaced by blue or white light sources. UV light is also emitted from fluorescence equipment and arc welding equipment, as well as sun-lamps and bactericidal lamps. For further details see ISBN 0 85951 063 8 from the National Radiological Protection Board. Protection against UV hazards is discussed in more detail in Chapter 2.

Blue light

Visible blue light (400–500 nm) sources activate diketones in dental composite materials and were developed to overcome the dangers of UV radiation. However, even blue light is not entirely safe, since it contains high energy photons with the potential for damage to the retina.[35,40-43] Blue light forms reactive free radicals in the eye and in the retina these produce peroxides that denature photoreceptors.[44] Blue light may therefore damage the retina.[44] Viewing blue light also disturbs vision for periods of up to 2 minutes afterwards. During this time, hue perception is impaired and repeated viewing of blue light sources used for curing some filling materials may lead to visual fatigue as well as cumulative damage to the retina. It may possibly also predispose to cataracts.[41]

Blue light emitters vary enormously in the amount of radiation emitted,[45] and exposure also depends on whether the light is viewed directly or is reflected from the mouth or teeth. Daily maximum permissible exposure for direct viewing can be as short as 12 minutes and for indirect exposure, 40 minutes.[43] Blue light damage is additive.[46] Protection against this hazard is discussed in Chapter 2.

White (visible) light

Visible white light (400 nm–700 nm) sources for photopolymerisation also emit minute amounts of both UV and blue light, and green light (490 nm–600 nm). Although the risks from this are very small, protective eyewear that absorbs these wavelengths should still be worn.[42]

Protection against this hazard is also discussed in Chapter 2.

Lasers

Laser is the acronym for *L*ight *A*mplification by *S*timulated *E*mission of *R*adiation. The wavelength of the photons (radiation) is controlled by the type of laser and lasing medium used. The effect of a laser on target tissue depends on the wavelength, beam power, degree of focus, duration of exposure and distance to target, as well as the absorption by the tissue.[37] In general, lasers rapidly heat and damage tissues. There are hundreds of different lasers in use, but really only four in surgical or dental practice, namely carbon dioxide, NdYAG (neodymium, yttrium, aluminium, garnet), krypton and argon-ion lasers (Table 4.6). Their use in dentistry is limited but expanding,[47-52] although the hazards involved in their use have received little attention.

The carbon dioxide laser emits light (wavelength 10·6 µm) which is absorbed by water-containing tissues and can be used to cut soft and hard tissues, including dental hard tissues. It cannot be transmitted by fibre-optics. Because the CO_2 laser is invisible it is used co-axially with a helium–neon laser to produce a visible red beam. CO_2 lasers are expensive and potentially very dangerous; they are rarely used in dentistry, except in surgery.

The NdYAG (wavelength 1·06 µm) and krypton lasers are also used clinically and have the great advantage that they can be transmitted down a fibre-optic path. The NdYAG (near infrared) laser is invisible and therefore used with a helium–neon laser. It is used in dentistry for cutting dentine and soft tissues. It is also used for photocoagulation.

The argon laser produces a blue-green light of 0·5 µm wavelength and can be transmitted by fibre-optics. It has applications in dentistry, mainly for polymerising some composite materials. It is also used for photocoagulation.

The helium–neon (He-Ne) laser, which produces light of 0·63 µm wavelength and the diode laser (0·90 µm wavelength) emit light in the near infrared or visible part of the spectrum and if restricted to only milliwatt powers, produce little if any heating or direct photochemical effect on tissues. For this reason they are known as 'soft' lasers. Indeed, the beam of a soft laser penetrates directly only to a depth of about 0·8 mm and soft lasers are of little proven benefit in dentistry.[53,54] However, the He-Ne laser makes a good projection screen pointer.

Lasers are therefore available with energies of different wavelengths which have specific absorptive characteristics in different

Table 4.6 Classification of medical lasers

Laser type	Wavelength μm	Typical class	Features
Helium–neon	0·63	1,2 or 3A or 3B	Little hazard to the eyes unless directly viewed intra-beam.
Gallium arsenide	0·85 0·90	3B	MPE can be exceeded unless viewed with diffuse reflector.
Argon ion	0·49 0·51	4	Direct intra-beam viewing and reflections are hazardous. Also a fire risk.
Krypton ion	0·53 0·57 0·65 0·68	4	Direct intra-beam viewing and reflections are hazardous. Also a fire risk.
NdYAG	1·06	4	Direct intra-beam viewing and reflections are hazardous. Also a fire risk.
Carbon dioxide	10·6	4	Direct intra-beam viewing and reflections are hazardous. Also a fire risk.
Dye for example Rhodamine 6G Rhodamine 640	0·59 0·63	4	Direct intra-beam viewing and reflections are hazardous. Also a fire risk.
Ruby	0·69	4	Direct intra-beam viewing and reflections are hazardous. Also a fire risk.

tissues.[55] The argon and NdYAG lasers, in particular, have wavelengths in the spectrum of visible light and are absorbed preferentially by pigmented tissues, especially by the retina which can be damaged if a laser is shone into the eye. The CO_2 laser emits energy in the infrared zone. This is invisible but damages tissue by the production of heat. The helium–neon laser is less damaging, but must still be used with care; even soft lasers are not without some hazard to the retina.

All lasers are potentially hazardous, particularly because of eye damage, burns and the risks of fire or electric shock.[37] The medical lasers used in practice (for example CO_2 and NdYAG) produce intense beams with power absorbed per unit area of tissue, many orders of magnitude greater than that from the sun. They can cause severe burns. The effects on tissues depend on the factors discussed above. Retinal tissues are burnt or photochemically damaged within seconds, often irreversibly, by the shorter wavelength light and near infrared radiation. Repeated exposures also have a deleterious cumulative effect on the retina. Ultraviolet and longer infrared radiations can burn the cornea or result in cataracts. Even the skin can be damaged by these various wavelengths. *All* lasers should therefore always be used with great care and *never* shone into the eyes, in unintended directions or onto brightly plated instruments which reflect the laser.[37,56]

Laser products are classified from 1 to 4, depending on the power output (Table 4.6). Class 1 lasers are virtually safe, but classes 3 and 4 must be used only under medical or dental supervision. Lasers should conform to BS 4803 (British Standard on Radiation Safety of Laser Products and Systems, 1983) and BS 5724 and users of class 3B and 4 lasers (Table 4.6) are required to consult the laser protection adviser and to register with the District Health Authority (Nursing Homes (laser) Regulations 1984).[57] Most dental lasers are Class 3B or 4.

Protection of the eyes against laser damage is discussed in Chapter 2. Guidelines on laser safety are available,[57] and are also summarised here (fig. 4.13).

The Health Authority or other employing Authority is responsible for the implementation of health and safety advice about lasers. Safety of lasers also requires the appointment of a Laser Protection Adviser (LPA) when class 3A, 3B or 4 lasers are in use (Table 4.6). Local Rules should be drawn up (Table 4.7) and a laser Controlled Area established, where maximum permissible exposure (MPE) may be exceeded (BS 4803: part 3: 1983). Warning signs (BS 4803: Part 3: 1983) must be provided at every entrance (fig. 4.14). All laser products must carry clearly visible labels, indicating the laser class, precautions required, maximum laser output, and wavelength (fig. 4.15).

A Nominated User, skilled in the safe use of the laser, should be present when a class 3B or 4 laser is used medically, and should be registered with the Health Authority. Class 3A, 3B and 4 lasers must have a master control that will only function when the key is inserted

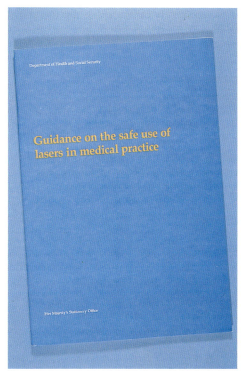

Fig. 4.13   Guidance on the safe use of lasers (HMSO, 1984).

and operated (fig. 4.16), and must give an audible or visible warning when the laser is switched on and operating or not discharged. Foot switches to operate the laser must be shrouded to prevent accidental operation. Class 3B and 4 lasers must have a red emergency shut-off switch in a prominent accessible position.

Medical lasers may produce damage at some distance from the working area if the beam is reflected out of, or is directly pointed away from, the area. Walls will block a laser but windows may not. The laser must therefore be aimed and fired only at the chosen tissue site. The operator should verbally warn staff in the vicinity that the laser is about to be fired, and all staff and patients should wear protective eyewear *suitable for the laser wavelength used* (*see* p 141).

Table 4.7 Example of Local Rules for laser use (Class 3B or 4)

(A) Description of laser system (wavelength/wattage) ....

(B) Laser class ....

(C) Safety measures
Safe use of the laser depends upon strict adherence to the following rules:

(1) Register
A register shall be kept of:

(a) Personnel authorised to operate the equipment.

(b) Personnel authorised to assist in the use of the equipment.

One authorised operator shall be nominated (eg a Laser Safety Supervisor) to ensure that the register is maintained and to assume overall control of the installation and its safe operation.

(2) Staff responsibilities
It is the responsibility of staff authorised to be present during use of the laser to be aware of the nature of the hazard involved, to be familiar with the Manufacturer's Operating Instructions and to ensure that the requirements for their own safety and for the patient's safety are being observed.

(3) Laser Controlled Area
The operating area in which the laser is to be used shall be designated Laser Controlled Area while the laser is in that area. In so far as is practicable, entry into the Laser Controlled Area shall be limited to personnel whose presence at the operation is essential.

Spectators shall not be permitted into the Laser Controlled Area unless appropriate supervisory approval has been obtained, and appropriate protective measures taken.

(4) Eye and skin protection
All personnel in the Laser Controlled Area shall wear proper laser protective eyewear when the laser apparatus is connected to the electrical mains supply. The one exception is the surgeon who uses the operating microscope during the firing of the laser. All protective eyewear shall be labelled clearly with the optical density value, the wavelength(s) against which protection is afforded and the maximum radiant exposure or irradiance to which the eyewear may be exposed. If the design of the eyewear leaves no room for this inscription, then the eyewear shall be labelled clearly with an identity mark traceable to a certificate bearing a statement of the above optical parameters.

While the maximum permissible exposure for skin is the same as that for eyes, it may not be practical to insist that staff wear protective gauntlets and it is the responsibility of the operator to ensure that the laser is fired only when it has been aimed at the operating site.

(5) Test procedure
The safety circuits should be tested at the beginning of each day's use. When testing, care must be taken to ensure that the beam is directed at non-flammable material sufficient to absorb all the energy emitted from the laser aperture, eg asbestos block or moist gauze.

Table 4.7—*continued*

---

(6) **Custody of the key**
When not in use the key will be kept in the custody of . . . .
. . . .

The key will be clearly labelled with the words:

'Laser. To be used by authorised personnel only'.

(7) **Procedure before activation of CO_2 laser**
The laser system incorporates a manual shutter at the laser head which can block off both visible and infra-red laser beams. This shutter shall be closed in order to block the beams except when the microscope-laser assembly has been positioned by the operator and aimed approximately at the target area. The shutter may then be opened in order to allow finer adjustment with the micromanipulator mirror and the red He-Ne laser spot. If the assembly is then to be positioned at a new site, the manual shutter must again be closed.
    The operator, each time he activates the laser source by stepping on the foot-switch, must clearly announce his intention to do so, in order to warn staff in the vicinity.
    The laser shall only be activated by the operator who is responsible for the safe custody of the master key to the system.
    The operator is responsible for ensuring that persons assisting in the procedures are fully trained in the safe performance of their duties, and is responsible for the safety of any visitors who may be present.
    When the laser is in operation the number of persons in the room shall be kept to a minimum.
    All personnel except the attending nurse and the operator should keep behind the laser/microscope and well clear of the operator. Appropriate laser safety goggles must be worn by all personnel except the operator who will be protected by the viewing microscope.
    The laser shall not be switched on unless it is directed towards the patient, a suitable thermal barrier or a power measuring instrument.

(8) **General precautions in the use of high power infra-red laser sources**
Care must be taken to avoid directing the laser beam at instruments: metallic surfaces reflect laser light.
    When working in the vicinity of the patient's face, or where laser light can reach the patient's eyes, eye protection is recommended. The patient's lips can be protected to some extent by moist gauze, an energy-absorbing material. It may be desirable to place moist gauze behind a target area when aiming the laser at an oblique target which has healthy tissue as a background. Consideration should be given to the possibility that the laser beam may penetrate completely through some tissue, creating a hazard to theatre staff. In this case, moist gauze should be positioned so as to absorb any exit radiation.

(9) **Operation of laser**
The following operating procedure shall be observed:

(a) Close the key switch and verify that the warning light outside the door is illuminated.
(b) Close the door.

Table 4.7—*continued*

(c) Carry out the manufacturer's recommended TEST procedure.
(d) Adjust the microscope for treatment, then press the ON switch. Verify that the aiming beam is present. Set the desired power level.
(e) Select the mode of operation. Advise all present that treatment is about to start and then proceed using the foot-switch.
(f) For a short pause in treatment press the *standby* switch to disable the foot-switch.
(g) When treatment of a patient is completed, or a change of equipment position is necessary press the OFF switch.
(h) At the end of the session of operation remove the key.

When the equipment is unattended by an authorised operator, the control panel must be switched off and the key withdrawn and placed in safe custody by the authorised operator.

Warning signs
The laser shall have attached to it a clearly displayed warning sign, bearing the words:

DANGER
VISIBLE AND INVISIBLE LASER RADIATION
AVOID EYE OR SKIN EXPOSURE TO DIRECT OR
SCATTERED RADIATION
CLASS 'X' LASER PRODUCT

and shall include statements of the maximum output of laser radiation and either the laser medium or the emitted wavelengths. In addition, a sign shall be clearly displayed on the outside of the door of the Laser Controlled Area.

Operators and assistants must sign that they have read and understood these Local Rules. The completed statement will be sent to the Secretary of the Radiological Safety Committee.

Explosion hazards

Plastic or rubber anaesthetic tubes may be pierced by the laser beam, with the consequent risk of a serious explosion hazard if flammable agents are being used. Such tubing must be protected with a coating which will reflect any incident CO_2 laser energy. Aluminium tape (3M No 425) has been recommended for this purpose. All such tubes in close proximity to the operating site must be protected before the laser is first activated.

Accidents

Any incident should be reported to the LPA who will investigate it (see also the Notification of Accidents and Dangerous Occurrences Regulations, 1980; Chapters 3 and 6).

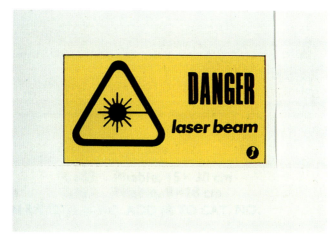

Fig. 4.14   Laser warning sign.

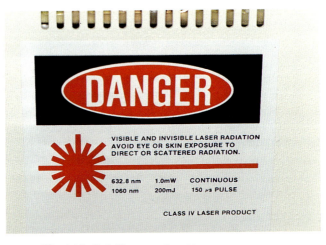

Fig. 4.15   Labelling on a dental NdYAG laser.

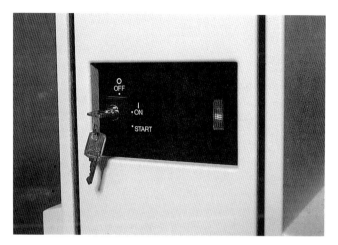

Fig. 4.16 Lasers must be key controlled.

Video display units (VDUs or monitors)

VDUs have now appeared in most workplaces, including many dental practices and there has been some concern about their potential for adverse effects on health. The chief hazard from VDUs is that of tripping over the cables, but eye strain, postural problems and, theoretically, radiation are also possible hazards (Table 4.8).

VDUs operate in the same way as television receivers. In addition to emission of light, which forms the image on the screen, excitation of the phosphors by the electron beam also causes emission of minute amounts of ultraviolet and infrared rays, and low energy x-rays. Very low frequency (VLF) and extremely low frequency (ELF) electro-

Table 4.8 Possible hazards and alleged complaints associated with office computers

Known hazards	Alleged hazards[a]
RSI (repetitive strain injury)	Miscarriages
Electric shocks or burns	Male reproductive problems
Stress from printer noise, cyberphobia, heat, etc.	Facial dermatitis
	Cancers
	Cataracts
	Photosensitive triggering of epilepsy

[a]Not proven.

magnetic radiation is also emitted. Measurement of the radiation from VDUs has, however, shown the level to be exceedingly low and often lower than from many domestic appliances.[58-61]

At least 15 million video display units (VDUs) are in use in offices and homes as computer screens, in North America. Cataracts, reproductive disorders, foetal congenital abnormalities and facial dermatitis have allegedly resulted from working with VDUs, but recent authoritative reviews of the evidence have shown that these are no more frequent than in those who are not exposed to VDUs.[60,61]

Reports of a rosacea-like dermatitis in VDU-operators have mainly been from northern Europe,[62-68] where the relative humidity in heated rooms is low and static electric fields can form. Electrostatic shielding using metal nets or metallised plastic effectively reduces this problem; polyamide carbon shields are less effective.[59] Some monitors (eg Taxan) have a particularly low level of electrostatic and electromagnetic emission. Other manufacturers, perhaps taking advantage of public concern, are now producing low-radiation VDUs. Shields such as Periphlex may be useful in other cases.

The possible production of cataracts through VDU use has been a source of concern, but there is no reliable evidence that this is a hazard.[60] Indeed, radiation-induced cataracts require some 10 000 times the exposure expected from a VDU. However, prolonged work at VDUs is fatiguing, particularly for those with minor sight defects, as correction for middle-distance viewing is rarely carried out adequately. This should be considered by dental staff who find computer work particularly tiring. Special spectacles may be needed, or existing spectacles may require modification for this purpose. If the eyesight cannot readily accommodate for reading computer monitors, and if appropriate spectacles have not been prescribed, it is possible that the resulting eyestrain may lead to blurred vision, tension and headaches. This in turn may lead to depression and some of the other symptoms ascribed to working with VDUs.

Spectacles such as Comput-irex are said to filter blue and UV light and diminish screen flicker. Lighting should also be carefully arranged to illuminate any documents being read but not to degrade the screen image. Screen flicker should no longer contribute to fatigue. If there is flicker, it is from one of the earlier screens or there is some fault. Currently available VDUs, even inexpensive ones, have no visible flicker owing to the use of persistent phosphors.

Eye disorders such as eyestrain, irritation and blurred vision, and headaches, may follow any work involving prolonged intensive use of the eyes. This is especially the case in older individuals, where lighting is poor, or where the person is not wearing proper spectacles, but these disorders are not increased in VDU operators. However, a rather strange but benign visual phenomenon (the McCullough effect), can follow long periods of viewing green characters on a black background, and consists of letters or lines on a contrasting background assuming a pink colour. The cause of the McCullough effect is unknown.

A further point of concern has been that the flickering of the VDU display might provoke epileptic attacks, but there is no good evidence for concern and, as mentioned previously, modern VDUs flicker less than conventional television screens.

Another anxiety is that of the possible musculoskeletal disorders and stress-inducing effects of VDUs—repetitive strain injury (RSI). There is some evidence that these can be genuine problems and that pains and stiffness in the neck, shoulders, back and wrists, and carpal tunnel syndrome (Chapter 3) are not uncommon.[60,70] These, however, are related more to poor posture and the elimination of tasks that once required office workers to get up and move around once in a while, rather than concentrating on the VDU itself. Sounds from cooling fans and daisywheel printers, though not responsible for hearing loss, can aggravate or tire VDU operators, even though the sound rarely exceeds 68 dB (Chapter 2). A few VDU operators do become stressed by the work, but these are operators who sit for very long hours at repetitive tasks under close monitoring.[60,71] Fear of the new technology (cyberphobia) is a rare but recognised cause of stress. Most VDU operators, however, have a better quality of life at work since automation has removed many of the more mundane, boring jobs.

Radiation and the eyes

Various types of radiation can damage the eyes, and although hazards to the eyes are discussed in Chapter 2, x-irradiation, lasers and some ultraviolet irradiation—electromagnetic radiations of shorter than 400 nm wavelength (fig. 4.12)—are particular hazards, especially to the lens. Less obvious dangers come from infrared radiation within the 400–1400 nm wavebands, which can burn or cause photochemical damage to the retina, and from sunlight. Holidays in the sunshine may well constitute a risk similar to or greater than that from some

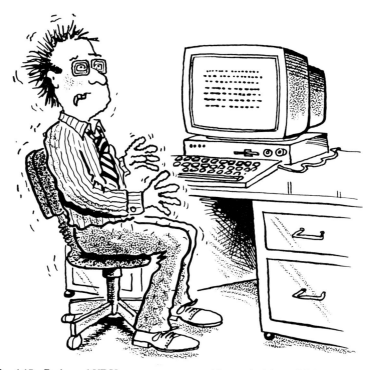

Fig. 4.17   Prolonged VDU use may cause repetitive strain injury (RSI), but there is no evidence of other occupational hazard.

dental light sources! Sunlight, particularly when viewed directly, can cause damage via a range of different wavelength radiations. Wavelengths below 315 nm are absorbed mainly by the cornea and can cause photokeratitis and cataracts; light between 315 nm and 400 nm is less damaging, but may be absorbed by, and damage, the lens. Visible (blue) light in the 400–500 nm range can produce retinitis, whereas infrared radiation of 700–1400 nm can thermally injure the retina and radiation from 1400 nm to 1500 nm wavelengths can damage the cornea or cause cataracts.

X-irradiation of sufficient level can not only induce cataracts but can also damage the developing eye in the foetus.

Pacemaker interference

Electromagnetic radiation is emitted from some dental equipment such as ultrasonic scalers and electrosurgical units, as well as diathermy units, microwave ovens, computer terminals and induction casting machines. Magnetic resonance imaging (MRI) or nuclear magnetic resonance (NMR) equipment can also interfere with pacemakers.

Electromagnetic radiation can interfere with older types of unshielded pacemakers and, if in doubt, the cardiologist concerned should be consulted or the above equipment not used. However, for all practical purposes, this is no longer a serious problem.

Hearing aid interference

A recent study has shown that dental x-rays do not have any adverse effect on hearing aids.[72] Nevertheless, patients should remove them before extra-oral radiography is carried out, as they may cast a shadow on the film.

References

1   Warren S, Lombard S. Survey of radiation exposure of Massachusetts dentists. *J Mass Dent Soc* 1966; **15**: 223–224.
2   Leading article. Dental x-rays, for caries or cash? The *Lancet* 1983; **2**: 609.
3   Kendall GM, Darby SC, Rae S. The level of dental radiography in Great Britain. *Br Dent J* 1981; **151**: 377–379.
4   Wall BF, Kendall GM. Collective doses and risks from dental radiology in Great Britain. *Br J Radiol* 1983; **56**: 511–516.
5   Sewerin I. Annual number of intra-oral radiographs in Denmark and other countries. *Community Dent Oral Epidemiol* 1986; **14**: 123.
6   Council on Dental Materials, Instruments and Equipment. Recommendations in radiographic practices: an update, 1988. *J Am Dent Assoc* 1989; **118**: 115–117.
7   Smith NJ. The hazards to the dentist and his staff from dental radiology. *Dent Pract Dent Rec* 1972; **22**: 409–413.
8   Kinkel HlH, Young M. Diagnosis, treatment and prognosis of Roentgen ray injuries to dentists. *J Am Dent Assoc* 1955; **51**: 1–7.
9   Jiraseh L, Jirashowa M. Occupational dermatitis in stomatological centre staff. *Cesk Dermatol* 1978; **53**: 50–57.
10   Arndt VD, Lenz U, Konig W. Platten epithel karzinom der Haut mit Toderfolge bei einem beruflich strahlen-exponierten stomatologen. *Berufsdermatosen* 1975; **23**: 201–207.
11   White SC, Frey NW. An estimation of somatic hazards to the United States population from dental radiology. *Oral Surg* 1977; **43**: 152–159.

12	Smith NJD. Risk assessment: the philosophy underlying radiation protection. *Int Dent J* 1987; **37**: 43–51.
13	Kaugars GE, Broga DW, Collett WK. Dental radiologic survey of Virginia and Florida. *Oral Surg* 1985; **60**: 225–229.
14	Monsour PA, Kruger BJ, Barnes A, Sainsbury A. Measures taken to reduce X-ray exposure of the patient, operator and staff. *Aust Dent J* 1988; **33**: 181–192.
15	Havukainen R. Survey of dental radiographic equipment and radiation doses in Finland. *Acta Radiol* 1988; **29**: 4.
16	Hewitt JM, Shutteworth PG, Nelthorpe PA, Hudson AP. Improving protection standards in dental radiography. *In* Goldfinch EP (ed). *Radiation protection— Theory and practice.* pp 81–84. Bristol: Institute of Physics, 1989.
17	Hicks HH. Hazards of radiation from x-ray exposure. *J Am Dent Assoc* 1967; **75**: 1194–1195.
18	Kerr RA. Indoor radon: the deadliest pollutant. *Science* 1988; **240**: 606–608.
19	Gratt BM, White SC, Halse A. Clinical recommendations for the use of D-speed film, E-speed film, and xeroradiography. *J Am Dent Assoc* 1988; **117**: 609–614.
20	Hirschmann PN, Lovelock DJ, Gravely JF, Senior WB. Reduction of the dose to patients during lateral cephalometric radiography. *Br Dent J* 1985; **158**: 415.
21	Sikorski PA, Taylor KW. The effectiveness of the thyroid shield in dental radiology. *Oral Surg* 1984; **58**: 225–236.
22	Bean LR, Devore WD. The effect of protective aprons in dental roentgenography. *Oral Surg* 1969; **28**: 505–508.
23	Triolo K, Konicki DL, Struba RJ. Radiation hygiene—an overview. *Dent Hygiene* 1979; **53**: 359–364.
24	Kaffe I, Littner MM, Kuspet ME. Densitometric evaluation of intraoral x-ray films. Ektaspeed versus Ultraspeed. *Oral Surg* 1984; **57**: 80–87.
25	Shira RE. Methods for reducing patient exposure combined with Kodak Ektaspeed dental X-ray film. *Dent Radiog Photo* 1981; **54**: 80–87.
26	British Institute of Radiology. Low attenuation materials and rare earth screens in radiodiagnosis. *Br J Radiol* 1986; **59**: 745.
27	The Ionising Radiations Regulations. Health and Safety Commission, 1985. ISBN 0-11-057-3331.
28	The Ionising Radiation (Protection of Persons undergoing medical examination of treatment) Regulations 1988. Health and Safety Commission, 1988. ISBN 0-11-086778-5.
29	The protection of persons against ionising radiation arising from work activity (Approved Code of Practice) Health and Safety Commission, 1985. ISBN 0-11-883838-5.
30	Guidance notes for the protection of persons against ionising radiations arising from medical and dental use. National Radiological Protection Board, 1988. ISBN 0-85951-299-1.
31	Radiation Protection in Dental Practice. Department of Health, 1988.
32	Abelson PH. Effects of electric and magnetic fields. *Science* 1989; **245**: 241.
33	National Radiological Protection Board. Advice on the protection of workers and members of the public from possible hazards of electric and magnetic fields with frequencies below 300 GHz. HMSO, 1986. ISBN 0-85951-267-3.
34	Servantie B. Damage criteria for determining microwave exposure. *Health Physics* 1989; **56**: 781–786.
35	Ham WT, Mueller HA, Sliney DG. Retinal sensitivity to short wavelength light. *Nature* 1976; **260**: 153–155.
36	Lerman S. Human ultraviolet radiation cataracts. *Ophthalmol Res* 1980; **12**: 303–314.
37	Sliney DM, Wolbarsht M. Effects of optical radiation on the eye. In: *Safety with*

lasers and other optical sources. A comprehensive handbook. pp 101–151. New York: Plenum Press, 1980.

38 Mills LF, Lytle CD, Anderson FA *et al.* A review of biological effects and potential risks associated with ultraviolet radiation as used in dentistry. Rockville, MA, US Department of Health, Education and Welfare, Public Health Service, Food and Drug Administration, Bureau of Radiological Health, 1975.

39 Peterson RW, Bostrom RG, Coakley JM *et al.* Measurements of the radiation emissions from the Nuva-lite dental appliance. Springfield, VA, National Technical Information Service, US Department of Commerce. Report No DHEW (FDA) 75-8081 1975.

40 Wolbarsht M, Allen R, Beatrice E *et al.* Letter to the editor. *Invest Ophthalmol Vis Sci* 1980; **19**: 1124.

41 Davis LG, Baker WT, Cox EA *et al.* Optical hazards of blue light curing units: preliminary results. *Br Dent J* 1985; **159**: 259–262.

42 Ellingson OL, Landry RJ, Bostrom RG. An evaluation of optical radiation emissions from dental visible polymerisation devices. *J Am Dent Assoc* 1986; **112**: 67–70.

43 Moseley H, Strang R, MacDonald I. Evaluation of the risk associated with the use of blue light polymerizing sources. *J Dent* 1987; **15**: 12–15.

44 Ligh RQ. Ocular concerns with light-curing units. *Hawaii Dent J* 1986; **17**: 31–32.

45 Cook WD. Spectral distributions of dental photopolymerising sources. *J Dent Res* 1982; **61**: 1436–1438.

46 Sliney DH. Standards for the use of visible and non-visible radiation on the eye. *Am J Optom Physiol Opt* 1983; **30**: 278–286.

47 Clayman L, Fuller T, Beckman H. Healing of continuous wave and rapid superpulsed carbon dioxide laser-induced bone defects. *Oral Surg* 1978; **36**: 932.

48 Tuffin JR, Carruth JAS. The carbon dioxide surgical laser. *Br Dent J* 1980; **149**: 255–258.

49 Horch HH, Gerlach KL. CO_2 laser treatment of oral dysplastic precancerous lesions. *Lasers Surg Med* 1982; **2**: 179–185.

50 Pecaro BC, Garehime WJ. The CO_2 laser in oral and maxillofacial surgery. *J Oral Maxillofac Surg* 1983; **41**: 725–728.

51 Frame J. Carbon dioxide laser surgery for benign oral lesions. *Br Dent J* 1985; **158**: 125–128.

52 Miserendino L, Neiburger E, Pick R. Current status of lasers in dentistry III. *Dent J* 1987; **56**: 254–256.

53 Wilder-Smith P. The soft laser: therapeutic tool or popular placebo? *Oral Surg* 1988; **66**: 654–658.

54 Strang R, Moseley H, Carmichael A. Soft lasers—have they a place in dentistry? *Br Dent J* 1988; **165**: 221–225.

55 American Medical Association Council on Scientific Affairs. Lasers in medicine and surgery. *J Am Med Assoc* 1986; **256**: 900–907.

56 Neiburger EJ, Miserendino L. Laser reflectance: hazard in the dental operatory. *Oral Surg* 1988; **66**: 659–661.

57 Guidance on the safe use of lasers in medical practice. DHSS, 1984. ISBN 0-11-320857-X.

58 Tuthill RW. Assessment of the literature on health effects related to video display terminals: final report to the Massachusetts Department of Public Health. Boston, Department of Health Statistics and Research, Massachusetts Department of Public Health, 1985.

59 Bureau of Radiological Health. An evaluation of radiation emission from video display terminals. US department of Health and Human services, 1981. Publication FDA 81-8153.

60   Beljan JR *et al.* Health effects of video display terminals. *J Am Med Assoc* 1987; **257**: 1508–1512.
61   Christian C. Are computers bad for your health. *Pract Comp* 1989; **April**: 60–62.
62   Rycroft RJG, Calnan CD. Facial rashes among visual display unit operators. *In* Pearce B (ed). *Health hazards of VDTs.* pp 13–15. Chichester: John Wiley and Sons, 1984.
63   Tjonn HH. Report of facial rashes among VDU operators in Norway. *In* Pearce B (ed) *Health hazards of VDTs.* pp 17–23. Chichester: John Wiley and Sons, 1984.
64   Nilsen A. Facial rash in visual display unit operators. *Contact Derm* 1984; **8**: 25–28.
65   Linden V, Rolfsen S. Video computer terminals and occupational dermatitis. *Scand J Work Env Health* 1981; **7**: 62–67.
66   Fisher A. 'Terminal' dermatitis due to computers. *Cutis* 1986; **38**: 153–154.
67   Liden C, Wahlberg J. Work with video display terminals among office employees. *Scand J Work Env Health* 1985; **11**: 489–493.
68   Liden C, Wahlberg J. Does visual display terminal work provoke rosacea? *Contact Derm* 1985; **13**: 235–241.
69   Berg M, Langlet I. Defective video displays, shields and skin problems. *Lancet* 1987; **1**: 800.
70   Keogh G. Injury time. *Pract Comp* 1989; *April*: 64–65.
71   Smith MH, Cohen BGF, Lambert W, Stammerjohn J. An investigation of health complaints and job stress in video display operators. *Human Factors* 1981; **23**: 387–400.
72   Jones AA, Dickens RL, Armbruster DL, Laughter JS. Dental X rays found to have no effect on hearing aids. *J Am Dent Assoc* 1986; **113**: 912–913.

National Radiation Protection Board: Chilton, Didcot, Oxon OX11 0RQ. Tel: 0235 831600.
Dental Monitoring Service: Northern Centre, Hospital Lane, Cookridge, Leeds LS16 6RW. Tel: 0532 679041.
Kodak Lanex: Kodak UK, PO Box 66, Station Road, Hemel Hempstead, Herts HP1 1JU.
3M Trimax: 3M House, PO Box 1, Bracknell, Berks RG12 1JU.
Fuji RX: Fuji Photofilm (UK) Ltd, Fuji Film House, 125 Finchley Road, London NW3 6JH.
X-Alert: Evident Dental Co. Ltd, 57 Wellington Court, Wellington Road, London NW8 9TD.
GXRI Alarm: Nesor Products, Claremont Hall, Pentonville Road, London N1 9HR.
Taxan monitors: Cookham Road, Brucknell, Berks, RG12 1RB.
Periphlex low-radiation VDU shields: Computer Marketing plc, 8 Frimley Road, Camberley, Surrey GU15 3HS.
Comput-irex spectacles: Jencon's Scientific, Cherrycourt Way Industrial Estate, Leighton Buzzard LUZ 8UA.

Appendix

Laser protective goggles and spectacles[a]

A G Electro-optics Tarporley Cheshire CW6 0TW	Fred Reed Optical Co Inc USA
Barr and Stroud Caxton Street Anniesland Glasgow	Glendale Optical Co (All wavelengths)
British-American Optical Co Ltd Radlett Road Watford Herts	
Green Cross Safety The Safety Centre 74 High Street Tring Herts HP23 4AF	

[a] Select and use those for the correct wavelength

5

Infectious Hazards in Dentistry

Dental staff may be exposed to contagious diseases clinically and in the laboratory, but most infective illness in dental staff is from respiratory viruses and is not strictly occupational. Serious occupation-related infection, apart from hepatitis B, appears to be surprisingly infrequently recorded in clinical dental staff and even this is probably now less of a hazard with immunisation and good infection control. Dental technical laboratory staff are at even lower risk.

Blood and serum are the sources most likely to transmit serious infection and dental instruments are often contaminated with these body fluids.[1] Furthermore, microorganisms are readily transmitted in the dental environment[2] by touch as well as by splatter and possibly aerosols (see Chapter 2). Health care facilities, particularly hospitals, are well recognised reservoirs of infection and may be responsible for a wide range of nosocomial (hospital) infections.

Infections to which clinical dental and possibly laboratory staff may be exposed, either in the community or in hospital facilities, include:

(1) Viruses
   (a) Hepatitis viruses B, D, and non-A non-B infections;
   (b) HIV;
   (c) Infections with herpes simplex, varicella-zoster, cytomegalovirus, Epstein-Barr virus, and herpesvirus 6;
   (d) The common cold and other respiratory viruses;
   (e) Hand, foot and mouth disease and herpangina;
   (f) Papillomavirus infections;
   (g) Parvovirus infections;
   (h) Human T cell lymphotropic virus I;
   (i) Human T cell lymphotropic virus II.

(2)   Bacteria
    (a) Tuberculosis;
    (b) Syphilis;
    (c) Gonorrhoea;
    (d) Legionellosis.

(3)   Other infections
    Rubella and other microbes

Fuller details of these and other relevant infections are available elsewhere;[3] this chapter outlines the points relevant to the possible occupational hazards in dentistry and their control.

The relative risks from these different infections vary widely as a result of such factors as the frequency with which they are encountered, their infectivity, the ability of the organism to survive outside the body, the severity of the resulting infection, the host response and the availability of effective treatment. Immunocompromised staff should take especial care in control of cross-infection.

Hand, foot and mouth disease is probably one of the most infectious and capable of causing minor epidemics among clinical dental personnel. However, it is usually so mild that it is of little importance. The HIV virus represents a complete contrast, in many respects, in that the risk of infection in a dental care setting appears to be extremely low but, should it happen, the consequences can be severe.

Certain high risk groups such as intravenous drug abusers (Table 5.1) can be recognised and are more likely to be infected with blood-borne microbes than the average patient. It should be remembered that such groups may carry multiple infective agents, including sexually transmitted diseases.

Vaccines are available against hepatitis B virus and tuberculosis, but not against others such as non-A non-B hepatitis or human immunodeficiency viruses (HIV). Protection against most infections therefore depends on good cross-infection control. Infected patients can by no means always be identified and thus *all* tissues and body fluids must be regarded as potentially infectious. Cross-infection control is crucial to protect staff and other patients. Important measures for clinical dental staff include the wearing of suitable protection, namely eye protection, masks and gloves and, especially, the avoidance of needle-stick or sharps injuries. A recent study showed that 84% of American dentists had experienced accidental

Table 5.1 The main high-risk groups for blood-borne viral infections (HBV, HDV, NANBH, HIV)[a]

Promiscuous male homosexuals and bisexuals[a]
Intravenous drug abusers[a]
Haemophiliacs and others who have received untreated blood products or infected blood
Persons from some Third World countries (particularly sub-Saharan Africa, South East Asia and South America)
Prostitutes (especially male) in some areas
Sexual contacts of any of the above

[a] Some persons in institutional care such as long-stay mental care facilities and prisons, fall into these groups and not infrequently there is more than one risk factor (eg prostitution to fund intravenous drug abuse) and more than one infection. Other viruses such as CMV, EBV and HTLV-1 may infect these groups, especially intravenous drug abusers, and sexually transmitted diseases are common.

skin punctures in a 5-year period[4] and this illustrates the level of care needed.

Under the terms of the Health and Safety at Work etc Act (1974) and Control of Substances Hazardous to Health (1988) Regulations, an employer in the UK has a legal obligation to protect persons attending or working in his/her practice or laboratory from infection as well as other hazards. The legal aspects are discussed mainly in Chapters 6 and 7, but there is clearly also a moral duty to practise good cross-infection control procedures.

Microbial agents of most concern in dentistry

Hepatitis viruses

Many viruses can cause hepatitis but the most important are hepatitis A, hepatitis B, hepatitis D, and non-A non-B hepatitis viruses. These all cause essentially similar clinical illnesses but, in brief, hepatitis A is transmitted by food and water and is a hazard particularly of visiting hot countries where sanitation is poor whilst the other hepatitis viruses are transmitted mainly via blood, blood products or sexually. Non-A non-B hepatitis (so-called because the viruses have not all clearly been identified) is the most common type of hepatitis transmitted by blood transfusions, but no specific precautions can be taken to prevent the spread of these viruses. Currently, hepatitis B virus (HBV) and the frequently associated delta agent, hepatitis D virus (HDV) are in many respects the greatest infective hazards to clinical dental staff. However, recent studies, carried out in the industrialised countries, of patients with hepatitis,[5] showed 14–47% to be caused by non-A non-B hepatitis (NANBH); it is therefore clear that NANBH is also an occupational hazard to health care workers.[6]

Hepatitis B
Hepatitis B is a relatively common infection and there are estimated to be over 200 million chronic carriers of HBV worldwide.[7] Hepatitis B virus is readily transmitted by blood, sexually, perinatally or, possibly, by saliva.[8] Although the early mortality is very low in most outbreaks, the infection is potentially lethal since chronic liver disease and cancer can follow. The delta agent which may be associated with the hepatitis B antigen can cause a particularly virulent infection (see below). Because it is so readily transmitted, hepatitis B (despite the outbreak of AIDS) is probably the most serious infective hazard faced in dentistry. However, fortunately, active immunisation is effective and safe.

The hepatitis B virus (HBV) is a DNA virus.[8,9] It replicates in hepatocytes and some lymphocytes and is found in the serum of patients with hepatitis B as the Dane particle (fig. 5.1). This particle is infectious and consists of a central core containing DNA, an enzyme termed DNA polymerase (DNA-P), the core antigen (hepatitis B core antigen; HBcAg) and an outer protein shell of surface antigen (hepatitis B surface antigen; HBsAg) (fig. 5.2). The Dane particle (and hence serum containing it) is infectious.

Also present in the serum of infected patients are spherical and tubular particles of HBsAg; these particles are, however, *non-infectious*. HBcAg is not present in serum but another antigen, termed the e antigen (hepatitis B e antigen; HBeAg) which appears to be a breakdown product of the core antigen may be found and implies that the patient is infectious.[8,9]

Three main serotypes of HBV exist and a variant HBV known as HBV-2 has recently been described in West Africa, Europe and the Far East.[10,11] Other variants are also appearing.

In the Third World, HBV infection is endemic and is common perinatally and in childhood. In industrialised nations, infection is less common, and acquired mainly in adult life, and usually parenter-

HEPATITIS B ASSOCIATED PARTICLES

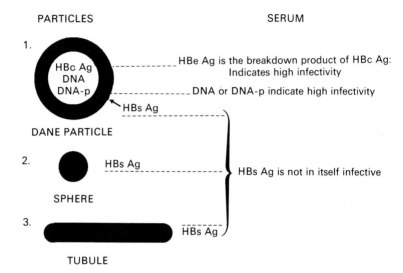

Fig. 5.1 Hepatitis B associated particles in serum.

HEPATITIS B

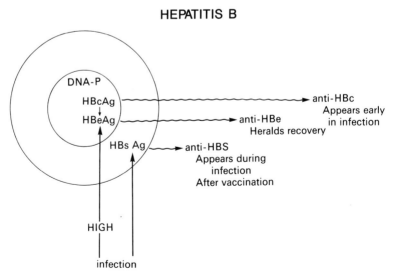

Fig. 5.2 Hepatitis B virus (HBV).

ally or by sexual contact.[12] Some 50% of HBV infections are subclinical and not associated with jaundice (anicteric infection). About 45% of individuals infected with HBV develop acute hepatitis with anorexia, malaise, nausea, and jaundice (fig. 5.3), pale fatty stools and dark urine. There may be pruritus. These features are not specific to HBV, but myalgia, arthralgia and a rash are all suggestive of HBV infection. The liver tends to become enlarged and tender. Liver enzymes (transaminases) such as aspartate aminotransferase (AST), alanine aminotransferase (ALT) and gamma glutamyl transpeptidase (GGT) appear in the serum, along with raised levels of bilirubin and often of alkaline phosphatase.[8,9]

Serological and biochemical evidence of HBV infection is present for a variable period from 1 to 6 months and serological evidence of previous HBV infection usually remains thereafter (see below).

Carrier state and complications. Most patients with acute hepatitis B recover spontaneously within a few weeks and have no sequelae. Some 4–5% of patients fail to clear HBV by 6 to 9 months and then become chronic carriers, characterised by persistence of HBV antigens in the serum. In the initial stages of the carrier state, patients develop chronic hepatitis and this may be complicated by cirrhosis. Later, the carrier state develops and, although termed the 'healthy' carrier state, other complications such as polyarteritis nodosa, glo-

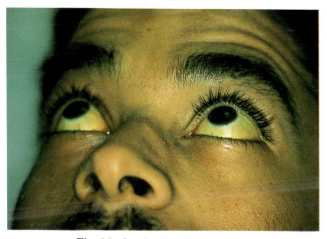

Fig. 5.3 Icteric sclerae in hepatitis B.

merulonephritis, mixed cryoglobulinaemia, or hepatocellular carcinoma may develop (fig. 5.4).

It is now generally recognised that, although there are intermediate forms, there are two main types of chronic hepatitis B carrier. Patients with chronic *persistent* hepatitis carry HBsAg but not HBeAg, and are not at great risk of severe liver damage. By contrast, patients with chronic *active* (or aggressive) hepatitis, carry both HBsAg and HBeAg for a long period, have biochemical evidence of liver damage, are chronically ill, and are at special risk of cirrhosis and possibly carcinoma of the liver. The carrier state most frequently follows anicteric hepatitis and neonatal infection and thus patients do not always give a history of jaundice. Many patients are therefore unsuspected carriers.

Although the early mortality rate of hepatitis B infection is low, of

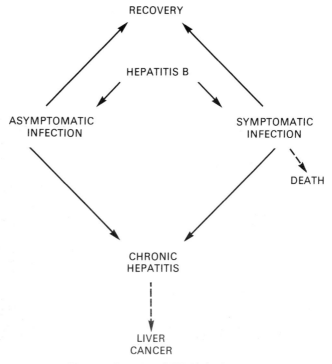

Fig. 5.4 Sequelae of HBV infection.

the order of 1%, a much higher mortality has been recorded in some outbreaks, particularly where there has also been infection with the delta agent (see below), and in male homosexuals.

Serological markers of hepatitis B

The surface antigen (HBsAg). HBsAg is found in the late incubation period when the patient may still be asymptomatic, in acute infection, and in chronic infection with HBV. A negative test for HBsAg usually, but not invariably, indicates that HBsAg is absent and that the patient is non-infectious, but absence of antibody to the core antigen (anti-HBc) is a more reliable test (see below) of non-infectivity. The presence of HBsAg indicates that the patient has been infected with HBV. However, unless HBeAg (the e antigen) is also present, the patient carrying HBsAg presents very little, if any, infective risk.

The surface antibody (Anti-HBs :HBsAb). Antibody to the surface antigen begins to appear in the serum as the patient starts to recover, but there may be a short period ('window') during which HBsAg has become undetectable and anti-HBs has yet to become detectable. At this time, both serological tests will be negative, despite the patient being infected. During recovery, anti-HBs is usually but not invariably detectable and rises in titre.

Anti-HBs also appears after immunisation with hepatitis B vaccines (see below). The presence of anti-HBs is usually taken to indicate immunity to further HBV infection; it is frequently long-lived and detectable for several years after HBV infection or immunisation.

The core antigen (HBcAg). This antigen is not present in serum but only in liver cells.

The core antibody (Anti-HBc; HBcAb). In contrast to surface antibody, anti-HBc appears at the onset of the disease and rises quickly in titre to remain for many years as an indicator of previous HBV infection. IgM class anti-HBc indicates recent infection; IgG class is seen in recovery or carrier states. Anti-HBc in high titres may indicate a chronic carrier state and is then often found in the absence of anti-HBs. This antibody is probably a better index of infection than HBsAg.

The e antigen (HBeAg). HBeAg appears in the serum simultaneously with HBsAg but disappears sooner during recovery. The presence of HBeAg is an indicator of high infectivity since e antigen is closely associated with HBV-DNA and DNA-P.

The e antibody (Anti-HBe; HBeAb). Antibody to e antigen appears in the serum soon after the appearance of HBeAg in most patients and its appearance usually heralds recovery. The *absence* of anti-HBe but carriage of antigen indicates high infectivity.

Carriers of HBsAg and also HBeAg but not anti-HBe are more likely to develop chronic active hepatitis (and the serious complications discussed above) and transmit infection, than those who carry anti-HBe but not HBeAg. However, up to 20% of those with anti-HBe from the Middle East and Mediterranean littoral have HBV-DNA in their serum and are an infectious risk.[13]

DNA polymerase (DNA-P). DNA polymerase in the serum is, like HBeAg, an indicator of high infectivity, since it is present in Dane particles.

Risk from hepatitis B to dental staff
The carriage rate of hepatitis B virus in the general population of North America and Western Europe is 0·1–0·5%.[12] However, it is considerably higher in hot climates such as in South East Asia, the Pacific rim and sub-Saharan Africa, where 5–40% of the population may be carriers[14] and where dental staff are consequently at higher risk.[15] There are also high risk groups such as drug abusers and promiscuous male homosexuals as well as *certain* immigrant groups. For instance, recent immigrants from Vietnam constitute one of the higher risk groups (Table 5.1).

In the USA, the risk to health care personnel is about four times greater than to the general population,[16] and dental surgeons have one of the highest infection rates of all health care workers.[16] A study of Australian health care workers in hospitals and institutions also showed dental staff to be the major risk group for hepatitis B infection[17] and a German study, conducted over 10 years ago, showed that 5% of dentists had suffered clinical hepatitis during the first 14 years of their professional work and that by 35 to 39 years of work in dentistry, 33% had suffered clinical hepatitis.[18] The fact that infection is more likely to be contracted the longer staff have been in dental practice has been confirmed in a Greek study.[19] Other studies have shown that the occupational risk is greatest in oral surgeons,[20] less in general dental practitioners,[21] usually lower in dental surgery assistants and hygienists[21-25] and lowest in clerical staff, dental laboratory technicians[21,23] and dental students[19,23,26,27] (Table 5.2).

The prevalence of hepatitis B virus markers in Danish dentists is double that of the general population, as assessed by testing blood donors[28] and the risk to British dental staff is probably of about the same order. The increased risk of hepatitis B to dental staff is clearly highest among those working surgically with adult patients in urban areas and with high risk groups (Table 5.2)[8,9,15-45] However, studies of British clinical dental staff revealed that only about 1% were hepatitis B carriers in one dental hospital, and there was no evidence of past or present HBV infection in staff in another.[44,45] Furthermore, the latest reports of hepatitis B in English health care staff revealed the average number of reported cases of acute hepatitis B in English dentists to be only about two to three per year, and there were no reported cases in 1987 or 1988.[46] Clearly there is at present only a low and falling risk to British dental staff, and immunisation should make this a risk of the past.

Transmission of hepatitis B
Dental staff who are carriers or incubating hepatitis B can transmit

Table 5.2 Risk to dental personnel from hepatitis B[a]

Dental group	Level of occupational risk	% showing serological evidence of HBV infection[b]
General practitioners	Greater than the general population: lower than hospital dentists	5–30
Oral surgeons	Highest amongst dentists	20–40
Hospital general dentists	Lower than oral surgeons	16
Paedodontists	Lower risk than other clinicians	2–8
Hygienists	Lower than most dentists	12–17
Surgery assistants	Lower than most dentists	0–13
Technicians	Lower than most dentists	4–14
Students	Lowest	0–9
Clerical	Lowest	0–9

[a] Based on references 13–43, all studies from industrialised countries. The risks are presumably higher in developing countries.
[b] Hospital personnel tend to have higher figures; those wearing gloves lower figures.

infection to patients and there have been at least 10 incidents, with occasional fatalities from infection transmitted in dental practice, some recorded over 30 years ago.[8,9,47-57] Transmission of infection to patients has also led to medicolegal claims (Chapter 7). These unfortunate episodes serve to emphasise the ease of transmissibility of HBV, since the attack rates of HBV in patients exposed to HBsAg positive dentists have varied from 1 in 40 to 1 in 400.[49] Those dentists implicated in transmission have been HBeAg and/or Dane particle positive.[50] The risk of infection increased with duration of exposure and degree of operative trauma, and dramatically decreased when gloves were worn.[50] Indeed, one dentist who infected at least 55 patients over a 3-year period when he did not wear gloves, failed to infect any of 8000 patients during a subsequent year when he wore gloves, even though he remained infectious.[51] Another dentist who did not wear gloves appeared to be the source of at least eight cases, of whom two died.[52]

The prevalence of HBV infection is highest in areas where standards of living are low, and in certain high risk groups (see above and Table 5.1) and is increasing in many areas.

Blood and blood products are the fluids most likely to be responsible for cross-infection. Minute quantities of blood, far less than 0·0001 ml, have transmitted the disease.[8,9] There have also been many reports of epidemics or clusters of cases related to the handling of blood and blood products, and many cases have followed infected needlestick injuries, injections and blood transfusion. The risk of HBV transmission following a needlestick injury involving infected blood appears to be about 20–25%.

Saliva from HBsAg-positive patients may contain HBsAg, Dane particles, HBV-DNA and DNA-P and might be infective, especially if the patient is HBeAg positive.[8,9,12,58-64] Saliva may also contain infected blood or serum.[65] There is some evidence of transmission of HBV to household contacts (presumably via saliva and saliva-contaminated objects)[66,67] and at least one report of transmission of HBV infection by a human bite.[68] However, social contact has a very low risk of transmission, even in children in day care centres,[69] unless there is biting or scratching. Oral exposure to infected saliva also appears to carry only a very low risk of transmission.[12,70,71] Primate experiments have confirmed the oral transmissibility of HBV infection by serum, semen and to some extent by saliva, although the infectivity relates mainly to the HBeAg status, and saliva appeared not to transmit the infection when given orally.[9,72-74] Indeed, in one study of 19 dental personnel exposed to oral secretions from HBV-infected persons, none of the dental personnel contracted infection.[75] The evidence regarding the risk of transmission of HBV via saliva is therefore conflicting, but an HBeAg carrier might infect non-immune dental staff via cuts or abrasions in the latter's hands.

Hepatitis B virus infection is more likely, therefore, in individuals who, for one reason or another, are exposed frequently to blood, blood products or to other infected individuals, but this is mainly if the exposure is intimate or involves close contact with body fluids. Sexual transmission of HBV is well documented both in heterosexuals, especially if promiscuous, and in homosexual males. Sexual transmission of HBV is now so important as to constitute the main risk factor in some areas. Male homosexuals and bisexuals, intravenous drug abusers, and others form obviously high-risk groups (Table 5.1), but, in terms of numbers, a greater occupational hazard in dentistry is presented by the unsuspected carrier. Occupational transmission of infection in dentistry is most likely to be from contact with infected blood. There is no real evidence of transmission by inhalation.[76]

The risk of infection from a person is related to the serological markers; patients who are HBeAg positive are highly infectious, but those who are HBeAg-negative are of extremely low infectivity. Infective carriers can only be *suspected* if there is a history of jaundice, or if they come from high-risk groups, but the great majority of hepatitis infections are subclinical. Many infectious patients will therefore be treated unknowingly in dental practice, as are carriers of the HIV virus and other infections.[77] Serological screening is little used in dentistry, since it cannot detect all patients. Moreover, studies of dental hospital patients showed that less than 1% were seropositive and even in studies of *high-risk* groups attending dental hospitals in Britain and America, less than 10% were seropositive and only 1 or 2% were HBeAg positive.[78-81]

In summary, therefore, the risks from hepatitis B (and NANBH see below) stem from the following facts:
(1) they are now widespread;
(2) a chronic carrier state is common;
(3) the viruses survive well outside the body on surfaces and instruments in the dental surgery, and are relatively resistant to disinfection;

(4) minute amounts of body fluids can transmit infection;
(5) infection can lead to chronic active hepatitis, cirrhosis and death from liver failure or liver cancer.

All dental patients should therefore be treated as infectious ('universal precautions'); the minimal precautions are that gloves should be worn for all clinical dental work, needlestick injuries must be avoided, and, most important of all, *clinical dental staff should be immunised against hepatitis B virus* (see page 180).

The delta agent: hepatitis D virus (HDV)

The delta agent is an RNA virus (fig. 5.5) that will only replicate in the presence of HBsAg (ie it is a 'defective' virus).[82] Delta infection is mainly transmitted parenterally with HBV and is increasing in prevalence. It is becoming a major problem for abusers of intravenous drugs and some haemophiliacs. HDV is also transmitted by sexual contact[83] (Table 5.1). In non-endemic areas such as the USA and Northern Europe, HDV is mainly confined to those exposed to blood or blood products. In endemic areas such as the Mediterranean littoral, HDV is endemic among those infected with HBV (superinfection) and there may sometimes be co-infection with several other

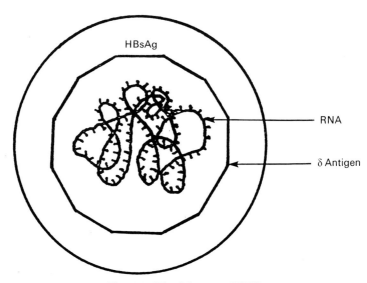

Fig. 5.5 The delta agent (HDV).

viruses. Delta infection either coincides with acute hepatitis B, or superinfects patients with chronic hepatitis B.[84] If the delta agent causes acute hepatitis, it may precipitate fulminant liver disease,[82] although there is resolution in most cases.

Serological tests (anti-HDV) are now available to detect delta infection[86] and it is clear that in some areas, up to 30% of HBsAg carriers are infected with HDV.[87] Some episodes of delta hepatitis have been reported in dental patients, with occasional deaths.[88]

Immunisation against hepatitis B also protects against the delta agent and this strengthens the need for immunisation.

Hepatitis A

Hepatitis A is the common form of infectious hepatitis. It is mainly transmitted by faecally-contaminated food such as raw shellfish, and is frequently acquired during a holiday abroad in the sun. Clinically, hepatitis A and hepatitis B infections are similar, except that full recovery is the general rule after hepatitis A.

There is little evidence that hepatitis A is transmitted during dental procedures.

Non-A non-B hepatitis (including hepatitis C)

Non-A non-B hepatitis (NANBH) is caused by several viruses.[5,8,9] Hepatitis C is the most common cause of hepatitis following blood transfusions. Some of these viruses have not yet been fully characterised, although particles similar to flaviviruses and togaviruses have been identified in serum.[89] The disease appears to be similar in most respects to hepatitis B, except that it is generally a less severe acute illness; however, chronic infection and chronic liver disease are *more* common.[5,90]

NANBH and hepatitis C (HCV) are at least as common and important an infection as HBV. Worldwide, NANBH causes at least 15–20% of clinical cases of viral hepatitis and is increasing in prevalence.[5,91] In some industrialised countries, up to 50% of viral hepatitis is NANBH,[5] although the carriage rate in the general population is only of the order of 1%.[89] There are, however, significant numbers of carriers of NANBH, mainly in the groups at high risk for hepatitis B and AIDS, especially intravenous drug abusers and haemophiliacs (Table 5.1). *However, most have not been recognised* because of the lack, until recently, of serological tests of NANBH infection. Diagnosis of NANBH infection has depended largely on the exclusion of all other known agents and the use of blood tests showing raised levels of so-called 'surrogate' serum markers such as anti-HBc or alanine transaminase which indicate hepatitis B (since commonly there is co-infection with HBV and NANBH) or liver damage.[5] A serological test for antibodies to HCV is now available.

Clinical types of NANBH hepatitis include parenteral (blood and blood-product borne), non-parenteral (sporadic) cases, and epidemic (usually water-borne). The incubation period is about 2–3 months for the parenteral form. The symptoms are similar to those of hepatitis B.

Epidemiological studies have been conducted largely in the USA, Scandinavia and the UK, predominantly on the parenteral type, since this is most commonly recognised. In health care workers, it is the parenterally transmitted types that are the main occupational risk.[5,6]

Blood or blood-product transmitted NANBH (parenteral NANBH). The principal route of transmission of NANBH in the present context is via blood or blood products and HCV is now the most common cause of post-transfusion hepatitis in both the USA and UK, although subclinical infection is more frequent.[5] Recipients of organ transplants, patients on haemodialysis and others frequently exposed to blood or blood products are also at high risk of acquiring HCV.

In several studies, the majority of cases of NANBH have been in intravenous drug abusers, who are also prone to multiple and chronic infections with NANBH and other microorganisms.[91–94] NANBH can also be transmitted sexually.[89]

NANBH and health care workers. NANBH has only occasionally been reported in health care workers, laboratory staff and persons handling blood or blood products, or among those in social contact with infected patients.[5,6,91] However, the incidence of asymptomatic infection is unknown. The risk of contracting NANBH infection via needlestick injuries *appears* to be less than that of HBV, but the evidence is tenuous.

Transmission of NANBH in dentistry. NANBH is transmitted in a similar way to HBV and thus is potentially transmissible in dentistry.[89,91] Indeed, there has been at least one outbreak that may have originated after dental treatment[95] and there is evidence of transmission of NANBH to close contacts and within households.[5,91] A recent report suggests that non-A non-B virus may be transmissible by saliva, although there is no evidence as yet that this is of clinical importance.[96] However, non-A non-B hepatitis can, at least theoretically, be transmitted in dental practice and the same precautions should be adopted as for hepatitis B, especially as there may be more than one causal agent and there is no vaccine or specific treatment available.

Human immune deficiency viruses and the acquired immune deficiency syndrome (AIDS)

AIDS is caused by RNA retroviruses termed human immune deficiency viruses (HIV). Although AIDS was first recognised in the early 1980s in the USA, cases have now been diagnosed retrospectively as early as 1968 in the USA and 1959 elsewhere.[97,98] By March 1990, there were some 3000 persons with AIDS reported in the UK. In contrast, there were over 100 000 AIDS patients reported in the USA by the summer of 1989. HIV is far more common and is spreading rapidly through most communities. Many cases are caused by HIV-1,[99] but HIV-2 is now spreading to Europe, the Americas and elsewhere from West Africa.[100-103]

HIV typically infects and damages CD4-positive cells (mainly some helper T lymphocytes, Langerhans cells, and macrophages) and can cause profound immunodeficiency and death (fig. 5.6). Early infection can produce a glandular fever type of illness, with fever and sore throat but then the patient may be asymptomatic for months or years before persistent generalised lymphadenopathy (PGL) or AIDS-related complex (ARC) is detected. Infections or neoplasms and full blown AIDS may then develop. Death is usually from

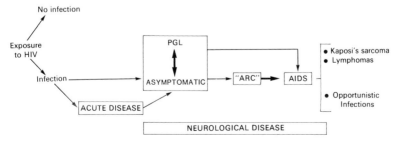

Fig. 5.6 Sequelae of exposure to HIV (Courtesy of S. Porter).

infection by a great variety of microbes ranging from viruses to parasites. One of the latter, *Pneumocystis carinii* causes an otherwise rare type of pneumonia which is the most common cause of death. Malignant neoplasms, also otherwise rare, namely lymphomas and Kaposi's sarcoma, are the other main complications. Another effect of the virus is brain damage, which can have a number of clinical manifestations but typically culminates in dementia and death. These latter symptoms need not necessarily be associated with typical AIDS.[104]

Human immunodeficiency virus (HIV)

HIV contains at its centre RNA and the enzyme reverse transcriptase, which the virus uses to multiply itself (fig. 5.7). Three core proteins p24, p18 and p15 are antigenic in natural infection and patients infected with HIV develop antibodies to HIV, especially antibodies to antigens p24 and gp 160. A coat glycoprotein gp120 derived from a gp 160 precursor is the major target for neutralising antibodies.[102]

The patterns of infection with HIV and consequent serological responses appear to fall into one of the following categories:[107]

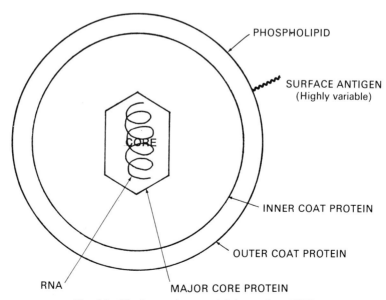

Fig. 5.7 The human immunodeficiency virus (HIV).

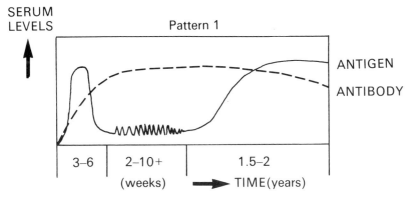

Fig. 5.8 Usual pattern of HIV infection.

(1) The most common pattern is where there is prolific viral replication within 3 to 6 weeks after exposure, HIV and HIV antigens are detected in blood, and there is an early immune response with antibodies to p24. These reach a high level in about 6 weeks and remain high and detectable by ELISA (Enzyme Linked ImmunoSorbent Assay) and Western blot tests (fig. 5.8; see below).

(2) A rare pattern is where a prolonged seropositive state is followed by loss of antiviral antibodies (ELISA and Western blot tests become negative) but HIV remains in the lymphocytes (fig. 5.9). Thus, the patient is HIV-antibody negative but probably infectious.

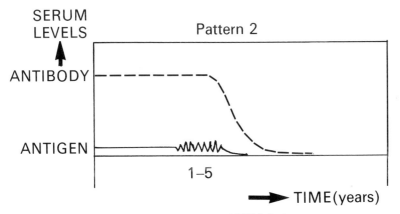

Fig. 5.9 Rare pattern of HIV infection.

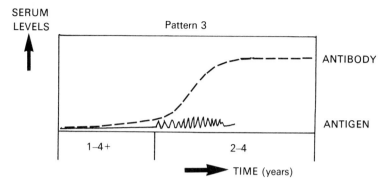

Fig. 5.10   Silent HIV infection.

(3) In up to 25% of some groups there is prolonged silent HIV infection; virus is present but antibodies may take up to 3 years to become detectable. The implications of this pattern are most disturbing (fig. 5.10), since again the patient is HIV-antibody negative but is probably infectious.

Serological markers of and tests for HIV

The ELISA screening test for serum *antibodies* to HIV has a sensitivity of about 98% and specificity of about 99% under optimal conditions. It is rapid and easy to use, but there may be false positive or negative results. Confirmatory assays such as Western blotting are thus also used and will detect HIV antibodies at the very earliest from 11 to 13 days after the onset of clinical symptoms. Antibodies may, however, in some cases, not appear until up to 3 years after infection.[108] There is some cross-reactivity between HIV-1 and HIV-2 on Western blotting[106] but, as HIV-2 spreads, assays for the latter become necessary.

Assays for HIV *antigens*, usually the p24 antigen, are now available and can often reveal HIV infection before antibodies have become detectable, but even antigen assays are occasionally negative. Fortunately, newer techniques that have become available to detect the DNA or RNA of HIV, such as the polymerase chain reaction (PCR), are more sensitive[109,110] and are able to detect HIV in infected seronegative persons.

Although HIV can also be detected by *viral culture*, this lacks the ease, sensitivity and reproducibility needed for clinical work. *Confidentiality is essential with respect to all aspects of testing for HIV.*

Oral lesions in HIV infection

Most AIDS patients have head and neck manifestations at some stage, and oral lesions are often early signs of HIV infection.[9,111-114] Oral lesions such as candidosis, hairy leukoplakia and orofacial zoster may be indicators of poor prognosis.

Few of the oral lesions seen in HIV-infected persons are specific, although hairy leukoplakia is virtually pathognomonic of HIV infection and oral Kaposi's sarcoma is also seen predominantly in AIDS and only occasionally in other immunocompromised persons in Britain and the USA. Other lesions such as oral candidosis and intra-oral herpes simplex virus infections often reflect underlying immunodeficiency states. Aphthous ulcers are common in otherwise normal persons, but onset or increased severity in adulthood should arouse suspicion of HIV infection.

In practical terms, any of these oral lesions should arouse suspicion of HIV, especially in a person from a group at high risk for HIV, namely homosexual or bisexual males, intravenous drug abusers, some haemophiliacs, those from areas of high prevalence and consorts of any of the aforementioned groups (Table 5.1).

Common non-specific manifestations possibly suggestive of HIV

Cervical lymph node enlargement

Lymphadenopathy is an almost invariable feature of AIDS-related complexes and AIDS.

Aphthous-type ulceration

Severe aphtha-like ulceration is common in HIV-infected individuals and severe necrotising ulceration involving the fauces has been observed in some AIDS patients. Thalidomide or zidovudine may control these ulcers.

HIV-related gingivitis and periodontitis

Severe gingivitis, sometimes resembling acute necrotising ulcerative gingivitis (ANUG; Vincent's gingivitis; trench mouth) is a common oral problem in HIV infection, despite a good standard of oral care in many cases. A characteristic feature of the HIV-gingivitis (HIV-G) is spontaneous haemorrhage and sometimes ulceration of the gingivae, and a failure to respond to conventional dental care. Rapid destruction of the periodontium and alveolar bone may lead to pain, and tooth mobility and loss (HIV periodontitis: HIV-P).

Candidosis

Oral candidosis is often present in HIV infection. Thrush is seen at some stage in over 75% of patients and may be the first manifestation. In a young adult male or other person from a high risk group, the development of thrush without a local cause, such as xerostomia or concurrent treatment with corticosteroids or antibiotics, is strongly suggestive of HIV infection. Severe oral thrush usually implies concurrent oesophageal candidosis and may indicate susceptibility to systemic opportunistic infection.

Other types of oral candidosis seen in HIV infection include erythematous candidosis and hyperplastic (candidal leukoplakia) types. The tongue is a commonly involved site, giving rise to a central red area, sometimes termed median rhomboid glossitis. Angular stomatitis (cheilitis), a lesion more usually a feature of otherwise healthy elderly denture-wearers must, if seen in a young individual, be treated with suspicion as HIV may be the underlying cause.

All forms of oral candidosis in HIV infection can be managed with conventional topical anti-fungal therapy, but ketoconazole or fluconazole may be required if the infection persists or there is oesophageal infection.

Herpes simplex and zoster viral infections

Oral herpes simplex (HSV) and varicella-zoster virus (VZV) infections can be especially severe and persistent and can be a marker of poor future prognosis.

Salivary gland involvement

Xerostomia (dry mouth) is not uncommon in HIV patients, but is of unknown aetiology. It may give rise to an increased risk of periodontal disease. Caries may also be accentuated in patients who eat large amounts of confectionery. Parotid gland enlargement (unrelated to xerostomia) is a common feature of paediatric AIDS and can also occasionally be seen in infected adults who may also develop cystic lesions in the parotids.

Manifestations specific or virtually specific to HIV infection

Kaposi's sarcoma

Kaposi's sarcoma may be oral or perioral in 50% of US male homosexuals with AIDS. Kaposi's sarcoma may be an early oral manifestation of symptomatic HIV infection and commonly presents as a red, blue or purple macule, papule or nodule, usually on the palate, especially at the junction of the hard and soft palates. Kaposi's sarcoma is virtually never seen in haemophiliacs or in children with AIDS.

Lymphomas and other neoplasms

Oral lymphomas can arise in HIV infection, often as a lump or ulcer. Oral squamous cell carcinoma has been reported in a few patients.

Hairy leukoplakia

Hairy leukoplakia appears to be virtually pathognomonic of HIV (it appears only rarely in other immunocompromised states) and may be a useful indication of poor prognosis. Hairy leukoplakia, which has been observed in infected patients from all at-risk groups, is characterised by soft, white, adherent plaques, particularly affecting the lateral margins and ventral aspects of the tongue. There is epithelial hyperplasia, giving rise to a hairy appearance although the surface more frequently appears corrugated. The white patches can also have a homogeneous plaque-like appearance.

Epstein-Barr virus (EBV) has been implicated in the aetiology of hairy leukoplakia since the virus replicates within lesional tissue. Furthermore, acyclovir can cause transient regression of lesions and long-term resolution has been observed in patients receiving ganciclovir or zidovudine.

Less common, non-specific but suggestive manifestations

Human papillomavirus (HPV) infections can occasionally appear in the mouths of HIV-infected individuals, usually as common warts, venereal warts or papillomas. Benign white patches on the lips can also develop (benign epithelial hyperplasia), and HPV-13 has been implicated in their aetiology.

Other infections include typical and atypical mycobacteria, Epstein-Barr virus, cytomegalovirus, *Cryptococcus neoformans*, *Escherichia coli* and histoplasmosis, any of which can also cause oral ulcers. Cranial neuropathies, affecting the V, VII, VIII and IX nerves, are rare features of HIV encephalitis.

Other, uncommon orofacial features of HIV infection include thrombocytopenic purpura or parotitis or, rarely, hyperpigmentation and cat-scratch infection.

Congenital HIV infection can give rise to a variety of facial malformations as well as opportunistic infections and neoplasms.[111-114]

Transmission of HIV

HIV, like hepatitis B and some other viruses, can be transmitted by infected blood and blood products, and sexual intercourse, but not by the airborne route. The prevalence of HIV infection is rapidly rising in most parts of the world, especially in urban areas, but few manifest clinical disease early on (fig. 5.11). The high-risk groups for AIDS

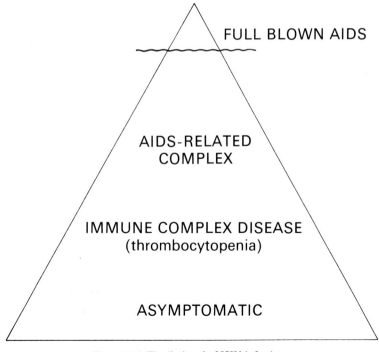

Fig. 5.11   The 'iceberg' of HIV infection.

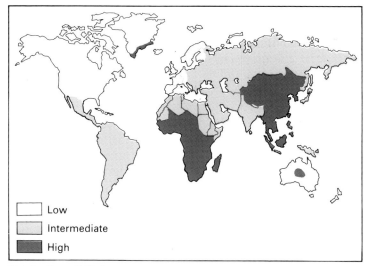

Distribution of HBsAg

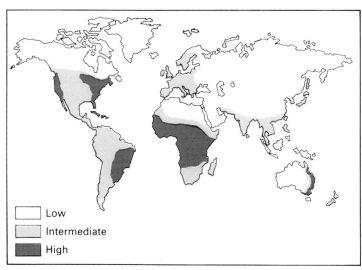

Distribution of HIV

Fig. 5.12   High risk areas for HIV and other blood-borne viruses.

are in most respects similar to those for hepatitis B, except that in most areas (outside Africa) sexually active male homosexuals and bisexuals still account for over 75% of cases.[115] Intravenous drug abusers form a large proportion of cases in many areas (fig. 5.12; Table 5.1) and there are often multiple risk factors. In Africa, and increasingly in some other areas, heterosexual spread is becoming important, particularly where anal intercourse is common.[99-104] Many prostitutes are now infected, especially in sub-Saharan Africa (Table 5.3) and increasingly in South America and elsewhere.[100] It has been estimated that heterosexual Britons may be 300 times more likely to acquire AIDS abroad than at home.[116] Eventually, it has been suggested that heterosexual spread will be numerically the main route of HIV infection.[117] Haemophiliacs and others who had received unscreened blood or untreated blood products were infected and many have died as a consequence. However, heat treatment of blood products and screening for AIDS antibodies in blood donors should now have virtually eliminated this risk. In the UK, only about one in one million blood donations were HIV-antibody positive in 1988. However, since screening for HIV antibodies does not exclude all HIV infected blood, the risk of transmission from blood transfusions, though small, must still exist.

Table 5.3 Transmission of HIV in different areas[a]

Area	Main mode of sexual transmission	Other main routes
N. America W. Europe Antipodes	Homosexual (50% male homosexuals may be HIV + ve)	IVDA[b] Blood
Sub-Saharan Africa Latin America	Heterosexual (25% adults now HIV + ve and up to 70% of prostitutes are HIV + ve)	Blood transfusion. Unsterile needles. Perinatal.
North Africa Middle East E. Europe Asia Pacific	Prostitutes (up to 60% may be HIV + ve)	Blood IVDA

[a] As of 1988–1989
[b] IVDA = intravenous drug abuse.

There are important differences between HIV and HBV, especially in that much larger quantities of blood appear to be needed to transmit HIV infection. The AIDS virus is also very much more fragile and less resistant to antiseptics and disinfectants (page 193). A mere prick from an infected needle readily transmits HBV but is unlikely to transmit HIV. Perhaps 0·5% of these injuries transmit HIV;[118–120] this is far lower than the risk from HBV and, probably, NANBH. Nevertheless, precautions against needlestick injuries are of the utmost importance (as discussed below), not least because HIV-positive patients are frequently infected with HBV and other microorganisms.

HIV in saliva

Although HIV may be present in whole saliva and in salivary glands, it is not always detectable in saliva from infected persons.[121–127] Furthermore, there is antiviral activity in the saliva.[128,129] It does not appear to be possible to transmit HIV by mere social contact or even by living in the same household (fig. 5.13), provided there is no sexual contact. Of approximately 100 000 American cases of AIDS, none were in family members who were not involved in high-risk be-haviour. Saliva is therefore most unlikely to constitute a significant vehicle for transmission of HIV. The disease can be transmitted by heterosexual intercourse, by blood transfusion, very occasionally by human bites, and from an infected woman to a foetus, but does not otherwise spread within families.[130]

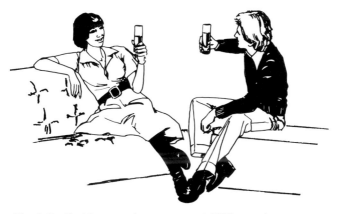

Fig. 5.13   Social contact does not transmit HIV: sexual contact can.

Occupational hazards from HIV

Needlestick or other sharps injuries are the greatest danger for occupational transmission of HIV. Human bites are a rare route of transmission and infection follows particularly when the biter has frank blood in the mouth.[131]

A few health care workers—including one dentist in the USA[132]— have acquired AIDS as a result of a needlestick or other injuries when treating an infected patient. Several published studies show that this dentist was the only person out of about 5000 dental clinical staff with no other known risk activity, who was positive for HIV antibodies (Table 5.4).[4,132–137] He worked in New York, an area of exceptionally high prevalence, he did not wear gloves, and he suffered several needlestick injuries. Others working with infected patients have not contracted HIV.[138] Although there are no known cases of UK dental staff being infected occupationally, at least one British surgeon has died from infection, apparently acquired in this way, and about 20 health care workers worldwide have been reported to have been occupationally infected with HIV, mostly from sharps injuries involving HIV-infected blood.[132,138–150] Considering that there is a very high frequency of sharps injuries among health care workers,[135,151,152] that the AIDS epidemic has been spreading for a decade or more, and that in areas of high risk such as New York City up to 1 in 10 needlestick accidents have been reported during the care of an AIDS patient,[153,154] the occupational risk appears *very* low. Even in areas of sub-Saharan Africa, where the prevalence of HIV is high, and hygiene and medical technology are limited, most infected hospital workers have acquired HIV non-occupationally.[155]

In view of a latent period of up to 3 years, negative HIV-antibody tests soon after needlestick injuries may yet prove to be misleading.

Table 5.4 Occupational risks of HIV to dental staff[a]

Country	Number tested	Number positive	Year
USA	10	0	1986
Denmark	961	0	1986
USA	255	0	1987
USA	1309	1	1988
USA	1195	0	1988
Germany	1807	0	1988
Various	167	0	1988

[a] Based on references 132–137

The possibility of occupational transmission cannot therefore be dismissed and adequate precautions must be taken, particularly as the incidence of infection rises. 'Universal precautions' against cross-infection are needed (see below), since blood and saliva from HIV patients may contain HBV and other microbial agents.

There are no documented cases of occupational transmission of HIV to non-clinical dental staff. The risks from sexual transmission are considerably greater, and many more dental staff have acquired HIV infection by this means, than from their occupation.

HIV-positive dentists

There is no proof of transmission of HIV from a health care worker during normal patient care.* However, in view of the concern that AIDS *might* be transmitted by an HIV-positive dentist to a patient, the GDC has issued a statement (January 13, 1988) to the effect that, first, dentists who suspect that they have been infected by HIV should seek medical advice and follow any consequent recommendations regarding modification of their practices necessary to protect their patients. Secondly, dentists who know or suspect that they are HIV-positive and who jeopardise the well-being of their patients by failing to obtain appropriate medical advice or by failing to act on such advice, are behaving unethically. Such behaviour may raise the question of professional misconduct (*see* Chapter 7).

Further advice is contained in *AIDS: HIV-infected health care workers* (HMSO, 1988. ISBN 0 11 321140 6).

Recognition of AIDS or HIV-positive patients

Oral infections and other features of AIDS or its prodromes may enable patients to be recognised. A young adult male who develops thrush for no apparent reason is likely to have AIDS; if he has oral Kaposi's sarcoma or hairy leukoplakia, these are virtually pathognomonic of the disease. Nevertheless, despite the frequency with which oral or perioral lesions are seen in AIDS or its prodromes, the majority of patients who are infective lack overt clinical signs to suggest the possibility. Indeed, there are many tens of thousands of HIV-antibody positive, potentially infective persons in the UK, and the number has been doubling every 9 months or so.

---

* One possible case has now been reported. *MMWR* 1990; **39**: 489–493.

Non-specific laboratory indicators of HIV infection
These include lymphopenia, low CD4 lymphocyte counts, and increased serum levels of ß2 microglobulin and neopterin.[156]

The 'AIDS test' for antibodies
This is the main way by which infectivity is assessed; enzyme-linked immunosorbent assays (ELISA) for HIV antibodies are prone to false positive results which must always therefore be confirmed with the Western blot HIV antibody test. As discussed above, there are a number of HIV-infected persons who do not carry antibodies but harbour the virus. They are seronegative but are still a potential source of infection.

Should patients be screened for HIV?
In the UK, it was not legally permissible until recently to carry out HIV tests merely for diagnostic purposes. Patients must always give consent before testing and should be counselled professionally if found to be positive. Such testing has quite dramatic and profound implications, however, and in any case, as discussed earlier, a minority (perhaps 25%) are infected but do not give a positive antibody test. There is usually a latent period which can sometimes be as long as 3 years after infection before antibodies appear. Also, in some cases, antibodies can disappear from the circulation late in the disease.

Overall, therefore, it is best that clinical dental staff treat *all* patients, their tissues, blood and secretions as potentially infective, as discussed at the end of this chapter.

In summary, it is simply not possible to identify all potentially infectious dental patients. Good cross-infection control measures are needed for all dental patients.

Herpetic infections

Herpes viruses are DNA viruses that, after primary infection, become latent.[9] The herpes viruses include herpes simplex virus (HSV), varicella-zoster virus (VZV), Epstein-Barr virus (EBV), cytomegalovirus (CMV) and human herpes virus 6 (HHV6). Several of the herpetic infections are common in immunocompromised persons and they pose a hazard, particularly to immune deficient persons, and to the foetus in the first trimester of pregnancy.[9] Most of these viruses can be found in saliva.[9] Dental staff in the West are now not infrequently non-immune, except to VZV, since they may not have been exposed to all the viruses in childhood. The infections are thus sometimes contracted in adulthood, occasionally occupationally.

Herpes simplex virus (HSV)

Herpes simplex is the most common herpes virus known to be transmitted to clinical dental staff.[9,157,158] HSV infection is now less common in children, resulting in less widespread immunity in adults. One study in the USA showed over 40% of dental students and hospital staff to be non-immune to HSV and thus at risk from infection.[159]

The primary oral infection is typically an acute vesiculating stomatitis with gingivitis; this was at one time a disease of infancy or childhood, but is now probably just as frequently seen in adults. After the primary oral infection, a minority of patients become susceptible to recurrent herpes labialis (cold sores) or, very rarely, recurrent intra-oral infection, often with ulcers. As mentioned earlier, herpetic stomatitis can be a feature of HIV disease and of other immunocompromised states such as leukaemia.[9,158]

Transmission of herpes simplex

The saliva from patients who have had a primary infection can contain the virus even when no oral lesions are seen. Vesicle fluid from recurrent infection is highly infected, and saliva is sometimes also infectious in asymptomatic persons, and is a common route of transmission.[160,161] Salivary shedding of HSV is increased in the immunocompromised and is also increased in patients with orofacial trauma or malignant disease, and those who are undergoing head and neck irradiation, or cytotoxic chemotherapy.[162,163]

Infection can be transmitted to clinical dental staff who are non-immune, and can cause primary herpetic stomatitis or an herpetic whitlow (fig. 5.14).[164] The latter is a painful, usually periungual infection on a finger. As with the oral lesions, such infections are characterised by vesicles which precede breakdown of the skin and crusting. This may interfere with the dental staff's work schedule or, if he or she soldiers on, can infect patients. However, most herpetic whitlows are found in persons with primary herpetic stomatitis or recurrent genital herpes;[165] occupational infection is fortunately now uncommon.

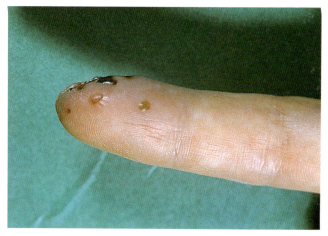

Fig. 5.14   Herpetic whitlow.

Another possibility (though it may be no more than theoretical) is to convey the virus to the eye to cause herpetic keratitis, with the possibility of impairment of vision. By contrast, genital herpes is frequently transmitted sexually.

Although HSV is an occupational hazard to clinical dental staff, herpes simplex is only moderately infectious and gloving provides adequate protection. It should be remembered that herpetic lesions in dental staff are also infectious and that outbreaks among patients have originated from clinical dental staff.[166]

If infection is acquired, acyclovir taken at the earliest possible moment is effective and will suppress recurrent infections if taken long-term.[3,9,158]

Varicella-zoster virus (VZV)

The varicella-zoster virus causes chickenpox in the non-immune (mostly children), whilst herpes zoster is a reactivation infection, usually in old age or in the immunocompromised patient.[8,167] The development of zoster in a young adult may suggest HIV infection. Chickenpox is typically a mild illness, but shingles can be a painful and debilitating disease, especially if the trigeminal region is attacked.

The lesions of chickenpox and shingles are infective, but most clinical dental staff are likely to be immune as a result of childhood infection, since chickenpox is highly contagious and spreads particularly by the airborne route.[168] Gloves and mask *may* confer some protection. Dental staff are more likely, therefore, to develop shingles after retirement and as a result of reactivation of endogenous virus rather than from a patient.

Acyclovir is effective treatment but must be given at the earliest possible moment and in large doses orally, or even intravenously.[3,9] It is particularly indicated for immunocompromised persons.

Cytomegalovirus (CMV)

Although there is no good evidence of occupational transmission of CMV to dental staff,[45] the virus can be transmitted to other health care workers in blood and can be a particular hazard to pregnant staff since it can cause foetal damage in those who have not acquired immunity.[9,169] In others, it causes a glandular fever type of syndrome but the Paul-Bunnell test is negative.

CMV is also transmitted in body fluids, particularly urine and saliva.[170–177] Between 25 and 60% of preschool children shed CMV without apparent symptoms.[178] CMV is found in large amounts in the saliva of immunocompromised patients.[9,170–176] Adults may not be immune in industrialised countries unless they have experienced infection as a child.[171,179] There is also no doubt that CMV can be transmitted by close social contact as well as sexually.[170,180,181] Occupational transmission to health care workers is rare,[181–183] although in day-care centres, persons caring for the children have a five-fold increased risk of infection.[177] Gloves and masks should confer protection in dentistry.

Epstein-Barr virus (EBV)

Epstein-Barr virus (EBV) causes asymptomatic infections, or glandular fever (infectious mononucleosis) with atypical mononuclear cells in the blood and, usually, a positive Paul-Bunnell test. EBV remains latent in salivary and oropharyngeal epithelium. The possible role of EBV in hairy leukoplakia has been discussed earlier.

Infectious mononucleosis is probably spread predominantly by kissing, but can also be transmitted in blood. Dental, and other, students are not infrequently affected. EBV can readily be cultured from saliva, especially from persons with infectious mononucleosis or immunocompromised patients,[9,184–190] but also intermittently from asymptomatic carriers. Most dental staff are probably immune and there appears to be no specific occupational risk,[45] but dental trainees are occasionally infected, probably through social contact, especially kissing. Again, gloves and masks should confer protection in dentistry.

Human herpes virus 6 (HHV-6)

HHV-6 is a newly recognised virus, which may cause a rash (exanthem subitum). Like all herpes viruses, it becomes latent, may be reactivated and may be found in saliva.[191–193] HHV-6 infects CD4 lymphocytes[194] and may modulate the course of HIV infection. No occupational hazard is known.

The common cold and other respiratory viruses

The route of infection by these viruses is probably by droplet or contact spread. Dental staff are at risk of infection from patients, but probably less so than commuters in crowded trains.

Gloves and masks should confer protection. However, when clinical dental staff acquire one of these infections, they should, for their own sake have an adequate period of bed rest or, if this is not possible, try to avoid treating patients who are elderly or who have chronic respiratory disease, for whom such infections can be dangerous.

Hand, foot and mouth disease and herpangina

As mentioned earlier these are highly infectious diseases, usually caused by Coxsackie viruses.[9] They are usually very mild and therefore of little significance. Typical manifestations of hand, foot and mouth disease are a mild stomatitis with one or two small ulcers and a vesiculating rash on the extremities. Herpangina typically causes similar lesions on the soft palate and pharynx, and a sore throat. Infection can be asymptomatic but may occasionally lead to myocarditis or encephalitis.

Coxsackie viruses can be found in saliva and can spread by contact and in aerosols.[195,196] Occasionally, clinical dental staff have acquired the infections from patients, and infection can spread among dental staff;[9,197,198] gloves and masks may be protective.

Papillomaviruses

Human papillomaviruses (HPV) are epitheliotropic DNA viruses which are the cause of infective warts, particularly in children who can, rarely, transmit the infection from a finger to the oral cavity,[9,199] and in male homosexuals and others who occasionally contract oral warts and other HPV-related lesions.[199,200] HPV are not a significant hazard to clinical dental staff, as they are likely to have adequate levels of immunity.[201] Gloves should be protective.

Parvoviruses

Parvoviruses are DNA viruses that infect a range of small mammals and are now known to infect man. Parvovirus B19 is the main human pathogenic parvovirus known and was first recognised in 1980 as causing illness in humans, usually in school children.[202,203] Infection is asymptomatic in about 20%; others develop fever and a rash, mainly on the face and extremities (erythema infectiosum: fifth disease). A few develop a transient arthropathy or, rarely, anaemia, especially immunocompromised persons. In pregnant women, infection very occasionally produces foetal damage. More than 50% of adults have serological evidence of past infection with parvovirus B19 and, presumably, the same would apply to dental staff, who will thus be immune.

Occupational transmission to health care workers has been reported; there is also clear evidence of transmission among household contacts[202,203] and, at least theoretically, some risk to dental staff. Blood and respiratory secretions of infected persons contain the virus, but faeces and urine do not. It is not clear whether B19 is present in saliva.

Human T lymphotropic virus I (HTLV-I)

HTLV-I is a retrovirus known to be transmitted by blood, especially blood transfusions. It is endemic in the Caribbean, parts of South America, Africa, and Southern Japan, and has also now been reported in intravenous drug abusers and others in North America, Europe and elsewhere.[100,204] In areas outside the USA and Europe, it is associated with adult T cell leukaemia in Japan and tropical spastic paraparesis in Caribbean countries.[204] HTLV-I is, like HIV, more prevalent in urban than rural areas and there may be co-infection, suggesting a sexual route of infection or drug abuse.[100] It is unclear whether there is any occupational hazard from HTLV-I although, theoretically at least, it may be transmissible like other blood-borne viruses.

Human T lymphotropic virus II (HTLV-II)

HTLV-II is a retrovirus that has been isolated from some patients with a T cell variant of hairy cell leukaemia.[204-206] Any occupational hazard from HTLV-II is unclear.

Tuberculosis

As is well known, tuberculosis is a communicable disease caused predominantly by *Mycobacterium tuberculosis*. The tubercle bacillus is highly resistant to chemical disinfectants and is one of the organisms most resistant to heat. Tuberculosis can be transmitted by inhalation, ingestion or direct inoculation.

Tuberculosis had become rare in the indigenous population of western countries, but is more common in the Third World. In the West, it is now prevalent among immigrants from Southeast Asia[3] and non-tuberculous mycobacterioses are also increasing.[207] Tuberculosis and nontuberculous ('atypical') mycobacterioses, particularly *M. avium-intracellulare* infection, are increasingly frequently seen in AIDS patients.[208-209] Exceedingly rare now, though a possibility in an AIDS patient, is oral tuberculous ulceration, which may lead to the recognition of open pulmonary tuberculosis or other mycobacteriosis.[210,211]

The main forms are tuberculous cervical lymphadenitis and pulmonary infection. Tuberculosis, if active and untreated (and occasionally mistaken for a smoker's cough), is a possible hazard to clinical dental staff, since the bacilli appear in sputum and saliva. In the UK in 1981–1982, 38 cases of pulmonary tuberculosis were reported among health care workers; 18 of these were nurses or doctors.[183] Clinical dental staff may also be at risk. A further potential source of infection is hospital and, occasionally, public water supplies. Several studies from the USA have demonstrated atypical mycobacteria, notably *M.xenopi*, *M.kansasii* and *M.avium* in hospital water supplies,[212-214] and patients have been infected as a result.[214] Public water supplies, at least in some parts of the USA, have also been shown to be infected with *M. avium-intracellulare*.[215]

Although a US study in 1978 showed a far higher seroconversion in dental students than among controls,[216] clinical dental staff and other health care workers have only rarely been known to have acquired tuberculosis from patients.[217-219] Tuberculosis has, however, been transmitted in recent years from a dental surgeon to patients and, in one case where the disease was not suspected, to no fewer than 15 patients.[220]

Gloves and mask and, possibly, immunisation with BCG should be adequate protection. Apart from routine cross-infection control measures (see below), inhalational anaesthetic or sedation equipment must be disinfected if it has been used on a tuberculous patient.

Syphilis

Syphilis, as is well known, is a sexually transmitted disease caused by the bacterium *Treponema pallidum*. About 3000 new cases of syphilis are reported annually in Britain. The primary and secondary stages are highly infective and can affect the mouth.[3, 221] However, such cases are either rarely seen in dental practice or (depressing thought) are frequently unrecognised. The mouth can also be affected in the tertiary stage, but this is mainly of historical interest and, in any case, infectivity is low by this stage. Syphilis is common among AIDS patients. It can then assume atypical forms, but the range of clinical manifestations under such circumstances is as yet uncertain.

Transmission of syphilis to clinical dental staff was not a major hazard even when the disease was more common and protective clothing was not worn. Sexually transmitted diseases are, by definition, far less contagious than infections such as chickenpox, and are transmitted predominantly by close contact of mucosae. They are not airborne infections. Gloves should be adequate protection.

Gonorrhoea

Approximately 50 000 cases of gonorrhoea are reported annually in Britain. The main effects are on the genito-urinary tract, but oral lesions have occasionally been reported.[222] Oropharyngeal carriage of the causal *Neisseria gonorrhoea* (gonococcus) is well recognised but often asymptomatic.

The rarity of oral gonorrhoea may be due to the reported inhibitory effect of amylase in the saliva on the gonococcus. Nevertheless, when there is pharyngeal gonorrhoea, the gonococcus can also be isolated from the saliva in nearly 60% of cultures.[223]

There seems to be little possibility of transmitting gonorrhoea in the course of normal clinical dental practice and gloves should provide adequate protection.

Legionellosis

Legionella are relatively recently discovered Gram-negative bacteria, ubiquitous in water and soil. Several species are recognised, including *L. pneumophila*, *L. micadadei*, *L. bozemanii* and *L. feelei*.[224-227]

Transmission of *Legionella* species is by an unusual route, mainly by aerosol dissemination of infected water, particularly from air-conditioning plants, but also from other sources and occasionally drinking water. Although the bacteria (usually *L. pneumophila*) appear to be ubiquitous and present in many natural collections of water, the reasons for the colonisation of and spread from particular artificial reservoirs remains unclear.

Many infections are subclinical, but pneumonia (Legionnaires' disease) or a non-pneumonic influenza-like illness (Pontiac fever) are typical effects. Many individuals, particularly young people, are asymptomatic antibody carriers as a result of asymptomatic infection. In the USA, the antibody carriage rate ranges from 5% to 25%, according to the area sampled.[228,229] Smokers and the elderly, particularly those with respiratory disease, are particularly at risk from infection and are liable to develop a pneumonia which can be fatal in about 15% of cases. Immunocompromised patients are also especially liable to infection.

There have been many outbreaks of *Legionella* infection in hotels, spas and even in health care facilities,[225,230-245] including one related to the drinking water.[233] An outbreak of Legionnaire's disease in London in 1988 was unusual in that young adults, some of whom were mere passers-by in the streets outside the affected building, were also infected. Some developed the non-pneumonic, influenza-like form of the disease (Pontiac fever). This outbreak has lead to the suspicion that more virulent strains of *Legionella* exist and that the infection may be considerably more common than was earlier believed.

The relevance of Legionnaires' disease in the present context is that water in dental units may also harbour *Legionella*. Dental units which sometimes stand idle for days, such as over the weekend or holidays, may allow proliferation of *Legionella*.[246] As this water can then be disseminated in aerosols from dental instruments, spread of legionellosis in the dental surgery seems to be at least a theoretical possibility.[247] As a consequence, hospital dental departments have been closed when *Legionella* has been found in the units, until they have been disinfected. The current disinfectant of choice is sodium hypochlorite.

There have been several outbreaks of legionellosis in hospitals, though there is as yet no direct evidence of transmission in dental hospitals or practices.[247] However, studies have shown serum antibodies to *Legionella* species to be more frequent in some US and European dental students and hospital dental staff than in the normal population.[248] Antibodies did not develop until after more than one year of work in the hospitals, and dentists showed the highest prevalence of antibodies, followed by dental surgery assistants and technicians. This suggests that repeated exposure to infected aerosols is a possible predisposing factor.[249–250]

It may be a wise precaution to flush through dental units with fresh water before and after use, and especially first thing in the morning, to clear out contaminants (*see* Chapter 2) before treating patients. This is likely to be most important if immunocompromised patients are to be treated.

There appears to be little evidence of a serious hazard to health care workers while caring for patients with legionellosis, although the evidence is somewhat controversial.[251,252]

Other infections

Organisms such as staphylococci are not uncommon in the skin flora and may cause tenosynovitis after penetrating wounds.[253] They have been transmitted to patients during surgery, and can produce wound infection, septicaemia, and endocarditis[254] (*see* Chapter 2). Skin infections are common in dental personnel, especially in those not wearing gloves routinely, and in those with chronic disease such as diabetes.[255]

Health care, especially clinical, workers in hospital infectious disease or paediatric units, can be exposed to a range of other microorganisms, including particularly rubella, but also diphtheria, measles, mumps, respiratory syncytial virus, chlamydiae, mycoplasma and various adenoviruses, as well as parasites (ie scabies).[256–269] Non-immune workers may be infected but routine cross-infection control measures such as vaccination (against diphtheria, tetanus, polio and pertussis, and measles, mumps and rubella using DTP,

MMR and polio vaccines) and the use of careful personal hygiene and gloves, mask and eye protection will significantly reduce the risk of most infections. Indeed, the low risk of cross-infection to dental staff of organisms such as *N. meningitidis* and adenoviruses has been demonstrated by one study on US naval dental officers.[270]

It would seem that 10–20% of American health care staff lack rubella antibodies and more than ten outbreaks of rubella have been reported among hospital staff.[269] Some women believed to be immune may in fact be susceptible because other viral infections which cause rashes have been mistaken for rubella. It is important, therefore, that female health care workers are warned of the possible dangers of rubella to the foetus. They should also receive rubella immunisation at least 4 months before stopping contraception;[269] there is also evidence that non-immune dental trainees may sometimes contract rubella during their course.[45]

Cross-infection control and the dental surgery

The advent of AIDS has re-emphasised the need for effective cross-infection control, although the hepatitis B virus, the delta agent, and non-A non-B viruses, as well as other microorganisms, probably constitute a greater real hazard than HIV.

Official guidelines for cross-infection control are now available in the UK, USA and other countries, and show a remarkable unanimity in approach to cross-infection control[270–275] (Tables 5.5, 5.8, 5.9 and 5.10). The reader is referred particularly to the 1988 report by the BDA Dental Health and Science Committee[271] (fig. 5.15) and to the 1988 ADA report.[274] The basic concept is that any tissue, blood or blood-contaminated saliva may be infected by viruses or other microorganisms, thereby constituting an infective risk. Infective material should not be spread about needlessly (fig. 5.16) and sharps injuries must be avoided. Where such materials are present, cross-infection control is always needed. The main points are summarised in Tables 5.5, 5.8 and 5.10.

Immunisation
Vaccination against HBV, tuberculosis (and rubella for females) are recommended for clinical dental staff and trainees, in addition to the routine immunisations discussed above. Further details are available

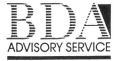

ADVISORY SERVICE

CONTROL OF CROSS INFECTION IN DENTAL PRACTICE

Fig. 5.15 BDA guidelines.

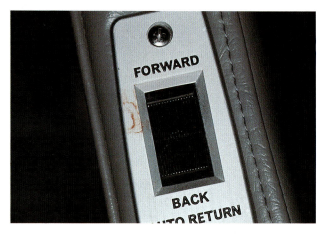

Fig. 5.16 Blood splatter on a dental chair control.

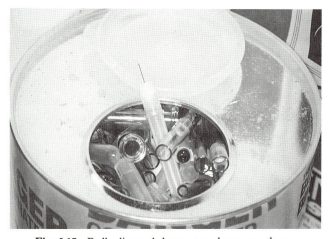

Fig. 5.17 Badly disposed sharps are a danger to others.

in '*Immunisation against infectious disease*' (HMSO, 1988. ISBN 011 3211 36 8).

Vaccination against HBV is indicated for all clinical dental staff and trainees.[272] Although some dental staff may have a lower risk of injuring themselves with contaminated instruments and are less exposed to blood than those undertaking surgery, it is clear that dental surgery assistants are at high risk from sharps injuries[276] and

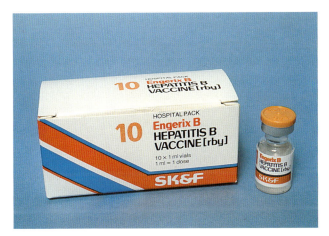

Fig. 5.18   Engerix B recombinant HBV vaccine (Smith, Kline and French).

that all practising clinical dental staff should have active immunisation against hepatitis B virus. The fear that the original vaccine (H-B-
Vax), prepared from carriers, could transmit HIV, can be dismissed
and, in any event, recombinant vaccines (eg Engerix*) are now
available (fig. 5.18). Three injections should be given, at intervals,
into the deltoid muscle. Side-effects are mild and rare, but a few
individuals (particularly those who are immunocompromised or
elderly, or seriously overweight) do not produce adequate antibody
(anti-HBs) levels after a normal course of vaccination and need to
have it repeated. In all persons, booster doses are needed, probably at
3–5-year intervals since, after 5 years, only about 75% of individuals
still have adequate antibody levels.[277,278]

Even after vaccination, common sense precautions against infection
should be maintained, since immunisation does not protect against
other agents. Those who are likely to have become infected as a result
of a wound while treating a high-risk patient and have not been
immunised, should have immediate passive immunisation with hepatitis B immune globulin (HBIG) as well as active immunisation, even
though the value of HBIG has recently been questioned (see later).

It is perhaps surprising that health care personnel do not always
follow guidelines for immunisation. For example, some 50% of

*Details can be found at the end of the chapter.

prospective hospital workers in New York had had inadequate diphtheria immunisation,[279] and immunisation against hepatitis B has, until recently, often not been taken up by dental staff. Infection control has also, until fairly recently, left much to be desired.[280–282] However, most dental students and clinical dental staff in Britain and North America, especially younger staff, are now being immunised against hepatitis B[283–287] and this is a major advance in protecting against most variants of HBV and delta agent.

Need for cross-infection control

Dental staff have a moral and legal obligation to practice effective measures for control of cross-infection. AIDS has been the spur to improve techniques and to develop appropriate equipment and other products. There is now clear evidence of improvements in all aspects of cross-infection control,[284,288–297] and it is obvious that these measures are acceptable to patients[298–301] and workable in general dental practice[302] and hospital practice.

There is no doubt that dental clinical instruments and the operator's hands[303] may be contaminated with potentially infected body fluids and microorganisms (including HBV[304,305], HSV[306,307] and HIV[308]). Some, particularly HBV, survive drying for several days.[309] HIV can survive in aqueous solution for more than 14 days at 20–22°C and for up to 11 days at 37°C but, in the dry, infectivity is lost after 6 days at room temperature.[310]

The evidence suggests not only that HIV is present in lower concentration in the blood of HIV-infected individuals than is HBV in the blood of HBV-infected persons,[311] but also that HIV is fairly fragile and readily destroyed by heat,[312] drying, and some chemicals (see below). Procedures virucidal to HBV are therefore probably effective against HIV and some other agents. Mycobacterial spores, by contrast, are considerably more resistant to heat and chemicals.

Patient examination and treatment

Personal hygiene is of paramount importance. For example, one study showed traces of blood under the fingernails of clinical personnel who did not wear gloves.[313] Handwashing facilities should have non-touch taps. Towels should be of the single use, disposable type or a hot air drier can be provided. In addition to the hands, clothes can be contaminated with hepatitis B virus and, presumably, other

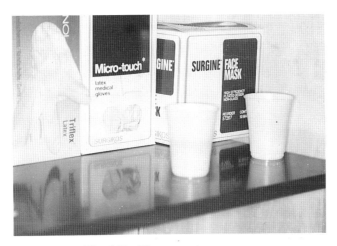

Fig. 5.19 The surgery is not a canteen.

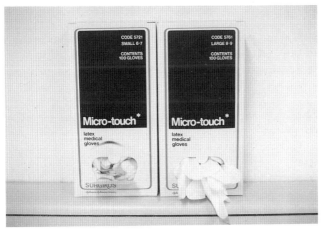

Fig. 5.20 Gloves must be worn for all clinical work and handling anything that has been in the mouth or in contact with body fluids or tissues.

viruses. Staff should also never eat, drink or smoke in clinical areas (fig. 5.19).

Oral examination or dental treatment of any patient, and the handling of instruments used in the mouth, should always be carried out while wearing gloves (fig. 5.20) and great care should be taken to avoid penetrating (sharps) injuries. Protective glasses or eye protec-

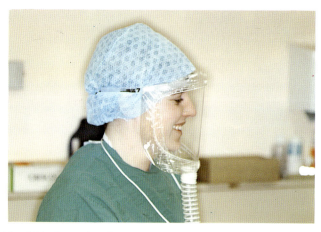

Fig. 5.21   Protective gloves or protective eyewear should be worn.

tion should be used during dental treatment of any patient (fig. 5.21); a facemask is advisable where splatter or aerosols are likely to be produced (figs 5.21 and 5.22). Disposable equipment should be used wherever possible and non-disposable equipment should be auto-claved.

The General Dental Council has recently issued statements that have a profound effect on this issue. 'A dentist has a duty to take

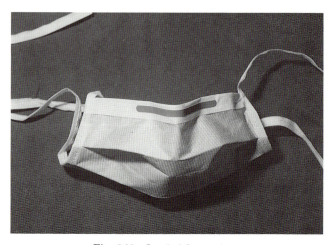

Fig. 5.22   Surgical facemask.

appropriate precautions to protect his staff and his patients from the risk of cross-infection in the dental surgery. Failure to provide and use adequate sterilisation facilities may render a dentist liable to proceedings for misconduct.

'There has been considerable public concern about the risk of contracting AIDS and, more recently, about the possibility that patients might be infected by doctors or dentists who are themselves suffering from AIDS or are HIV-positive. There is no known instance of transmission of the AIDS virus from dentist to patient in the course of treatment. The risk of cross-infection in the dental surgery has always existed. Dentists have a duty to understand the risk and the precautions which must be taken to avoid it.'

'It is the ethical responsibility of dentists who believe that they may have been infected with HIV to obtain medical advice and, if found to be infected, to submit to regular medical supervision. Their medical supervision will include counselling, in particular in respect of any changes in their practice which might be considered appropriate in the best interests of protecting their patients. It is the duty of such dentists to act upon the medical advice they have been given, which may include the necessity to cease the practice of dentistry altogether or to modify their practice in some way.

'Dentists who know that they are, or believe that they may be, HIV-positive and who might jeopardise the well-being of their patients by failing to obtain appropriate medical advice or to act upon the advice that has been given to them are behaving unethically and contrary to their obligations to patients. Behaviour of this kind may raise a question of serious professional misconduct.'

In the UK there are also legal requirements under the Health and Safety at Work etc Act that need to be met (*see* Chapter 6) and patients have made successful claims against dentists after acquiring hepatitis B (*see* Chapter 7).

Sterilisation of equipment
Single use disposable equipment should be used where possible, but as far as other equipment is concerned, the aim is to achieve sterilisation, that is the removal or destruction of all living micro-organisms and spores. Microorganisms vary in their susceptibility to heat but, in general, bacteria are more resistant than viruses, and spores are the most difficult to kill. Spores are produced particularly by clostridia and can cause tetanus or gas gangrene.

As late as 1985, one survey showed some 20% of British general dental practitioners to be using boiling water to 'sterilise' instruments, even though laboratory testing has shown this method to be inadequate in practice.[313] Current recommendations for sterilisation are to clean instruments (wearing heavy duty rubber gloves) and then autoclave them (figs 5.23 and 5.24), preferably unwrapped, at 30 psi (2·068 bar) at 134°C for 3·5 minutes (Table 5.6). Instruments can also be effectively sterilised if placed in autoclave bags, provided that most of the air is removed and the bags are not stacked.[314] Sterilisation should be checked with an indicator system (eg TST strips, sensor sheets or Brown steriliser control tubes or Kavo Steril Indicator Strips) (fig. 5.25).[315] It is important to sterilise not only instruments that are to be soon used again but also those to be sent for maintenance or repair (*see also* Chapter 6).

Portable steam sterilisers are now available but should meet BS 3970 (BSI, 1988). Further details of portable steam sterilisers are available in '*An evaluation of portable steam sterilisers for unwrapped instruments and utensils*' from Health Equipment Information No 185, July 1988, (*see* p 230 for address). Only five out of the eleven models tested combined the basic instrumentation and acceptable performance criteria. They were: Instaclave 20/35 (Alapro), Little Sister II (Surgical Equipment Supplies), Stericube (Cabburn), Sterimate (model SMA) (CMI) and 2000 (Surgical Equipment Supplies).

Guidance from the DH Procurement Directive is reproduced here

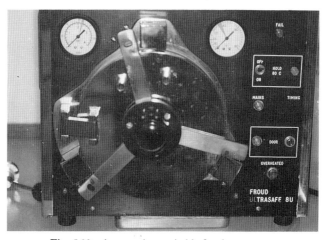

Fig. 5.23   An autoclave suitable for the surgery.

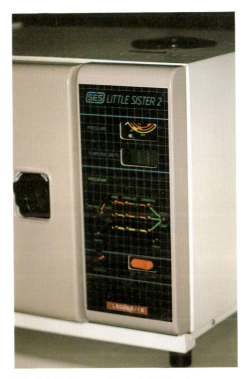

Fig. 5.24 An autoclave suitable for the surgery.

Table 5.5 Ten main points to minimise cross-infection in the dental surgery

---

(1) Avoid needlestick or other sharps injuries.
(2) Use effective sterilisation and disinfection procedures.
(3) Have clinical staff immunised, particularly against hepatitis B.
(4) Have patients use 0·2% chlorhexidine mouthrinse pre-operatively to decrease the number of oral microbes present.
(5) Use rubber dam to isolate tooth or treatment area; use high speed evacuation.
(6) Avoid causing oral bleeding wherever possible.
(7) Wear protective gloves, masks, eyewear, and/or face shields and follow good hygiene procedures.
(8) Wear clean clinical attire; change clothes before leaving the clinic.
(9) Minimise the working area, use a tray system, or cover surfaces and equipment with disposable plastic, paper or foil wraps. Uncovered surfaces and equipment should be wiped with absorbent towelling and then disinfected following work activities.

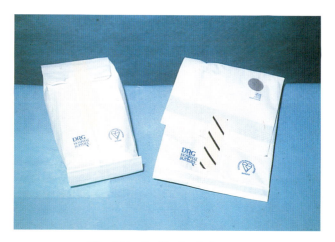

Fig. 5.25   Sterilisation indicator.

in some detail. The requirements being used for the evaluation are based on the current draft British Standard for small bench top steam sterilisers.

The main requirements in the selection of an autoclave are:

(1) The steriliser should have a preset automatic cycle.

(2) The operating cycle should achieve a sterilising temperature of 134°C for a minimum hold-time of 3 minutes.

(3) During the sterilisation hold period, the temperature differential between the chamber discharge or vent and the load should not exceed 2°C.

(4) Attainment and maintenance of satisfactory conditions during the sterilisation stage should be monitored using a temperature sensor separate from the autoclave's thermometer and thermostat.

(5) The steriliser should provide separate indications of the temperature and of the pressure within the chamber. A single pressure gauge marked with a temperature scale is not acceptable.

(6) The door or lid should be provided with an interlock or locks to prevent (a) release of the door or lid mechanism until the gauge pressure in the chamber is 200 mbar or less; (b) the door or lid being opened until the chamber has been effectively vented to atmospheric pressure.

(7) The temperature of external surfaces which may be inadvertently touched when operating the steriliser should not exceed 100°C. The

temperature of surfaces which must be touched during operation of the steriliser should not exceed 55°C.

(8) The pressure vessel should be acceptable for insurance purposes to a competent inspection authority, eg the AOTC—The Associated Offices Technical Committee or The Independent Engineering Insurers' Committee.

(9) The vessels should be fitted with an over-pressure protection device complying with either BS 2915 or BS 6759: pt 1.

(10) The steriliser should be electrically safe.

(11) If provided with a water reservoir, this should be easily drained and provide easy access for cleaning.

Small steam sterilisers of the type used in dental surgeries are intended for the sterilisation of unwrapped instruments and not for wrapped equipment, because the efficacy of air removal from packages is affected by the loading density and pattern within the steriliser chamber.

Since these factors are variable, the efficacy of air removal from packages will be unpredictable and the assurance of sterility uncertain. A further factor is that small steam sterilisers do not provide for an evacuation stage at the end of the sterilisation period to produce a dry load. The storage of an inadequately dried pack presents an opportunity for entry of microorganisms. Further study of the use of bags is essential in order to clarify this point.

Autoclaves need to be regularly examined by a competent person, since they are pressure vessels (*see* Chapters 3 and 6).

Preparation for autoclaving
Proper care of autoclaves is essential for their effectiveness and longevity (*see also* Chapter 3). All instruments should be thoroughly rinsed or cleaned ultrasonically before being placed on the autoclave trays, in order to remove amalgam, cements or other filling materials,

Table 5.6 Temperature/time relationships for sterilisation by autoclave[a]

Temperature	Time	Temperature	Time
115–118°C	30 minutes	126–129°C	10 minutes
121–124°C	15 minutes	134–138°C	3 minutes

NB: Figures taken from British Pharmacopeia 1980 Addendum 1983. The figures mean that the articles to be sterilised must be heated at the particular temperature for not less than specified holding time.
[a] For unwrapped instruments.

cotton wool or fibrous cleaning materials. This avoids clogging up the chamber and impairing the operation of the solenoid and air vent valve. It also reduces the chance of gasket failure and resulting steam leaks.

The contact surfaces of the chamber and gasket should be cleaned and a silicone compound should be regularly applied to the gasket. Extraneous chemicals, such as disinfectants and cleansers, should be rinsed off so that contaminated water in the reservoir will not cause the air vent valve to fail. Particular care should also be taken only to use distilled water since the accidental use of some chemicals may affect the operation of the valves and filter and can be very dangerous. The reservoir should not be overfilled, or filled during the cycle, since this causes flooding at the end of the cycle.

Trays should not be overloaded since, if instruments fall on to the bottom of the chamber, brown rust deposits may 'spot' the instruments and contaminate the water and the chamber.

Some equipment is damaged by autoclaving. For example, ultrasonic scalers can be difficult to autoclave; air/sonic scalers may therefore be preferred.[316] Dental handpieces have posed a particular problem, although autoclavable handpieces are now available (eg Kavo).

Hot air ovens can be used to sterilise some instruments, but in practice are a poor alternative because of the time needed (at least 180°C for 30 minutes or 160° for 60 minutes) and the possibility of disrupting the cycle and therefore sterilisation.

Endodontic instruments
It is better to sterilise endodontic instruments in a hot air (eg 'Safe Air') dental heater rather than a glass bead apparatus.[317]

Water supply (see Chapter 2)

Non-sterilisable equipment and materials
Some items cannot withstand autoclaving. Such equipment should be disposable where possible and *never re-used*.

Local anaesthetics
Local anaesthetic cartridges and needles (see below) should be discarded and not re-used; those practitioners who are not complying with this recommendation would be regarded as being guilty of

negligence and responsible for any resulting infection (see below for 'sharps injuries').

Working surfaces
Working areas should be minimised or zoned; surfaces likely to be touched should be covered with a disposable protective cover such as clingfilm (fig. 5.26) or, better, a tray system used. Surfaces are then disinfected with one of the chemicals discussed below.[271–274, 318–331]

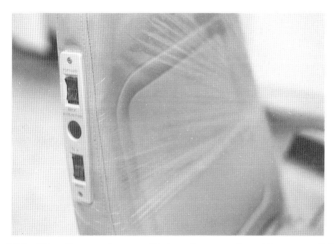

Fig. 5.26   Cling-film covering areas likely to be contaminated by operator's hands.

Disinfection

Glutaraldehyde may cause skin irritation and burns or other adverse effects (*see also* Chapter 2) but as an alkaline solution is one of the most effective virucidal agents and is widely used to disinfect contaminated surfaces, 3-in-1 syringes, impression materials and anaesthetic equipment (figs 5.27 and 5.28). Alkaline 2% glutaraldehyde must be made up freshly at least fortnightly, though at least three products (Cidex Long Life, Totacide 28 and Asep Extra Life) have double this active life. Alkaline glutaraldehyde acts to kill many viruses in 5–10 minutes, although it takes up to 10 hours to *sterilise* metal instruments (Table 5.7).[272, 320, 326]

Sodium hypochlorite (1000 ppm available chlorine, ie 1:100 dilution of household bleach) or *sodium dichloroisocyanurate* (eg Presept tablets;

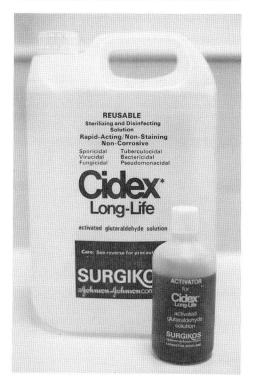

Fig. 5.27 Glutaraldehyde, with an active life of 28 days.

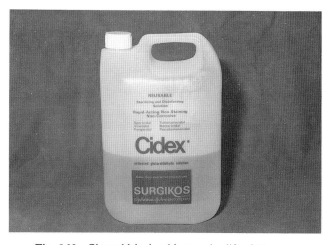

Fig. 5.28 Glutaraldehyde with an active life of 14 days.

Table 5.7 Chemical disinfection in dentistry

Agent	Comments
Glutaraldehyde 2% alkaline	One of the most effective disinfectants. Solution stable for 2 to 4 weeks only. Irritant to skin, eyes and respiratory tract. Virucidal in 10 minutes but takes 3 to 8 hours to destroy spores. Stains slightly and may be corrosive[a]
Sodium hypochlorite 1%	Fairly effective disinfectant. Fairly stable solution. Irritant to skin and eyes. Corrosive to many metals: discolours plastics: bleaches fabrics. Virucidal in 10 minutes but weakly effective against mycobacteria.
Iodophors (Betadine)	Less effective disinfectants than the above. Long shelf-life. Safe to handle. Stains slightly and may corrode some metals. Virucidal in 60 minutes. Now preferred to glutaraldehyde by some.
Sodium dichloroiso-cyanurate	Available as tablets or granules that dissolve to form hypochlorous acid. Bactericidal, including against *M. tuberculosis*. Virucidal

[a]Totacide 28 contains a corrosion inhibitor.

Surgikos) can be used[330,321] (fig. 5.29). Hypochlorite, however, bleaches fabrics and is somewhat corrosive, especially to aluminium.

Iodophors, such as povidone–iodine, are now advocated for surface disinfection, in view of the adverse effects of glutaraldehyde.[328,331]

Although HIV may be inactivated by alcohol, 70% industrial methylated spirit and ethanol fail to disinfect surfaces within 20 minutes,[326] even though they may partially wash the surface and dilute organisms, and are effective in aqueous solution.[321,322] Glutaraldehyde in 2% alkaline concentration is effectively virucidal against HIV within 2 minutes.[320,326] It must be made up freshly at regular, frequent intervals of no longer than 14 to 28 days, depending on the particular product, since re-use and serum proteins reduce its activity.[326] HIV is, reportedly, also inactivated within 10 minutes by some iodophors such as 0·5% povidone–iodine,[332–334] and by chlorhexidine, even at a concentration of 0·2% in alcohol,[334] though the assay for HIV infectivity used was relatively crude.[334]

Spillages of blood should be covered either with sodium dichloroisocyanurate granules or disposable towels and then with 10 000 ppm sodium hypochlorite for at least 10 minutes before wiping up.[321]

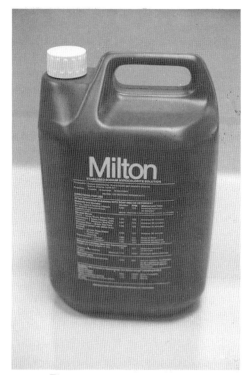

Fig. 5.29   Sodium hypochlorite.

General anaesthetic and relative analgesia masks

These are well documented sources of infection[335-338] and there have been occasional reports of outbreaks of infection spread by masks to patients and operators.[339-342].

Wiping with alkaline glutaraldehyde can effectively disinfect but not sterilise masks and is irritant,[339] and an iodophor is probably better. Autoclaving damages the rubber. Microwaves for 4 minutes have been recommended for sterilisation.[343]

Waste

Clinical waste should be carefully disposed of, in order to ensure that there is no risk of injury to staff or other persons. Sharps *must* be discarded into clearly labelled, rigid sharps containers (eg Dentanurse 'Safeguard'; DRG 'Sharpak'; 'Septodont' Disposi Needles) and incinerated (figs 5.30 to 5.32). Cardboard containers are not adequate as

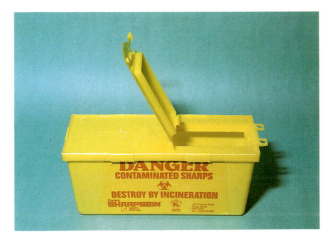

Fig. 5.30   Sharps container.

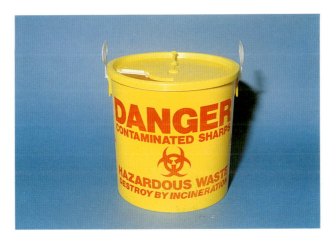

Fig. 5.31   Sharps container.

they may be perforated by sharps (fig. 5.33). Some companies such as Mediwaste and Rentokil will collect such waste at regular intervals.

Needles should neither be resheathed manually nor removed and discarded manually since it is at these times that needlestick injuries are likely. Several devices are available to aid needle disposal (eg Septodont: Aim-safe: Dentanurse: figs 5.34 to 5.37) and there is no doubt that the frequency of sharps injuries can be reduced through increased care by the user.

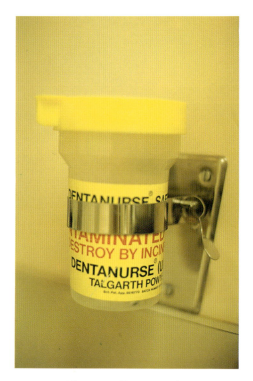

Fig. 5.32   Sharps container

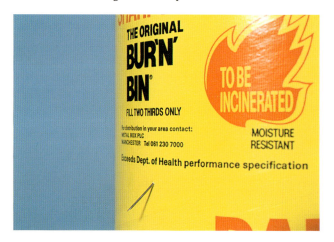

Fig. 5.33   Cardboard 'sharps' container that was perforated by a needle.

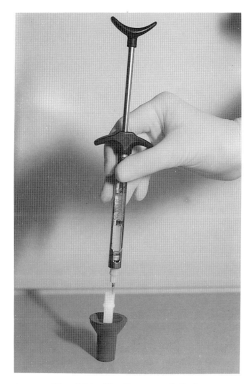

Fig. 5.34 Needle removal device.

Impressions

Impressions should be rinsed in running water to remove debris, blood and saliva, and disinfected before being sent to the laboratory (Table 5.8) in an impervious container, appropriately marked if there is a biohazard (fig. 5.38). The ADA and FDI recommend 10 to 90 minutes exposure to glutaraldehyde, depending on the type of impression material,[274,344] but UK recommendations are for 3 hours.[271] Elastomer impressions are easiest to disinfect. Immersion in 2% alkaline glutaraldehyde for one hour causes little dimensional change in silicone and polysulphide impressions, but may affect surface detail of alginates[327,345–357] It seems likely that one hour's exposure to fresh glutaraldehyde will be virucidal for impressions, as this is at least double the time needed to inactivate HBV.[358,359]

It is possible that materials such as Blueprint Asept (alginate) and Unosil (silicone rubber) may have some antimicrobial activity.

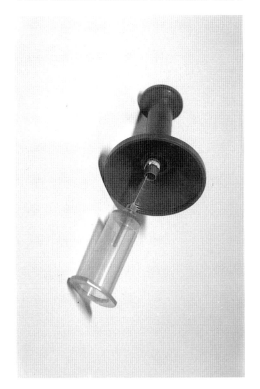

Fig. 5.35   Needle removal device.

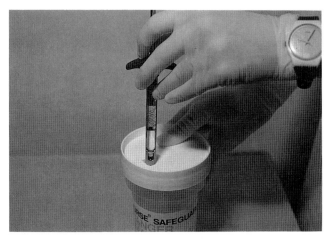

Fig. 5.36   Needle removal device.

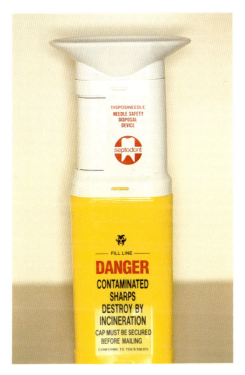

Fig. 5.37   Needle removal device.

Protective wear (*see also* Chapter 2)

Gloves should be worn for contact with clinical materials.[360] Aerosols and splatter should be minimised. Rubber dam will minimise aerosols and splatter containing body fluids and high volume aspiration is required. Protective eyewear or a face shield (fig. 5.21) will confer some protection against splatter, infected tooth or calculus fragments and foreign material and aerosols. Fresh gowns should be worn daily and discarded before leaving work.

Gloves

Gloves must be worn to prevent skin contact with blood, mucous membranes, tissues or saliva (Table 5.9). Without gloves, blood and microorganisms can be harboured beneath the nails for days. Dental staff who did not routinely wear gloves have contracted infection with

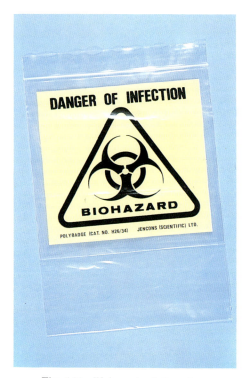

Fig. 5.38   Biohazard polythene bag.

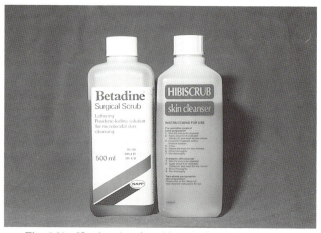

Fig. 5.39   Handscrubs of povidone–iodine and chlorhexidine.

Table 5.8 Control of cross-infection in clinical dentistry

Immunisation	Recommended against at least hepatitis B, tetanus, tuberculosis
Treatment	(1) *Treat all patients as potentially infectious* (2) Take a full relevant medical history. (3) Wear gloves, protective eyewear, gown or coat and particularly if using rotating or ultrasonic instruments, wear a mask. (4) Avoid sharps injuries: handle sharps carefully, do not resheath, discard into sharps bin. (5) Minimise splatter and aerosols, use rubber dam for restorative work and use high volume vacuum evacuation.
After treatment	(1) Remove and discard gloves and wash hands. (2) Wear heavy duty (eg Marigold-type) rubber gloves for instrument cleaning and disinfection/sterilisation procedures. (3) Clean all instruments of debris/blood. (4) Clean handpieces/air–water syringe/ultrasonic scalers and sterilise (otherwise disinfect). (5) Disinfect surfaces and change any surface covers. (6) Sterilise all instruments that have come into contact with blood, saliva, tissues or mucosa. (7) Dispose of waste safely. (8) Rinse in water and disinfect impressions or other materials or appliances to be sent to the laboratory.

herpes simplex, hepatitis B virus, and HIV, although needlestick injuries are probably the main route of transmission (see above). Hands should be washed thoroughly using chlorhexidine or some other suitable antiseptic[361-363] since soap alone is not virucidal[364] (fig. 5.39). Gloves can effectively protect against many microorganisms, including viruses such as HIV.[365,366] However, gloves will not protect if perforated; up to 80% of gloves perforate during surgery and up to 50% become permeable to bacteria after several hours' use.[367-375] Even fresh gloves that meet the British Standard BS4005 cannot be relied on to be free of micropunctures (fig. 5.40) and visual inspection cannot detect this type of defect.[373] Defective gloves have resulted in transmission of infections to patients[243] and may be one reason why gloves appeared not to confer protection against hepatitis B in one study on US oral surgeons.[376] Other studies, however, have shown protection of dental staff by glove use, or at least a lower infection rate in those wearing gloves.[377] Failure to wear gloves can also transmit

Table 5.9 Glove use in dentistry

Glove type	Use	Comments
Clean, protective latex gloves	Whenever putting fingers into the mouth of patients or handling blood- or saliva-contaminated instruments, equipment or appliances. When handling disinfectants or sterilants.	Re-use after disinfection with chlorhexidine possible but inadvisable.
Orthopaedic type	When anticipating a procedure that may tear or cut usual latex or vinyl exam gloves, or when carrying out surgery.	Gloves should cover the cuffs of a long sleeved gown to minimise skin exposure. Orthopaedic gloves are more resistant to tearing and cutting than many standard latex exam gloves. New gloves should be worn for treatment of each patient. Remove gloves, wash hands, and reglove with fresh gloves before treating the next patient. Do not attempt to disinfect gloves.
Heavy duty utility glove	During clean-up tasks	

HSV, HBV and other agents to dental patients.[51,52] Gloves should ideally be changed between each patient.[273]

Gloves are relatively easy to use in clinical dentistry.[378-380] Although, in the past, few dental practitioners wore them, the situation has radically changed and there is now wide usage of gloves in both hospital and general practice. Patients find this and other cross-infection control measures quite acceptable and most practitioners readily accept glove-wearing.[300,301] Problems such as allergic reactions of staff or patients to latex gloves, or antioxidants such as mercaptobenzothiazole, are very rare[381] and, in such cases, polyvinyl chloride or special hypoallergenic synthetic rubber gloves can usually be safely used (Table 5.9; Chapter 2). A spray-on microfilm may be of

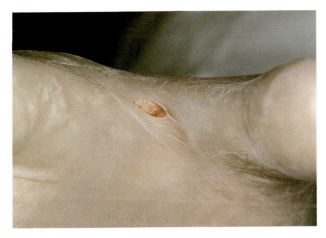

Fig. 5.40 An obvious defect in a new pair of gloves. Microdefects may be found even in some new gloves.

some value to reduce allergies (Invisible Skin +) as may skin creams (eg Skin Friend cream). Latex (polyisoprene) is mainly derived from *Hevea brasiliensis*, and contains proteins, lipids, nucleotides and co-factors; it is unclear which of these are responsible for the rare instances of contact allergy, rhinitis and even anaphylaxis.[382-384] Synthetic rubber (such as neoprene) appears not to cause cross-reactions in those sensitive to latex. Elastyrene disposable gloves contain zinc dithiocarbamate as antioxidant, and cause fewer skin reactions, as do other hypoallergenic gloves. Indeed, the use of gloves probably reduces sensitisation to various dental materials that might be handled. Various non-sterile gloves are available (*see* p 229).

The major problems encountered in glove usage include difficulties in handling endodontic instruments, a danger of the gloves catching in rotating instruments or catching light in a Bunsen burner flame, an effect on the setting of some impression materials and the fact that they are not puncture-resistant. New flameless heaters, as alternatives to Bunsen burners, overcome the ignition hazard (for example Safe Air: Carbolite Furnaces; Chapter 3). Natural latex gloves (but not synthetic gloves such as Biogel D, or vinyl gloves) may retard the setting of vinyl polysiloxane putty impression materials (eg Repro-sil),[385-387] since these gloves may contain traces of sulphur-containing rubber accelerators such as zinc diethyl dithiocarbamate. However, these materials should not normally be directly handled sufficiently for this to be of practical importance. A greater risk of delay in setting is from contact with rubber dam.

New developments in gloves include cut-resistant gloves incorporating a metal mesh, and gloves treated with silver sulphadiazine, which inhibits many microorganisms, including HIV. However, the effectiveness of the latter is not yet clear.

Mask and eye protection (see also Chapter 2)
It is important to minimise splatter and aerosols by the use of rubber dam and high-speed evacuation of the operating area. High-speed aspirators should exhaust externally in order to reduce aerosols in the surgery. The wearing of a facemask such as a surgical mask (fig. 5.22) or face shield, and eye protection is recommended in most current cross-infection control guidelines, despite the fact that mask efficacy is sometimes low and that airborne transmission of HBV[388] and HIV is unlikely. Moreover, tubercle bacilli[389] can occasionally be present in dental aerosols and HBV can be transmitted across the conjunctiva.[390] Avoiding talking may well be as effective as a mask in preventing cross-infection to the patient.[391] The filtering efficiency of surgical facemasks ranges from 14% to 99% and particles of 5 μm or less can penetrate them. Microorganisms pass so readily through the mask that the useful life is probably only 30–60 minutes. Paper or gauze masks are especially ineffective.[392–400]

Clothing
Protective attire should be worn only in the surgery or laboratory and not taken to eating areas. Clothing thought to be contaminated should be handled carefully and, if possible, autoclaved before laundering. In practice, clothing should be washed in a well-maintained machine, rinsed initially in the cold rinse cycle, then in the hot wash cycle at least at 80°C. Hospital clothing, if contaminated, is treated according to the Department of Health circular (Hospital laundry arrangements for used and infected linen (DHSS, 1987)).

Cross-infection control and the dental technical and other laboratories

In the USA, dental technicians have a *slightly* higher carriage of hepatitis B than dental clerical staff but lower than dental clinical staff.[21] Cross-infection is therefore at least theoretically possible, but most unlikely from the clinic to the clinical laboratory (and vice versa) and within the laboratory. Pathology and microbiology laboratories by their nature are more likely to present infectious hazards. The occupational risks in any laboratory are far less from infection than from accidents or other hazards.

There is no doubt that oral microorganisms can be transferred to the dental laboratory on clinical material such as dental impressions and occlusal records,[401-404] but there are only very rare reports of these as a source of infection, for example of *Mycoplasma pneumoniae*,[267] to laboratory personnel. Nevertheless, impressions received from the clinic should be washed in running water and then disinfected (Table 5.10). Any known infectious material must be clearly labelled as a biohazard and transported in an impervious container. Infected material, such as pumice, exists in laboratories but there is little evidence of a significant infective risk to technicians,[405-412] despite the fact that there may be infected aerosols.[413] Clearly, however, masks and eye protection are needed where splatter or aerosols are generated.

There is also little risk of cross-infection from the dental laboratory to the surgery, despite the fact that prostheses can be contaminated, probably mainly from dental pumice. The latter can be infected with oral and non-oral bacteria, including species of streptococci, staphylococci, *Escherichia coli*, acinetobacter, Bacillus, *Pseudomonas alcaligenes*, enterobacteriaciae, moraxella and micrococci.[407,414,415] The Gram-negative organism *Acinetobacter calcoaceticus* is especially

Table 5.10 Control of cross-infection in the dental laboratory

Immunisation	Recommended against tetanus, tuberculosis and possibly hepatitis B.
Material received	(1) Handle in gloves and laboratory coat in a special receiving area. (2) Disinfect material received that has not already been disinfected. (3) Dispose of contaminated waste safely.
Laboratory safety	(1) Wear safety glasses and mask when working with rotating instruments. (2) Avoid sharps injuries. (3) Make up fresh pumice for each case. (4) Autoclave ragwheels and polishing brushes. (5) Disinfect prostheses for surgical patients.

prevalent in pumice,[408] and dentures supplied from laboratories are often contaminated by acinetobacter. Bacillus species, *Klebsiella pneumoniae*, *Pseudomonas stutzeri*, *Enterobacter cloacae* and moraxella may also be found.[414]

Many of these organisms could theoretically cause disease in immunocompromised individuals, but there is no hard evidence of transmission via dental prostheses. Nevertheless, acinetobacter may infect surgical wounds in the head and neck[416,417] and it seems wise to decontaminate prostheses with hypochlorite before giving them to early post-operative or to immunocompromised patients.

Pumicing may also produce an infected splatter and aerosol.[405–409] Zephiran chloride 1:750 (benzalkonium) effectively decontaminates pumice,[406] but the best method of reducing contamination is to use 5 parts sodium hypochlorite to 100 parts distilled water with 3 parts green soap and to mix aliquots of pumice specifically for individual cases.

Management of needlestick and sharps injuries

Many needlestick and sharps injuries can be avoided. However, in the event of a needlestick injury, the best course currently available is as follows:

(1) *Immediately* wash the wound in running tap water and non-mucosal surfaces with soap.

(2) Record the accident.

(3) Have hepatitis B immune globulin *and* active immunisation if not already vaccinated against HBV. Vaccination at 0, 2 and 6 weeks (accelerated vaccination) may be most effective; the efficacy of immune globulin has not been established.[418]

(4) Have a booster of vaccine against HBV if already immunised but more than 3 years before.

(5) If HIV is likely to be involved, expert counselling of the wounded person and the patient is almost certainly required. Testing the patient on whom the instrument has been used, for HIV, should be considered and it may be advisable for the wounded person to have the HIV antibody test. If HIV-infected blood has been involved, the wounded person should avoid donating blood and should be tested at 3 or 6 months for HIV antibody.[419,420] As discussed previously, following infection with HIV, antibodies usually appear within 3 months but may not appear for up to 3 years. If health care workers

become HIV-positive, then they and their family should be counselled. Obviously, no reliable treatment is available but the advent of zidovudine opens the possibility for active intervention. A specialist physician should be consulted.

(6) Should an exposure of this type result in an illness then it will need to be reported formally by the employer to the Health and Safety Executive under the Health and Safety (The Reporting of Injuries, Diseases and Dangerous Occurrences) Regulations (RIDDOR), 1985. Illnesses acquired as a result of work with pathogens which present a hazard to human health fall within the requirements of the RIDDOR Regulations (*see* Chapter 3).

(7) The PHLS Communicable Disease Surveillance Centre (CDSC) and the Communicable Diseases (Scotland) Unit (CD(S)U) are conducting a national surveillance of accidental injury and other forms of contamination with HIV occurring in the United Kingdom.

References

1 Simpson JP, Whittaker DK. Serum contamination of instruments in dental practice. *Br Dent J* 1979; **146**: 76.

2 Autio KL, Rosen S, Reynolds NJ. Studies on cross-contamination in the dental clinic. *J Am Dent Assoc* 1980; **100**: 358–361.

3 Scully C, Cawson RA. *Medical problems in dentistry.* 2nd ed. Bristol: Wright, 1987.

4 Siew C, Gruninger SE, Hojvat SA. Screening dentists for HIV and hepatitis B. *New Engl J Med* 1988; **318**: 1400–1401.

5 Iwarson SA. Non-A, non-B hepatitis. In: *Recent advances in infection.* pp 119–129, 1989.

6 Skinhoj P, Vinterberg H, Aldershvile J, Kryger P. Hepatitis A, B and non-A, non-B in Danish hospital nursing staff. *J Clin Pathol* 1984; **37**: 763–766.

7 Murray-Lyon IM. Strategies for preventing hepatitis B. *Quart J Med* 1989; **71**: 277–278.

8 Scully C. Hepatitis B: an update in relation to dentistry. *Br Dent J* 1985; **159**: 321–328.

9 Scully C. Infectious diseases. *In:* Millard HD, Mason DK (eds). *1988 World workshop on oral medicine.* pp 131–212. Chicago: Yearbook Publishers, 1990.

10 Coursaget P, Yvonnet B, Bourdil C. HBsAg positive reactivity in man not due to hepatitis B virus. *Lancet* 1987; **2**: 1354–1358.

11 Budkowska A, Dubrenil P, Ouattara A, Pillot J. Hepatitis B virus type 2. *Lancet* 1988; **1**: 990.

12 Davis LG, Weber DJ, Lemon SM. Horizontal transmission of hepatitis B virus. *Lancet* 1989; **1**: 889–893.

13 Harrison TJ, Bal V, Wheeler EG, Meacock TJ, Harrison JF, Zuckerman AJ. Hepatitis B virus DNA and e antigen in serum from blood donors positive in HBsAg. *Br Med J* 1985; **290**: 260–261.

14 Sobeslavsky O. Prevalence of markers of hepatitis B virus infection in various countries: a WHO collaborative study. *Bull WHO* 1980; **50**: 621–628.

15   Mori M. Status of viral hepatitis in the world community: its incidence among dentists and other dental personnel. *Int Dent J* 1984; **34**: 115–121.

16   West DJ The risk of hepatitis B infection among health professionals in the United States: a review. *Am J Med Sci* 1984; **287**: 26–33.

17   Bennet NM, Carson JA, Fish BS, George LJ, Puszet PJ, Rankin DW, Wilkinson P, Norman AF, Stevens K, Maynard JH. An assessment of the prevalence of hepatitis B among health care personnel in Victoria. *Med J Aust* 1985; **143**: 495–499.

18   Eisenburg J, Holl J, Kruis W, Weinzierl M, Grunst J, Puttkammer D, Wendl N. Hepatitis risk to dentists. Studies on the frequency of hepatitis in dentists in the Munich region and in the district of Upper Bavaria. *Fortschr Med* 1977; **95**: 1249–1258.

19   Panis B, Ronmeliotou-Karayannis A, Papaevangelou G, Richardson SC, Mitsis F. Hepatitis B virus infection in dentists and dental students in Greece. *Oral Surg* 1986; **61**: 343–345.

20   Feldman RE, Schiff ER. Hepatitis in dental professionals. *J Am Med Assoc* 1975; **232**: 1228–1230.

21   Schiff ER, de Medina MD, Kline SN, Johnson GR, Chan Y-K, Shorey J, Calhoun N, Irish EF. Veterans administration cooperative study on hepatitis and dentistry. *J Am Dent Assoc* 1986; **113**: 390–396.

22   Amerena V, Andrew JH. Hepatitis B virus: the risk to Australian dentists and dental health care workers. *Aust Dent J* 1987; **32**: 183–189.

23   Savage CM, Christopher PJ, Murphy AM, Crewe EB, Lossin C. The prevalence of hepatitis B markers in dental care personnel at the United Dental Hospital of Sydney. *Aust Dent J* 1984; **29**: 75–79.

24   James SP, Sampliner RE. Hepatitis B in the dental setting. *J Maryland State Dent Assoc* 1978; **32**: 183–189.

25   Faoagali JL. Hepatitis B markers in Canterbury dental workers: a sero-epidemiological survey. *NZ Med J* 1986; **99**: 12–14.

26   Goebel WM, Gitnick GL. Hepatitis B virus infection in dental students: a two year evaluation. *J Oral Med* 1979; **34**: 33–36.

27   Hollinger FB, Grander JW, Nickel FR. Hepatitis B prevalence within a dental student population. *J Am Dent Assoc* 1977; **94**: 521–527.

28   Scheutz F, Melbye M, Esteban JI, Aldershvile J, Ebbesen P, Alter HJ. Hepatitis B virus infection in Danish dentists: a case-control and follow-up study. *Am J Epidemiol* 1988; **128**: 190–196.

29   Reed BE, Barrett AP. Hepatitis B virus carrier groups and the Australian community. *Aust Dent J* 1988; **33**: 171–176.

30   Epstein JB, Bucher BK, Bouchard S. Hepatitis B and Canadian dental professionals. *J Canad Dent Assoc* 1984; 7: 555–559.

31   Siew C, Gruninger SE, Mitchell EW, Burrell KH. Survey of hepatitis B exposure and vaccination in volunteer dentists. *J Am Dent Assoc* 1987; **114**: 457–459.

32   Aldershvile J, Brock A, Dietrichson O *et al.* Hepatitis B virus infections in Danish dentists. *J Infect Dis* 1978; **137**: 63–66.

33   Hardt F, Aldershvile, J, Dietrichson O *et al.* Hepatitis B virus infection in Danish surgeons. *J Infect Dis* 1979; **140**: 972–974.

34   Mosley JW, Edwards VM, Casey G, Redeker AG, White E. Hepatitis B virus infection in dentists. *New Engl J Med* 1975; **293**: 729–734.

35   Bass BD, Andors L, Pierri LK, Pollock JJ. Quantitation of hepatitis B viral markers in a dental school population. *J Am Dent Assoc* 1982; **104**: 629–632.

36   Feldman RE, Schiff ER. Hepatitis in dental professionals. *J Am Med Assoc* 1975; **232**: 1228–1230.

37 Glenwright HE, Edmondson HD, Whitehead FIH, Flewett TH. Serum hepatitis in dental surgeons. *Br Dent J* 1974; **136**: 409–413.
38 Goubran GF, Cullens H, Zuckerman AJ, Eddleston ALWF, Williams R. Hepatitis B virus infection in dental surgical practice. *Br Med J* 1976; **2**: 559–560.
39 Nicholas, NK. Viral hepatitis among practising dentists. *NZ Med J* 1977; **588**: 413–416.
40 Kreider SD, Lange WR. Hepatitis B vaccine. *New Engl J Med* 1984; **310**: 466.
41 Hofmann H, Tuma W, Heinz, FX, Frisch-Niggemeyer W, Kunz C. Infectivity of medical staff for hepatitis B. *Infection* 1988; **16**: 171–174.
42 Smith JL, Maynard JE, Berquist KR *et al.* Comparative risk of hepatitis B among physicians and dentists. *J Infect Dis* 1976; **133**: 705–706
43 Hurlen B, Iversen SB, Jonsen J. Frequency of hepatitis in dental health personnel in Norway. *Acta Odontol Scand* 1979; **37**: 189.
44 Cumming CG, Peutherer JF, Smith GLF. The prevalence of hepatitis B serological markers in dental personnel. *J Infect* 1986; **12**: 157–159.
45 Jones DM, Tobin JO'H, Turner EP. Australia antigen and antibodies to Epstein-Barr virus, cytomegalovirus and rubella virus in dental personnel. *Br Dent J* 1972; **132**: 489–491.
46 Polakoff S. Acute viral hepatitis B, laboratory reports 1985–8. *Commun Dis Rep* 1989: 26–29.
47 Foley FF, Gutheim RN. Serum hepatitis following dental procedures: a presentation of 15 cases including 3 fatalities. *Ann Intern Med* 1956; **45**: 369.
48 Gerety RJ. Hepatitis B transmission between dental or medical workers and patients. *Am J Intern Med* 1981; **95**: 229–231.
49 Hadler SC, Sorley DJ, Acree KH, Webster HM, Schable CA, Francis DP, Maynard JE. An outbreak of hepatitis B in a dental practice. *Am J Intern Med* 1981; **95**: 133–138.
50 Galambos JT. Transmission of hepatitis B from providers to patients. How big is the risk? *Hepatology* 1986; **6**: 320–325.
51 Rimland D, Parkin WE, Miller GB, Schrack WD. Hepatitis B outbreak traced to an oral surgeon. *New Engl J Med* 1977; **296**: 953–958.
52 Shaw FE, Barrett CL, Hamm R, Peare RB, Coleman PJ, Hadler SC, Fields HA, Maynard JE. Lethal outbreak of hepatitis B in a dental practice. *J Am Med Assoc* 1986; **255**: 3260–3264.
53 Reingold AL, Kane MA, Murphy BL *et al.* Transmission of hepatitis B by an oral surgeon. *J Infect Dis* 1982; **145**: 262–268.
54 Centers for Disease Control, Atlanta, Georgia, USA. Hepatitis B among dental patients—Indiana. *MMWR* 1985; **34**: 73–74.
55 Williams SV, Pattison CP, Berquist KR. Hepatitis B transmission by dentists. *J Am Med Assoc* 1974; **228**: 1231–1233.
56 Levin ML, Maddrey WC, Wands JR, Mendeloff AI. Hepatitis B transmission by dentists. *J Am Med Assoc* 1974; **228**: 1139–1140.
57 Centers for Disease Control. Outbreak of hepatitis B associated with an oral surgeon—New Hampshire. *Morbid Mortal Week Rep* 1987; **36**: 132–133.
58 Macaya G, Visona KA, Villarejos VM. Dane particles and associated DNA-polymerase activity in saliva of chronic hepatitis B carriers. *J Med Virol* 1979; **4**: 291–301.
59 Jenison SA, Lemon SM, Baker LN, Newbold JE. Quantitative analysis of hepatitis B virus DNA in saliva and semen of chronically infected homosexual men. *J Infect Dis* 1987; **156**: 299–307.
60 Davison F, Alexander GJM, Trowbridge R, Fagan EA, Williams R. Detection of hepatitis B virus DNA in spermatozoa, urine, saliva, and leucocytes, of chronic

HBsAg carriers. A lack of relationship with serum markers of replication. *J Hepatol* 1987; **4**: 37–44.

61 Broderson M. Salivary HBsAg detected by radioimmunoassay. *Lancet* 1974; **1**: 675.

62 Heathcote J, Cameron CH, Dane DS. Hepatitis B antigen in saliva and semen. *Lancet* 1974; **1**: 71.

63 Hurlen B. Salivary HBsAg in hepatitis B infection. *Acta Odontol Scand* 1980; **38**: 51–55.

64 Karayiannis P, Novick DM, Lok ASF. Hepatitis B virus DNA in saliva, urine and seminal fluid of carriers of hepatitis B e antigen. *Br Med J* 1985; **290**: 1853–1857.

65 Boucek CD. Blood in the mouth. *New Engl J Med* 1988; **319**: 1607.

66 Beasley RP, Hwang L-Y. Postnatal infectivity of hepatitis B surface antigen-carrier mothers. *J Infect Dis* 1983; **147**: 185–190.

67 Leichtner AM, Leclair J, Goldman DA, Schumacher RT, Gewold IH, Katz AJ. Horizontal nonparenteral spread of hepatitis B among children. *Ann Intern Med* 1981; **94**: 346–349.

68 Cancio-Bello TP, de Medina M, Shorey J, Valledor MD, Schiff ER. An institutional outbreak of hepatitis B related to a human biting carrier. *J Infect Dis* 1982; **146**: 652–656.

69 Shapiro ED. Lack of transmission of hepatitis B in a day care center. *J Pediatr* 1987; **110**: 93.

70 Glaser JB, Nadler JP. Hepatitis B virus in a cardiopulmonary resuscitation training course. *Arch Intern Med* 1985; **145**: 1653–1655.

71 Osterholm MT, Max BJ, Hanson M, Polisky HF. Potential risk of salivary-mediated viral hepatitis type B transmission from oral exposure to fomites. *J Hyg Camb* 1979; **83**: 487–490.

72 Bancroft WH, Snitbhan R, Scott RM *et al.* Transmission of hepatitis B virus to gibbons by exposure to human saliva containing hepatitis B surface antigen. *J Infect Dis* 1980; **135**: 79–85.

73 Scott RM, Snitbhan R, Bancroft WH, Alter HJ, Tingpalapong M. Experimental transmission of hepatitis B virus by semen and saliva. *J Infect Dis* 1980; **142**: 67–71.

74 Alter HJ, Purcell RH, Gerin JL *et al.* Transmission of hepatitis B to chimpanzees by hepatitis B surface antigen-positive saliva and semen. *Infect Immunol* 1977; **16**: 928–933.

75 SyWassink JM, Lutwick LI. Risk of hepatitis B in dental care providers: a contact study. *J Am Dent Assoc* 1983; **106**: 182–184.

76 Peterson NJ. An assessment of the airborne route in hepatitis B transmission. *Ann NY Acad Sci* 1980; **353**: 157–166.

77 Scholle R. Hepatitis B: changing our perceptions. *J Am Dent Assoc* 1985; **110**: 612–631.

78 Tullman MJ, Boozer CH, Villarejos VM, Feary TW. The threat of hepatitis B from dental school patients. *Oral Surg* 1980; **49**: 214–216.

79 Smith HM, Alexander GJM, Birnbaum W, Williams R. Does screening high risk dental patients for hepatitis B virus protect dentists? *Br Med J* 1987; **295**: 309–310.

80 Matthews RW, Hislop WS, Scully C. The prevalence of hepatitis B markers in high-risk dental out-patients. *Br Dent J* 1986; **161**: 294–296.

81 Boozer CH, Shopper TP, Weinberg R. The presence of anti-HBc in a dental school patient population. *J Am Dent Assoc* 1986; **112**: 854–856.

82 Rizzetto M. The delta agent. *Hepatology* 1983; **3**: 729–737.

83   Editorial. Hepatitis delta infections. *Br Med J* 1985; **290**: 1370–1371.

84   Caredda F, Antimori S, Pastecchia C, Monoui M. HBV/HDV coinfection. *Lancet* 1987; **2**: 455.

85   Hadler S, Monzon M, Ponzeto A. Virus infection and severe hepatitis: an epidemic in the Yucpa indians of Venezuela. *Ann Intern Med* 1984; **100**: 339–344.

86   Aragona M, Macagno S, Caredda F. Serological response to the hepatitis delta virus in hepatitis D. *Lancet* 1987; **1**: 478–480.

87   Hershaw RC, Chamel BB, Graham DR, Schyve PM, Mandel EJ, Kane MA, Fields HA, Hadler SC. Hepatitis D virus infection in Illinois state—facilities for the developmentally disabled. *Ann Intern Med* 1989; **110**: 779–785.

88   Cottone JA. Delta hepatitis: another concern for dentistry. *J Am Dent Assoc* 1986; **112**: 47–49.

89   Porter SR, Scully C. Non-A, non-B hepatitis and dentistry. *Br Dent J* 1990; **168**: 257–261.

90   Dienstag JL, Alter HJ. Non-A, non-B hepatitis: evolving epidemiologic and clinical perspectives. *Sem Liver Dis* 1986; **6**: 67–81.

91   Alter MJ. Non-A, non-B hepatitis: sorting through a diagnosis of exclusion. *Ann Intern Med* 1989; **110**: 583–585.

92   Alter MJ, Gerety RJ, Smallwood LA *et al.* Sporadic non-A, non-B hepatitis: frequency and epidemiology in an urban US population. *J Infect Dis* 1982; **145**: 886–893.

93   Norkrans G, Forsner G, Hermodsson S, Iwarson S. Clinical, epidemiological and prognostic aspects of hepatitis non-A non-B—a comparison with hepatitis A and B. *Scand J Infect Dis* 1979; **11**: 259–264.

94   Bartolotti F, Bertaggia A, Cadrobbi P, Realdi G. Epidemiological aspects of acute viral hepatitis in drug abusers. *Infection* 1982; **10**: 277–279.

95   Vagelli G. Non-A, non-B hepatitis in a dialysis population: spread by dental surgery? *Clin Nephrol* 1984; **22**: 268.

96   Abe K, Kurata T, Shickata T, Sugitani M, Oda T. Experimental transmission of non-A, non-B hepatitis by saliva (letter). *J Infect Dis* 1987; **155**: 1078–1079.

97   Nahmias AJ, Weiss, J, Yao X *et al.* Evidence for human infection with an HTLV-III/LAV-like virus in central Africa 1959. *Lancet* 1986; **1**: 1279–1280.

98   Garry RF, Witte MH, Gottlieb A, Elvin-Lewis M, Gottlieb MS, Witte CL, Alexander SS, Cole WR, Drake WL Jr. Documentation of an AIDS virus infection in the United States in 1968. *J Am Med Assoc* 1988; **260**: 2085–2087.

99   Centers for Disease Control. Update: Acquired immunodeficiency syndrome—United States 1981–1988. Morbidity and Mortality Weekly Report. *J Am Med Assoc* 1989; **261**: 2609–2617.

100   Cortes E, Detels R, Aboulafia D, Li XL, Mougdil T, Alam M, Bonecker C, Gonzaga A, Oyafuso L, Tondo M, Boite C, Hammershlak N, Capitani C, Slamon DJ, Ho DD. HIV-1, HIV-2 and HTLV-1 infection in high risk groups in Brazil. *New Engl J Med* 1989; **320**: 953–958.

101   Clavel F, Mansinho K, Chamaret S *et al.* Human immunodeficiency virus type 2 infection associated with AIDS in West Africa. *New Engl J Med* 1987; **316**: 1180–1185.

102   Centers for Disease Control. AIDS due to HIV-2 infection—New Jersey. *Morbid Mortal Weekly Rep* 1988; **37**: 33–35.

103   Horsburgh CR Jr, Holmberg SD. The global distribution of human immunodeficiency virus type 2 (HIV-2) infection. *Transfusion* 1988; **28**: 192–195.

104   British Medical Bulletin. HIV 1988, Volume 44.

105   Weber JN, Weiss RA. The virology of human immunodeficiency viruses. *Br Med Bull* 1988; **44**: 20–37.

106 Tedder RS, O'Connor T, Hughes A, N'je H, Corrah T, Whittle H. Envelope cross-reactivity in Western blot for HIV-1 and HIV-2 may not indicate dual infection. *Lancet* 1988; **2**: 927–930.

107 Haseltine WA. Silent HIV infections. *New Engl J Med* 1989; **320**: 1487–1488.

108 Imagawa D. HIV type 1 infection in homosexual men who remain seronegative for prolonged periods. *New Engl J Med* 1989; **320**: 1458–1462.

109 Hart C, Spira T, Moore J, Sininsky J, Schochetman G, Lifson A, Galphin J, Ou C-Y. Direct detection of HIV RNA expression in seropositive subjects. *Lancet* 1988; **2**: 596–599.

110 Ou C-Y, Kowk S, Mitchell SW *et al*. DNA amplification for direct detection of HIV-1 in DNA of peripheral blood mononuclear cells. *Science* 1988; **239**: 295–297.

111 Greenspan D, Greenspan JS, Pindborg JJ, Schiodt, M. *AIDS and the dental team*. Copenhagen: Munksgaard, 1986.

112 Scully C, Porter SR. Leading article. Orofacial manifestations of HIV infection. *Lancet* 1988; **1**: 976–977.

113 Scully C, Porter SR, Greenspan D. Secondary immunodeficiencies. *In* Jones JH, Mason DK (eds). *Oral manifestations of systemic disease*. pp 162–182. 2nd ed. London: Baillière Tindall Cox, 1990.

114 Scully C. Head and neck manifestations of HIV infection. *In*: McCarthy GM, Hamilton JT (eds). *AIDS research in dentistry*. pp 45–59. Ontario: University of Western Ontario Press, 1988.

115 Centers for Disease Control. Update: acquired immunodeficiency virus syndrome (AIDS)—worldwide. *Morbid Mortal Weekly Rep* 1988; **37**: 286–295.

116 Feachem RG, Phillips-Howard PA. Risk to UK heterosexuals of contracting AIDS abroad. *Lancet* 1988; **2**: 394–395.

117 Moss AR, Bacchetti P. Natural history of HIV infection. *AIDS* 1989; **3**: 55–61.

118 Wormser GP, Rabkin CS, Joline C. Frequency of nosocomial transmission of HIV infection among health care workers. *New Engl J Med* 1988; **319**: 307–308.

119 Lifson AR, Castro KG, McCray E *et al*. National surveillance of AIDS in health care workers. *J Am Med Assoc* 1986; **256**: 3231–3234.

120 Schupbach J. Human retrovirology facts and concepts. *Current topics in microbiology and immunology* 142. p 33–36. London: Springer-Verlag, 1989.

121 Archibald D *et al*. Antibodies to human T-lymphotropic virus type III (HTLV-III) in saliva of acquired immunodeficiency syndrome (AIDS) patients and in persons at risk for AIDS. *Blood* 1986; **67**: 831–834.

122 Groopman JE *et al*. HTLV-III in saliva of people with AIDS-related complex. *Science* 1984; **226**: 447–449.

123 Ho D *et al*. Infrequency of isolation of HTLV-III virus from saliva in AIDS. *New Engl J Med* 1986; **19**: 1606.

124 Lecatsas G *et al*. Retrovirus-like particles in salivary glands, prostate, and testes of AIDS patients. *Proc Soc Exp Biol Med* 1985; **178**: 653–655.

125 Tucker B, Schaeffer LD, Berson R, Mungo R, Miller R, Gomperts E, Warfield D. A comparison of HIV antibody and HIV viral findings in blood and saliva of HIV antibody-positive juvenile hemophiliacs. *Pediatr Dent* 1988; **10**: 283–286.

126 Levy JA, Greenspan D. HIV in saliva. *Lancet* 1988; **2**: 1248.

127 Fox PC, Baum BJ. Isolation of HTLV-III virus from saliva in AIDS. *New Engl J Med* 1986; **314**: 1387.

128 Fultz PN. Components of saliva inactivate human immunodeficiency virus. *Lancet* 1986; **2**: 1215.

129 Fox PC, Wolff A, Yeh C-K, Atkinson JC, Baum BJ. Saliva inhibits HIV-1 infectivity. *J Am Dent Assoc* 1986; **116**: 635–637.

130 Friedland GH, Klein RS. Transmission of the human immunodeficiency virus. *New Engl J Med* 1987; **317**: 1125–1135.

131 Scully C, Epstein J. Human bites (in press).

132 Klein RS, Phelan JA, Freeman K *et al.* Low occupational risk of human immunodeficiency virus infection among dental professionals. *New Engl J Med* 1988; **318**: 86–90.

133 Flynn NM, Pollet SM, Van Horne JR, Elvebakk R, Harper SD, Carlson JR. Absence of HIV antibody among dental professionals exposed to infected patients. *West J Med* 1987; **146**; 439–442.

134 Ebbesen P, Melbye M, Scheutz F, Bodner AJ, Biggar RJ. Lack of antibodies to HTLV-III/LAV in Danish dentists. *J Am Med Assoc* 1987; **256**: 2199.

135 Reichart PA, Bommerer M, Lange W, Koch MA. Absence of antibodies to HIV-1 among West-Berlin dental personnel. *AIDS-Forsch* (AIFO) 1988; **6**: 333–334.

136 Dobloug JH, Gerner NW, Hurlen B, Bruun JN, Skaug K. HIV and hepatitis B infection in an international cohort of dental hygienists. *Scand J Dent Res* 1988; **96**: 448–450.

137 Lubick HA, Schaeffer LD, Kleinman SH. Occupational risk of dental personnel survey. *J Am Dent Assoc* 1986; **113**: 10–11.

138 Centers for Disease Control. Update: human immunodeficiency virus infections in health-care workers exposed to blood of infected patients. *Morbid Mortal Weekly Rep* 1987; **36**: 285–289.

139 Michelet C, Cartier F, Ruffault A, Camus C, Genetet N, Thomas R. Needlestick HIV infection in a nurse. Presented at the Fourth International Conference on AIDS, Stockholm, June 12–16 (abstract), 1988.

140 Barnes DM. Health workers and AIDS: questions persist. *Science* 1988; **241**: 161–162.

141 Wallace MR, Harrison WO. HIV seroconversion with progressive disease in a health care worker after needlestick injury. *Lancet* 1988; **1**: 1454.

142 Anonymous. Needlestick transmission of HTLV-III from a patient infected in Africa. *Lancet* 1984; **2**: 1376–1377.

143 Oksenhendler E, Harzic M, Le Roux J-M, Rabian C, Clauvel JP. HIV infection with seroconversion after a superficial needlestick injury to the finger. *New Engl J Med* 1986; **315**: 582.

144 Neisson-Vernant C, Arfi S, Mathex D, Leibowitch J, Monplaisir N. Needlestick HIV seroconversion in a nurse. *Lancet* 1986; **2**: 814.

145 Gioannini P, Sinicco A, Carti G, Lucchini A, Paggi G, Giachino O. HIV infection acquired by a nurse. *Euro J Epidemiol* 1988; **4**: 119–120.

146 Ramsay KM, Smith EN, Reinarz JA. Prospective evaluation of 44 health care workers exposed to HIV-1 with one seroconversion. *Clin Res* 1988; **36**: 22A.

147 Weiss SH, Goedert JJ, Gartner S. Risk of human immunodeficiency virus (HIV-1) infection among laboratory workers. *Science* 1988; **239**: 681–687.

148 Centers for Disease Control. Update: acquired immunodeficiency syndrome and human immunodeficiency virus infection among health-care workers. *Morbid Mortal Weekly Rep* 1988; **37**: 229–239.

149 Marcus R. Surveillance of health care workers exposed to blood from patients infected with the human immunodeficiency virus. *New Engl J Med* 1983; **319**: 1118–1123.

150 Stricof RL, Morse DL. HTLV-III/LAV seroconversion following a deep intramuscular needlestick injury. *New Engl J Med* 1986; **314**: 1115.

151 Hamory BH. Under-reporting of needlestick injuries in a university hospital. *Am J Infect Control* 1983; **11**: 174–177.

152 Jagger J, Hunt EH, Brand-Elinaggar J, Pearson RD. Rates of needlestick injury

caused by various devices in a university hospital. *New Engl J Med* 1988; **319**: 284–288.

153   Weiss SH, Saxinger WC, Rechtman D *et al*. HTLV-III infection among health care workers: association with needle-stick injuries. *J Am Med Assoc* 1985; **254**: 2089–2093.

154   Krasinski K, LaCourture R, Holzman RS. Effect of changing needle disposal system on needle puncture injuries. *Infect Control* 1987; **8**: 59–62.

155   N'Galy B, Ryder RW, Bila K, Maundagalirwa K, Colebunders R, Francis H, Mann JM, Quinn TC. Human immunodeficiency virus infection among employees in an African hospital. *New Engl J Med* 1988; **319**: 1123–1127.

156   Moss AR. Predicting who will progress to AIDS. *Br Med J* 1988; **297**: 1067–1068.

157   Corey L, Spear PG. Infections with herpes simplex viruses. *New Engl J Med* 1986; **314**: 686–681, 749–757.

158   Scully C. Orofacial herpes simplex virus infections: Current concepts on the epidemiology, pathogenesis and treatment and disorders in which the virus may be implicated. *Oral Surg* 1989; **68**: 701–710.

159   Brooks SL *et al*. Prevalence of herpes simplex virus disease in a professional population. *J Am Dent Assoc* 1981; **102**: 31–34.

160   Spruance SL. Pathogenesis of herpes simplex labialis: excretion of virus in the oral cavity. *J Clin Microbiol* 1984; **19**: 675–679.

161   Hatherly LI, Hayes K, Jack I. Herpes virus in an obstetric hospital. Asymptomatic virus excretion in staff members. *Med J Aust* 1980; **2**: 273–275.

162   Kameyama T, Futami M, Nakayoshi N, Sujak UC, Yamamoto S. Shedding of herpes simplex virus type 1 into saliva in patients with orofacial fracture. *J Med Virol* 1989; **28**: 78–80.

163   Kameyama T, Kabashima M, Futami M, Yoshitake M, Hieda T, Sujaku C, Yamamoto S. Isolation of herpes simplex virus from saliva in patients operated. *J Jap Dermatol Soc* 1985; **34**: 397–402.

164   Rowe NH, Heine CS, Kowalski CJ. Herpetic whitlow: an occupational disease of practicing dentists. *J Am Dent Assoc* 1982; **105**: 471–473.

165   Gill MJ, Arlette J, Buchan K. Herpes simplex virus infection of the hand. *Am J Med* 1988; **84**: 89–93.

166   Manzella JP, McConville JH, Valenti W, Menegus MA, Swierkosz EM, Arens M. An outbreak of herpes simplex virus 1 gingivostomatitis in a dental hygiene practice. *J Am Med Assoc* 1984; **252**: 2019–2022.

167   Straus SE, Ostrove JM, Inchauspe G. Varicella-zoster virus infections. *Ann Intern Med* 1988; **108**: 221–237.

168   Leclair JM, Zaia JA, Levin MJ. Airborne transmission of chickenpox in a hospital. *New Engl J Med* 1980; **302**: 450–453.

169   Weller TH. The cytomegaloviruses: ubiquitous agents with protean clinical manifestations. *New Engl J Med* 1971; **285**: 203–214, 267–274.

170   Adler SP. Molecular epidemiology of cytomegalovirus: viral transmission among children attending a day care center, their parents and caretakers. *J Pediatr* 1988; **112**: 366–372.

171   Volpi A, Pica F, Cauletti M, Pana A, Rocchi G. Cytomegalovirus infection in day care centers in Rome, Italy: viral excretion in children and occupational risk among workers. *J Med Virol* 1988; **26**: 119–125.

172   Jones LA, Duke-Duncan PM, Yeager AS. Cytomegaloviral infections in infant-toddler centers: Centers for the developmentally delayed versus regular day care. *J Infect Dis* 1985; **151**: 953–955.

173   Pass RF, August AM, Dworsky M, Reynolds DW. Cytomegalovirus infection in a day care center. *New Engl J Med* 1982; **307**: 477–479.

174 Pass RF, Hutto C, Reynolds DW, Polhill RB. Increased frequency of cytomegalovirus infection in children in group day care. *Pediatrics* 1984; **74**: 121–126.

175 Stagno S, Reynolds DW, Pass RF, Alford CA. Breast milk and risk of cytomegalovirus infection. *New Engl J Med* 1980; **302**: 1073–1076.

176 Strangert K, Carlstrom G, Jeansson S, Nord CE. Infections in preschool children in group day care. *Acta Paediatr Scand* 1976; **65**: 455–463.

177 Adler SP. Cytomegalovirus and child day care. *New Engl J Med* 1989; **321**: 1290–1296.

178 Centers for Disease Control. Prevalence of cytomegalovirus excretion from children in five day care centers. *MMWR* 1985; **34**: 49–51.

179 Taber LH, Frank LA, Yow MD, Bagley A. Acquisition of cytomegaloviral infections in families with young children. A serological study. *J Infect Dis* 1985; **151**: 948–952.

180 Dworsky ME, Welch K, Cassady G *et al*. Occupational risk for primary cytomegalovirus infection among pediatric healthcare workers. *New Engl J Med* 1983; **309**: 950–953.

181 Young AB, Reid D, Grist NR. Is cytomegalovirus a serious hazard to female hospital staff? *Lancet* 1983; **1**: 975–976.

182 Committee on Infectious Diseases and Immunization. Cytomegalovirus: an occupational hazard? *Canad Med Assoc J* 1984; **131**: 730.

183 Gestal JJ. Occupational hazards in hospitals: risk of infection. *Br J Industr Med* 1987; **44**: 435–442.

184 Morgan DG, Niederman JC, Miller G, Smith MW, Dowaliby JM. Site of Epstein-Barr replication in the oropharynx. *Lancet* 1979; **2**: 1154–1157.

185 Lemon SM, Huth LM, Shaw JE. Replication of EBV in epithelial cells during infectious mononucleosis. *Nature* 1977; **268**: 268–270.

186 Niederman JC, Miller G, Pearson MA, Pagano JS, Dowaliby JM. Infectious mononucleosis: EBV shedding in saliva and the oropharynx. *New Engl J Med* 1976; **294**: 1353–1359.

187 Stranch B, Andrews LL, Siegal N. Oropharyngeal excretion of Epstein-Barr virus by renal transplant recipients and other patients treated with immunosuppressive drugs. *Lancet* 1974; **1**: 234–237.

188 Alsip GR, Ench Y, Sumaya CV, Boswell RN. Increased Epstein-Barr virus DNA in oropharyngeal secretions from patients with AIDS, AIDS-related complex, or asymptomatic human immunodeficiency virus infections. *J Infect Dis* 1988; **157**: 1072–1076.

189 Waterson AP. Virus infection (other than rubella) during pregnancy. *Br Med J* 1979; **2**: 564–566.

190 Miller G. Epstein-Barr virus. *In* Fields BN, Krupe DM *et al. Virology*. 2nd ed. 192–195. New York: Raven Press, 1990.

191 Yamanishi K, Okuno T, Shiraki K *et al*. Identification of human herpes virus-6 as a causal agent for exanthem subitum. *Lancet* 1988; **1**: 1065–1067.

192 Andre M, Matz B. Human herpes virus 6. (Letter). *Lancet* 1988; **2**: 1426.

193 Pietroboni GR, Harnett GB, Bucens MR, Honess RW. Antibody to human herpesvirus 6 in saliva. *Lancet* 1988; **1**: 1059.

194 Takahashi K, Sonoda S, Higashi K, Kondo T, Takahashi H, Takahashi M, Yamanishi K. Predominant CD4 T-lymphocyte tropism of human herpes virus 6-related virus. *J Virol* 1989; **63**: 3161–3163.

195 Couch RG, Douglas RB, Lindgren KM. Airborne transmission of respiratory infection with Coxsackie virus A type 21. *Am J Epidemiol* 1970; **91**: 78–86.

196 Gerone PJ, Couch RG, Keefer GV. Assessment of experimental and natural viral aerosols. *Bacteriol Rev* 1966; **30**: 576.

197 Southam JC. Bacterial and viral diseases and the oral mucosa. *In* Dolby AE (ed).

Oral mucosa in health and disease. pp 371–414. Oxford: Blackwell Scientific, 1975.

198 Cawson RA, McSwiggan DA. An outbreak of hand, foot and mouth disease in a dental hospital. *Oral Surg* 1969; **27**: 451.

199 Scully C, Cox M, Prime SS, Maitland NJ. Papillomaviruses: the current status in relation to oral disease. *Oral Surg* 1988; **65**: 526–532.

200 Greenspan D, de Villiers EM, Greenspan JS, DeSouza YG, zur Hausen H. Unusual HPV types in oral warts in association with HIV infection. *J Oral Pathol* 1988; **17**: 482–487.

201 Genner J, Scheutz F, Ebbesen P, Melbye M. Antibody to human papillomavirus in Danish dentists. *Scand J Dent Res* 1988; **96**: 118–120.

202 Ware R. Human parvovirus infection. *J Pediatr* 1989; **114**: 343–348.

203 Anderson LJ, Torok TJ. Human parvovirus B19. *New Engl J Med* 1989; **321**: 536–538.

204 Rosenblatt JD, Chen IS, Wachsman W. Infection with HTLV-1 and HTLV-II: evolving concepts. *Sem Hematol* 1988; **25**: 230–246.

205 Rosenblatt JD, Golde DW, Wachsman W *et al.* A second isolate of HTLV-II associated with atypical hairy-cell leukemia. *New Engl J Med* 1986; **315**: 372–377.

206 Kalyanaraman VS, Sarngadharan MG, Robert-Guroff M *et al.* A new sub-type of human T-cell leukemia virus (HTLV-II) associated with a T-cell variant of hairy cell leukemia. *Science* 1982; **218**: 571–573.

207 du Moulin GC, Stottmeier KD, Pelletier PA, Tsang AY, Hedley-Whyte J. Concentration of *Mycobacterium avium* by hospital hot water systems. *J Am Med Assoc* 1988; **260**; 1599–1601.

208 Horsburgh CR, Cohn DL, Roberts RB. *et al. Mycobacterium avium-intracellulare* isolates from patients with or without acquired immunodeficiency syndrome. *Antimicrob Agents Chemother* 1986; **30**: 955–957.

209 Zakowski P, Fligel S, Berlin OG *et al.* Disseminated *Mycobacterium avium-intracellulare* infection in homosexual men dying of acquired immunodeficiency. *J Am Med Assoc* 1982; **248**: 2980–2982.

210 Volpe F, Schwimmer A, Barr C. Oral manifestations of disseminated *Mycobacterium avium-intracellulare* in a patient with AIDS. *Oral Surg* 1985; **60**: 567–570.

211 Olsen WL, Jeffrey RB, Sooy CD, Lynch MA, Dillon WP. Lesions of the head and neck in patients with AIDS. *Am J Neuroradiol* 1988; **9**: 693–698.

212 McSwiggan DA, Collins CH. The isolation of *M. kansasii* and *M. xenopi* from water systems. *Tubercle* 1974; **55**: 291–297.

213 du Moulin GC, Stottmeier KD. Waterborne mycobacteria: an increasing threat to health. *ASM News* 1986; **52**: 525–529.

214 Stine TM, Harris AA, Levin S *et al.* A pseudoepidemic due to atypical mycobacteria in a hospital water supply. *J Am Med Assoc* 1987; **258**: 809–811.

215 Pelletier PA, du Moulin GC, Stottmeier KD. Mycobacteria in public water supplies: comparative resistance to chlorine. *Microbiol Sci* 1988; **5**: 147–148.

216 Miller RL, Micik RE. Air pollution and its control in the dental office. *Dent Clin North Am* 1978; **22**: 453.

217 Woodruff G. Tuberculosis and the dentist. *Aust Dent J* 1977; **2**: 61–66.

218 Craven RB, Wenzel RP, Atuk AO. Minimizing tuberculosis risk to hospital personnel and students exposed to unsuspected disease. *Ann Intern Med* 1975; **82**; 628–632.

219 Joint Tuberculosis Committee of the British Thoracic Society. Control and prevention of tuberculosis. *Br Med J* 1983; **2**: 1118–1121.

220 Smith WHR. Intra-oral and pulmonary tuberculosis following dental treatment. *Lancet* 1982; **1**: 842–844.

221 Manton SL, Egglestone SI, Alexander I, Scully C. Oral presentation of secondary syphilis. *Br Dent J* 1986; **160**: 237–238.

222   Chue PWY. Gonorrhoea: its natural history, oral manifestations, diagnosis, treatment and prevention. *J Am Dent Assoc* 1975; **91**: 829–835.

223   Guinta JL, Finmara NJ. Facts about gonorrhoea and dentistry. *Oral Surg* 1986; **62**: 529.

224   Reingold AL, Thomason BM, Brake BJ, Thacker L, Wilkinson HW, Kuritsky JN. *Legionella pneumonia* in the United States: the distribution of serogroups and species causing human illness. *J Infect Dis* 1984; **149**: 819.

225   Parry MF, Stampleman L, Hutchinson JH, Folta D, Steinberg MG, Krasnogor LJ. Waterborne *Legionella bozemanii* and nosocomial pneumonia in immunosuppressed patients. *Ann Intern Med* 1985; **103**: 205–210.

226   Edelstein PH. Control of Legionella in hospitals. *J Hosp Infect* 1986; **8**: 109–115.

227   Herwaldt LA, Gorman GW, McGrath T *et al.* A new Legionella species, *Legionella feeleii* species nova, causes pontiac fever in an automobile plant. *Ann Intern Med* 1984; **100**: 333–338.

228   Glick TH, Gregg MB, Berman B *et al.* Pontiac fever: an epidemic of unknown aetiology in a health department I. Clinical and epidemiologic aspects. *Am J Epidemiol* 1978; **107**: 149–160.

229   Wilkinson HW, Reingold AL, Brake BJ, McGiboney DL, Gorman GW, Broome CV. Reactivity of serum from patients with suspected legionellosis against 29 antigens of legionellaceae and *Legionella*-like organisms by indirect immunofluorescence assay. *J Infect Dis* 1983; **147**: 23–31.

230   Boldour I, Ergaz M. A prevalence study of *Legionella* species in geriatric institutions. *J Hyg Camb* 1984; **92**: 37–43.

231   Stout J, Yu LV, Vickers RM, Zuravleff JJ, Best M, Brown A, Yee RB, Wadowsky R. Ubiquitousness of *Legionella pneumophila* in the water supply of a hospital with endemic Legionnaires' disease. *New Engl J Med* 1982; **306**: 466–468.

232   Kirby BD, Snyder KM, Meyer RD, Finegold SM. Legionnaires' disease: report of sixty five nosocomially acquired cases and review of the literature. *Medicine* 1980; **59**: 188–205.

233   Arnow PM, Chou T, Weil D, Shapiro EN, Kretzchmar C. Nosocomial legionnaires' disease caused by aerosolized tap water from respiratory devices. *J Infect Dis* 1982; **146**: 460–467.

234   Meenhorst PL, Groothuis DG, Wilkinson HW, Feeley JC, van Furth R. Water-related nosocomial pneumonia caused by *Legionella pneumophila* serogroups 1 and 10. *J Infect Dis* 1985; **152**: 356–363.

235   Shands KN, Ho JL, Meyer RD *et al.* Potable water as a source of Legionnaires' disease. *J Am Med Assoc* 1985; **253**: 1412–1416.

236   Helms C, Massanari R, Zeitler R *et al.* Nosocomial Legionnaires' disease at University of Iowa hospital. *Clin Res* 1982; **30**: 777A.

237   Fischer-Hoch SP, Tobin JO'H, Nelson AM *et al.* Investigation and control of an outbreak of Legionnaires disease in district general hospital. *Lancet* 1981; **1**: 932–936.

238   Helms CM, Massanari RW, Wenzel RP, Pfaller MA, Moyer NP, Hall N. Legionella Monitoring Committee. Legionnaires' disease associated with hospital water system: 5 year progress report on continuous hyperchlorination. *J Am Med Assoc* 1988; **259**: 2423–2428.

239   Myerowitz RL, Pasculle AW, Dowling JN *et al.* Opportunistic lung infection due to 'Pittsburgh pneumonia agent'. *New Engl J Med* 1979; **301**: 953–958.

240   Rogers BH, Donowitz GR, Walker GK, Harding SA, Sande MA. Opportunistic pneumonia: a clinicopathological study of five cases by an unidentified acid-fast bacterium. *New Engl J Med* 1979; **301**: 959–961.

241   Farr BM, Tartaglino JC, Gratz, JC, Getchell-White SI, Groschell DHM.

Evaluation of ultraviolet light for disinfection of hospital water contaminated with legionella. *Lancet* 1988; **2**: 669–672.

242   Haley CE, Cohen ML, Halter J, Meyer RD. Nosocomial legionnaires disease: a continuing common source epidemic at Wadsworth Medical Centre. *Ann Intern Med* 1979; **90**: 583–586.

243   Fraser DW, Tsai TR, Orenstein W *et al*. Legionnaires disease, description of an epidemic of pneumonia. *New Engl J Med* 1977; **297**: 1189–1197.

244   Gestal JJ. Enfermedad de los legionarios, epidemiologia y profilaxis. I. *Med Galaica* 1981; **14**: 23–26.

245   Gestal JJ. Enfermedad de los legionarios, epidemiologia y profilaxis. II. *Med Galacia* 1981; **15**: 6–18.

246   Reinthaler F, Mascher F. Nachweis von *L. pneumophilia* in Dentaleinheiten. *ZBL Bakt Hyg I Abt Orig* B 1986; **183**: 86–88.

247   Scully C. The control of cross-infection in dentistry. *Br Dent J* 1989; **166**: 198–199.

248   Fotos PG, Westfall HN, Snyder IS, Miller RW, Mutchler BM. Prevalence of Legionella-specific IgG and IgM antibody in a dental clinic population. *J Dent Res* 1985; **64**: 1382–1385.

249   Reinthaler F, Mascher F, Stunzner D. *Legionella pneumophila*: seroepidemiologische Untersuchungen bei Zahnarzten und zahnarztlichen Personal in Osterreich. *ZBI Bakt Hyg II Abt Orig* B 1987; **1985**: 164–170.

250   Reinthaler FF, Mascher F, Stunzner D. Serological examinations for antibodies against Legionella species in dental personnel. *J Dent Res* 1988; **67**: 942–943.

251   Saravolatz L, Arking L, Wentworth B, Quinn E. Prevalence of antibody to the legionnaires' disease bacterium in hospital employees. *Ann Intern Med* 1979; **90**: 601–603.

252   Josephson A. Legionella pneumophila antibody in hospital employees. *Ann Intern Med* 1979; **91**: 653–654.

253   Koppel AC, Hackleman GL. Acute tenosynovitis after puncture wound of a finger by a dental bur. *J Am Dent Assoc* 1968; **76**: 828.

254   Van den Broek PJ, Lampe AS, Berbee GAM, Thompson J, Mouton RP. Epidemic of prosthetic valve endocarditis caused by *Staphylococcus epidermidis*. *Br Med J* 1985; **291**: 949–950.

255   Bleicher JN, Blinn DL, Massop D. Hand infections in dental personnel. *Plast Reconstr Surg* 1987; **80**: 420–422.

256   St Geme JW. Jr. Susceptibility of medical students to mumps: dubious value of currently available skin test antigens. *Pediatrics* 1972; **49**: 314–315.

257   Cembrero GC, Sanchez MR, Jimenex MT, Dominguez CM. Estudio del nivel inmunitario frente a la rubeola del personal femenino en un hospital. *Rev Med Univ Navarra* 1976; **1**: 99–106.

258   Hall CB, Geiman JM, Douglas RG, Meagher MP. Control of nosocomial respiratory syncytial viral infections. *Pediatrics* 1978; **62**: 728–732.

259   Sims DG, Downham APS, Webb JKG, Gardner PS, Weightman D. Hospital cross-infection on children's wards with respiratory syncytial virus and the role of adult carriage. *Acta Paediatr Scand* 1975; **64**: 5114–5144.

260   Hall CB, Douglas RG, Geiman JM, Messner MK. Nosocomial respiratory syncytial virus infections. *New Engl J Med* 1975; **293**: 1343–1346.

261   Ditchburn RK, McQuillin J, Garder PS, Courts BM. Respiratory syncytial virus in hospital cross-infection. *Br Med J* 1971; **2**: 671–673.

262   Faden H, Gallagher M, Ogra, P, McLoughlin S. Nosocomial outbreak of pharyngoconjunctival fever due to adenovirus type 4. *Ann Intern Med* 1974; **81**: 274.

263   Levandowsky RA, Rubenis M. Nosocomial conjunctivitis caused by adenovirus type 4. *J Infect Dis* 1981; **143**: 28–31.

264   Laibson PR, Ortolan G, Dupre-Strachan S. Community and hospital outbreak of epidemic keratoconjunctivitis. *Arch Ophthalmol* 1968; **80**: 467–473.

265   Dawson C, Darrell R. Infections due to adenovirus 8 in the United States. *New Engl J Med* 1963; **268**: 1031–1034.

266   Midulla M, Sollecito D, Feleppa F, Assensio AM, Ilari S. Infection by airborne *Chlamydia trachomatis* in a dentist cured with rifampicin after failures with tetracycline and doxycycline. *Br Med J* 1987; **294**: 742.

267   Sande MA, Gadot F, Wenzel RP. Point source epidemic of *Mycoplasma pneumoniae* infection in a prosthodontics laboratory. *Am Rev Resp Dis* 1975; **112**: 213–217.

268   Anonymous. Patient source of scabies among hospital personnel. *J Am Med Assoc* 1983; **250**: 1817–1818.

269   Centers for Disease Control. Rubella in hospitals. *Morbid Mortal Weekly Rep* 1983; **32**: 37–39.

270   Shreve WB, Tow HD. Bacteriological and serological surveillance of dentists exposed to dental aerosols. *Bull Tokyo Dent Coll* 1981; **22**: 151–157.

271   British Dental Association. The control of cross-infection in dentistry. *Br Dent J* 1988; **165**: 353–354.

272   Recommended infection-control practices for dentistry. Centers for Disease Control 1986; **35**: 237–246.

273   Department of Health and Social Security. Acquired immune deficiency syndrome (AIDS) Booklet 3: guidance for surgeons, anaesthetists, dentists and their teams in dealing with patients infected with HTLV III. Heywood (Lancashire), 1986.

274   Council on Dental Materials, Instruments and Equipment: Council on Dental Practice, Council on Dental Therapeutics. Infection control recommendations for the dental office and the dental laboratory. *J Am Dent Assoc* 1988; **116**: 241–249.

275   Advisory Committee on Dangerous Pathogens. HIV—the causative agent of AIDS and related conditions. 2nd revision. Department of Health and Health and Safety Commission. London, 1990.

277   Jacobsen IM, Dienstag L. Viral hepatitis vaccines. *Ann Rev Med* 1985; **37**: 241–261.

278   Scully C. Hepatitis B immunisation of dental students in 14 UK dental schools. *Br Dent J* 1989; **167**: 94.

279   Schneider WJ, Dykan M. The preplacement medical evaluation of hospital personnel. *J Occup Med* 1978; **20**: 741–744.

280   DiAngelis AJ, Little JW, Martens LV, Hastreiter RJ. Infection control in Minnesota dental practices. *Northwest Dent* 1987; **66**: 36–37.

281   Mitchell R, Cumming CG, MacLennan WD, Ross PW, Peutherer, JF, Baxter PMF. The use of operating gloves in dental practice. *Br Dent J* 1983; **154**: 372–374.

282   Yablon P, Spiegel RS, Wolf MW *et al.* Dentists' attitudes concerning infection control and occupational hazards. *J Am Coll Dent* 1988; **55**: 35–40.

283   Scully C. Hepatitis B immunisation of dental students in the 14 UK dental schools. *Br Dent J* 1989; **166**: 360.

284   Matthews RW, Scully C, Dowell TB. Acceptance of hepatitis B vaccine by general dental practitioners in the United Kingdom. *Br Dent J* 1986; **161**: 371–373.

285   Samaranayake LP, Scully C, Dowell TB, Lamey PJ, MacFarlane TW, Mat-

thews RW, MacDonald KC. New data on the acceptance of the hepatitis B vaccine by dental personnel in the United Kingdom. *Br Dent J* 1988; **164**: 74–77.

286   Matthews RW, Scully C, Dowell TB. Acceptance of hepatitis B vaccination by auxillary dental personnel in the United Kingdom. *Health Trends* 1987; **19**: 25–27.

287   Scully C, Pantlin L, Samaranayake LP, Dowell TB. Increasing acceptance of hepatitis B vaccine by dental personnel but reluctance to accept hepatitis B carrier patients. *Oral Surg* (in press).

288   Gerbert B. AIDS and infection control in dental practice: dentists' attitudes, knowledge and behavior. *J Am Dent Assoc* 1987; **114**: 311–314.

289   Mitchell R, Russell J. The elimination of cross-infection in dental practice—a 5-year follow-up. *Br Dent J* 1989; **166**: 209.

290   Matthews RW, Scully C, Dowell TB. Use of rubber gloves. *Br Dent J* 1987; **163**: 6.

291   Pitts NB, Nuttall NM. Blood borne viruses: precautions against cross-infection in routine dental practice in Scotland. *Br Dent J* 1988; **165**: 183–187.

292   Howard C. A survey of cross-infection control in general dental practice in England. *Health Trends* 1989; **21**: 9–10.

293   Matthews RW, Scully C, Dowell TB. Attitudes and practices regarding control of cross-infection in general dental practice. *Health Trends* 1989; **21**: 10–12.

294   Glenwright HD, Shovelton DS. The prevention of cross-infection. Progress in the West Midlands. *Br Dent J* 1989; **166**: 125–127.

295   Dowell TB, Matthews RW, Scully C. Attitudes and practices regarding control of cross-infection. *Br Dent J* 1988; **164**: 237.

296   Yablon P, Spiegel RS, Wolf MC. Changes in dentists' attitudes and behavior concerning infection control practices. *Quint Int* 1989; **20** 279–284.

297   Verrusio AC, Neidle EA, Nash KD, Silverman S Jr, Horowitz AM, Wagner KS. The dentist and infectious diseases: a national survey of attitudes and behavior. *J Am Dent Assoc* 1989; **118**: 553–562.

298   Yoder KS. Patient attitudes toward the routine use of surgical gloves in a dental office. *J Indiana Dent Assoc* 1985; **64**: 24–28.

299   Rothwell PS, Dinsdale RW, Brook IM, Rustage K, Clark A. Infection control in general dental practice. *Br Dent J* 1987; **162**: 134.

300   Girdler NM, Matthews RW, Scully C. Use and acceptability of rubber gloves for outpatient dental treatment. *J Dent* 1987; **15**: 209–212.

301   Bowden JR, Scully C, Bell CJ, Levers H. Cross-infection control: attitudes of patients toward the wearing of gloves and masks by dentists in the United Kingdom in 1987. *Oral Surg* 1989; **67**: 45–48.

302   Worthington LS, Rothwell PS, Banks N. Cross-infection control in dental practice. (2) A dental surgery planned with cross-infection control as the design priority. *Br Dent J* 1988; **165**: 226–228.

303   Allen AL, Organ RJ. Occult blood accumulation under fingernails: a mechanism for the spread of blood borne infections. *J Am Dent Assoc* 1982; **105**: 455–459.

304   Piazza M, Guadaynino V, Picciotto L. Contamination by hepatitis B surface antigen in dental surgeries. *Br Med J* 1987; **295**: 473–474.

305   Favero MS. Hepatitis B antigen on environmental surfaces. *Lancet* 1973; **2** 1455.

306   Nerurkas LS. Survival of herpes simplex virus in water specimens collected from hot tubs in spa facilities and on plastic surfaces. *J Am Med Assoc* 1983; **250**: 3081–3083.

307   Thomas LE, Sydiskis RJ, De Vore DT, Krywolap GN. Survival of herpes simplex virus and other selected microorganisms on patients charts. *J Am Dent Assoc* 1985; **111**: 461–464.

308   Resnick L, Veren K, Salahuddin SZ, Trondreau S, Markham PD. Stability and

inactivation of HTLV III/LAV under clinical and laboratory environments. *J Am Med Assoc* 1986; **255**: 1887–1891.

309 Bond WW, Favero MS, Petersen NJ, Gravelle CR, Ebert JW, Maynard JE. Survival of hepatitis B virus after drying and storage for one week (letter). *Lancet* 1981; **1**: 550–551.

310 Piszkiewicz D, Kingdom H, Apfelzweig R. Inactivation of HTLV-III/LAV during plasma fractionation. *Lancet* 1985; **2**: 1188–1189.

311 Centers for Disease Control. Recommendations for preventing transmission of infection with human T lymphotrophic virus type III/lymphadenopathy associated virus in the workplace. *Morbid Mortal Weekly Rep* 1985; **34**: 682–686.

312 McDougal JS, Martin LS, Cort SP, Mozen, Heldebrant CM, Evatt BL. Thermal inactivation of the acquired immunodeficiency syndrome virus, human T lymphotrophic virus-III/lymphadenopathy-associated virus, with special reference to antihemophilic factors. *J Clin Invest* 1985; **76**: 875–877.

313 Martin MV, Bartzokas CA. The boiling of instruments in general dental practice: a misnomer for sterilisation. *Br Dent J* 1985; **159**: 18–20.

314 Wood PR, Martin MV. A study of the use of autoclave bags in non-vacuum autoclaves. *J Dent* 1989; **17**: 148–149.

315 Field EA, Field JK, Martin MV. Time, steam, temperature (TST) control indicators to measure essential sterilisation criteria for autoclaves in general dental practice and the community service. *Br Dent J* 1988; **164**: 183–186.

316 Walmsley AD, Walsh TF, Laird WRE. Ultrasonic instruments in dentistry. (1) The ultrasonic scaler. *Dent Update* 1988; **15**: 321–326.

317 Forrester N, Douglas CWI. Use of the 'Safe air' dental heater for sterilising endodontic reamers. *Br Dent J* 1988; **165**: 290.

318 ADA Council on Dental Therapeutics. Quarternary ammonium compounds not acceptable for disinfection of instruments and environmental surfaces. *J Am Dent Assoc* 1978; **97**: 855.

319 Kobayashi H *et al*. Susceptibility of hepatitis B virus to disinfectants or heat. *J Clin Microbiol* 1984; **20**: 214–216.

320 Spire B, Barre-Sinoussi F, Montagnier L, Chermann JC. Inactivation of lymphadenopathy associated virus by chemical disinfectants. *Lancet* 1984; **2**: 899–901.

321 Hopkins R. Evaluation of a new disinfectant and the antigenicity and morphology of hepatitis B surface antigen. *Med Lab Sci* 1981; **38**: 419–420.

322 Molinari JA, Gleason MJ, Cottone JA, Barrett ED. Cleaning and disinfectant properties of dental surface disinfectants. *J Am Dent Assoc* 1988; **117**: 179–181.

323 Martin LS, McDougal JS, Loskoski SL. Disinfection and inactivation of the human T lymphotrophic virus type III/LAV. *J Infect Dis* 1985; **152**: 400–403.

324 Croughan WS, Behbehani AM. Comparative study of inactivation of herpes simplex virus types 1 and 2 by commonly used antiseptic agents. *J Clin Microbiol* 1988; **26**: 213–215.

325 Kurth R, Werner A, Barrett N, Dorner F. Stability and inactivation of the human immunodeficiency virus (HIV): a review. *AIDS-Forsch* 1986; **11**: 601–608.

326 Hanson PJV, Gor D, Jeffries DJ, Collins JV. Chemical inactivation of HIV on surfaces. *Br Med J* 1989; **298**: 862–864.

327 Thomasz FGV, Chong MP, Tyas MJ. Virucidal chemical glutaraldehyde on alginate impression materials. *Aust Dent J* 1986; **31**: 295.

328 Runnells RR. Infection control in the wet finger environment. Salt Lake City: Publishers Press, 1984.

329 Runnells RR. Heat and heat/pressure sterilisation. *Canad Dent Assoc* 1985; **13**: 46–49.

330   Mitchell EW. Chemical disinfecting/sterilizing agents. *Canad Dent Assoc* 1985; **13**: 64–67.

331   Cottone JA, Molinari JA. Selection for dental practice of chemical disinfectants and sterilants for hepatitis and AIDS. *Aust Dent J* 1987; **32**: 368–374.

332   Kaplan JC, Crawford DC, Durno AG, Schooley RT. Inactivation of human immunodeficiency virus by Betadine. *Infect Control* 1987; **8**: 412–414.

333   Asanaka M, Kurimura T. Inactivation of human immunodeficiency virus (HIV) by povidone–iodine. *Yonago Acta Med* 1987; **30**: 89–92.

334   Harbison MA, Hammer SM. Inactivation of human immunodeficiency virus by Betadine products and chlorhexidine. *J Acquired Immune Def Synd* 1989; **2**: 16–20.

335   Joseph JM. Disease transmission by ineffectively sanitized anesthetizing apparatus. *J Am Med Assoc* 1952; **149**: 1196–1198.

336   Tinne JE, Gordon AM, Bain WH, Mackey WA. Cross-infection by *Pseudomonas aeruginosa* as a hazard of intensive surgery. *Br Med J* 1967; **4**: 313–315.

337   Olds JW, Kisch AL, Eberle BJ, Wilson JN. *Pseudomonas aeruginosa* respiratory tract infection acquired from a contaminated anesthesia machine. *Am Rev Resp Dis* 1972; **105**: 628–632.

338   Jenkins JRE, Edgar WM. Sterilisation of anaesthetic equipment. *Anaesthesia* 1964; **19**: 177–190.

339   Hunt LM, Yagiela JA. Bacterial contamination and transmission by nitrous oxide sedation apparatus. *Oral Surg* 1977; **44**: 367–373.

340   Russell EA Jr, Gross A. Extent of bacterial contamination in a nonrebreathing inhalation sedation machine. *Oral Surg* 1979; **48**: 211–213.

341   Walter CW. Cross-infection and the anesthesiologist. *Anesth Analg* 1974; **53**: 631–644.

342   Yagiela JA, Hunt LM, Hunt DE. Disinfection of nitrous oxide inhalation equipment. *J Am Dent Assoc* 1979; **98**: 191–195.

343   Young SK, Graves DC, Rohrer MD, Bulard RA. Microwave sterilization of nitrous oxide nasal hoods contaminated with virus. *Oral Surg* 1985; **60**: 581–585.

344   FDI Recommendations for hygiene in dental practice, including treatment for the infectious patient. Technical Report No 10. *Int Dent J* **37**: 142–145.

345   Johnson GH, Drennan DG, Lynn Powell G. Accuracy of elastomeric impressions disinfected by immersion. *J Am Dent Assoc* 1988; **116**: 525–530.

346   Herrera SP, Merchant VA. Dimensional stability of dental impressions after immersion disinfection. *J Am Dent Assoc* 1986; **113**; 419–422.

347   Minagi S, Fukushima K, Maeda N, Satomi K, Ohkawa S, Akagawa Y, Miyake Y, Suginaka H, Tsuru H. Disinfection method for impression materials: freedom from fear of hepatitis B and acquired immunodeficiency syndrome. *J Prosthet Dent* 1986; **56**: 451–454.

348   Minagi S, Yano N, Yoshida K, Tsuru H. Prevention of acquired immunodeficiency syndrome and hepatitis B. II. Disinfection method for hydrophilic impression materials. *J Prosthet Dent* 1987; **58**: 462–465.

349   Kwok WM, Ralph WJ. The use of chemical disinfectants in dental prosthetics. *Aust Dent J* 1984; **29**: 180–183.

350   Merchant VA, Herrera SP, Dwan JJ. Marginal fit of cast gold MO inlays from disinfected elastomeric impressions. *J Prosthet Dent* 1987; **58**: 276–280.

351   Merchant VA, McNeight MK, Ciborowski CJ, Molinari JA. Preliminary investigation of a method for disinfection of dental impressions. *J Prosthet Dent* 1984; **52**: 877–879.

352   Storer R, McCabe JF. An investigation of methods available for sterilising impressions. *Br Dent J* 1981; **151**: 217–219.

353   Johansen RE, Stackhouse JA. Dimensional changes of elastomers during cold sterilisation. *J Prosthet Dent* 1987; **57**: 233–234.
354   Durr DP, Novak EV. Dimensional stability of alginate impressions immersed in disinfecting solutions. *ASDC J Dent Child* 1987; **54**: 45–48.
355   Bergman B, Bergman M, Olsson S. Alginate impression materials, dimensional stability and surface detail sharpness following treatment with disinfectant solutions. *Swed Dent J* 1985; **9**: 255–262.
356   Bergman M, Olsson S, Bergman B. Elastomeric impression materials. Dimensional stability and surface detail sharpness following treatment with disinfectant solutions. *Swed Dent J* 1980; **4**: 161–167.
357   Jones ML, Newcombe RG, Barry G, Bellis H, Bottomley J. A reflex plotter investigation into the dimensional stability of alginate impressions following disinfection by varying regimens employing 2·2 per cent glutaraldehyde. *Br J Orthod* 1988; **15**: 185–192.
358   Bond WW, Favero MS, Peterson NJ, Ebert JW. Inactivation of hepatitis B virus by intermediate to high level disinfectant chemicals. *J Clin Microbiol* 1983; **18**: 535–538.
359   Centers for Disease Control. Hepatitis surveillance. Report 41, 1977.
360   Centers for Disease Control. Recommendations for prevention of HIV transmission in health care settings. *Morbid Mortal Weekly Rep* 1987; **36**: Suppl 25, 15–18s.
361   Holderman RD, Parlette HL, Terezhalmy GT, Pelleu GB, Taybos GM. An evaluation of the efficacy and irritability of Sporicidin as a hand dip. *Oral Surg* 1986; **62**: 142–144.
362   Gobetti JP, Cerminaro M, Shipman C Jr. Hand asepsis: the efficacy of different soaps in the removal of bacteria from sterile, gloved hands. *J Am Dent J* 1986; **113**: 291–292.
363   Field EA, Martin MV. Disinfection of dental surgeons' hands with detergent preparations of triclosan and chlorhexidine. *J Dent* 1986; **14**: 7–10.
364   Eggers HJ. Handwashing and horizontal spread of viruses. *Lancet* 1989; **1**: 1452.
365   Leclair JM, Freeman J, Sullivan BF, Crowley CM, Goldmann DA. Prevention of nosocomial respiratory syncytial virus infections through compliance with glove and gown isolation precautions. *New Engl J Med* 1987; **317**: 329–334.
366   Zbitnew A, Greer K, Heise-Qualtiere J, Conly J. Vinyl versus latex gloves as barriers to transmission of viruses in the health care setting. *J Acquired Immune Def Synd* 1989; **2**: 201–204.
367   Nakazawa M, Sato MA, Mizuno K. Incidence of perforations in rubber gloves during ophthalmic surgery. *Ophthal Surg* 1984; **15**: 236–240.
368   Skaug N. Micropunctures of rubber gloves used in oral surgery. *Int J Oral Surg* 1976; **5**: 220–225.
369   Russell TR, Roque FE, Miller FA. A new method for detection of the leaky glove. *Arch Surg* 1966; **93**: 245–249.
370   Ritter M, French M, Eitzen H. Evaluation of microbial contamination of surgical gloves during actual use. *Clin Orthod Res* 1976; **117**: 303–306.
371   McCue SF, Berg EW, Saunders EA. Efficacy of double-gloving as a barrier to microbial contamination during total joint arthroplasty. *J Bone Joint Surg* 1981; **63**: 811–813.
372   Otis LL, Cottone JA. Prevalence of perforations in disposable latex gloves during routine dental treatment. *J Am Dent Assoc* 1989; **118**: 321–324.
373   Morgan DJ. Permeability studies on protective gloves used in dental practice. *Br Dent J* 1989; **166**: 11–13.
374   Penikett EJK, Gorrill RH. The integrity of surgical gloves tested during use. *Lancet* 1958; **2**: 1042–1043.

375 Furuhashi M, Miyamae T. Effect of preoperative hand scrubbing and influence of pinholes appearing in surgical rubber gloves during operation. *Bull Tokyo Med Dent Univ* 1979; **26**: 73–80.

376 Reingold AL, Kane MA, Hightower AW. Failure of gloves and other protective devices to prevent transmission of hepatitis B virus to oral surgeons. *J Am Med Assoc* 1988; **259**: 2558–2560.

377 Gonzalez E, Naleway C. Assessment of the effectiveness of glove use as a barrier technique in the dental operatory. *J Am Dent Assoc* 1988; **117**: 467–469.

378 Brantley CF, Heymann HO, Shugars DA, Vann WF. The effect of gloves on psychomotor skills acquisition among dental students. *J Dent Educ* 1986; **50**: 611–613.

379 Uldricks JM, Caccamo P, Beck FM, Schmakel D. Effect of surgical gloves on preclinical scaling skills. *J Dent Educ* 1985; **49**: 316–317.

380 Burke FJT, Watts DC, Wilson NHF. Some physical factors influencing tactile perception with disposable non-sterile gloves. *J Dent* 1989; **17**: 72–76.

381 Turjanmaa K, Laurila K, Makinen-Kiljunen S, Renunala T. Rubber contact urticaria: allergenic properties of 19 brands of latex gloves. *Contact Derm* 1988; **19**: 362–367.

382 Turjanmaa K, Reunala T. Contact urticaria from rubber gloves. *Dermatol Clin* 1988; **6**: 47–51.

383 March PJ. An allergic reaction to latex rubber gloves. *J Am Dent Assoc* 1988; **117**: 590–591.

384 Meding B, Fregert S. Contact urticaria from natural latex gloves. *Contact Derm* 1984; **10**: 52–53.

385 Neissen LC, Strassler H, Levinson PD, Ward G, Greenbaum J. Effect of latex gloves on setting time of polyvinylsiloxane putty impression material. *J Prosthet Dent* 1986; **55**: 128–129.

386 Welfare RD. Problems with addition-cured silicone putty. *Br Dent J* 1986; **160**: 268–269.

387 Rosen M, Touyz LZG, Becker PJ. The effect of latex gloves on setting time of vinyl polysiloxane putty impression material. *Br Dent J* 1989; **166**: 374–375.

388 Petersen NJ, Bond WW, Favero MS. Air sampling for hepatitis B surface antigen in a dental operatory. *J Am Dent Assoc* 1979; **99**: 465–467.

389 Belting CM, Haberfield GC, Juhl LK. Spread of organisms from dental air rotor. *J Am Dent Assoc* 1964; **68**: 34–47.

390 Bond WW, Petersen NJ, Favero MS, Ebert JW, Maynard JE. Transmission of type B viral hepatitis B via eye inoculation of a chimpanzee. *J Clin Microbiol* 1982; **15**: 533–434.

391 Orr NWM. Is a mask necessary in the operating theatre? *Ann Royal Coll Surg Engl* 1981; **63**: 390–391.

392 Micik RE, Miller RL, Leong AC. Studies on dental aerobiology. III. Efficacy of surgical masks in protecting dental personnel from airborne bacterial particles. *J Dent Res* 1971; **50**: 626–630.

393 Craig DC, Quayle AA. The efficacy of face-masks. *Br Dent J* 1985; **158**: 87–90.

394 Greene VW, Vesley D. Method for evaluating effectiveness of surgical masks. *J Bacteriol* 1962; **83**: 663–667.

395 Nicholes PS. Comparative evaluation of a new surgical mask medium. *Surg Gynaecol Obstet* 1964; **118**: 579–583.

396 Thomas CGA. Efficiency of surgical masks in use in hospital wards. *Guy's Hosp Rep* 1961; **110**: 157–167.

397 Guyton HG, Buchanan LM, Lense FT. Evaluation of respiratory protection of contagion masks. *Appl Microbiol* 1956; **4**: 141–143.

398 Freake R, Abbott L. Method for testing bacteriological efficiency of surgical masks in the operating theatre. *Lancet* 1966; **1**: 78–79.

399 Ford CR, Peterson DE. The efficiency of surgical face masks. *Am J Surg* 1963; **106**: 954–957.

400 Bailey R, Giglio P, Blechman H, Nunez C. Effectiveness of disposable face masks in preventing cross contamination during dental procedures. *J Dent Res* 1968; **47**: 1062–1065.

401 Ray KC, Fuller ML. Isolation of mycobacterium from dental impression material. *J Prosthet Dent* 1963; **13**: 93–94.

402 Posti JJ. Contamination between the dental surgery and dental laboratory. *Suom Hammaslaak Toim* 1970; **66**: 49–55.

403 Posti JJ. Bacterial contamination between the dental surgery and the dental laboratory. *Zahntechnik* 1970; **28**: 358–359.

404 Rowe AHR, Forrest JO. Dental impressions: the probability of contamination and a method of disinfection. *Br Dent J* 1978; **145**: 184–186.

405 Miller RL, Burton WE, Spore RW. Aerosols produced by dental instrumentation. Proceedings of the First International Symposium on Aerobiology. Berkeley, 1963.

406 Larato DC. Disinfection of pumice. *J Prosthet Dent* 1967; **18**: 534-535.

407 Katberg JW Jr. Cross-contamination via the prosthodontic laboratory. *J Prosthet Dent* 1974; **32**: 412–419.

408 Williams HN, Falker WA, Hasler JF, Libonati JP. The recovery and significance of nonoral opportunistic pathogenic bacteria in dental laboratory pumice. *J Prosthet Dent* 1985; **54**: 725–730.

409 Clark FP, Micik RE, Thomas RL. Environmental study of dental laboratories. Department of Health, Education and Welfare, 1970.

410 Williams HN, Falkler WA, Hasler JF. Acinetobacter contamination of dental laboratory pumice. *J Dent Res* 1983; **62**: 1073.

411 Clark JP, Micik RE, Thomas RL. Environmental study of dental laboratories. *J Calif Dent Assoc* 1971; **47**: 1.

412 Henderson CW *et al.* Evaluation of the barrier system, an infectious control system for the dental laboratory. *J Prosthet Dent* 1987; **58**: 517–521.

413 Ragniamo RP *et al.* Airborne microorganisms collected in preclinical dental laboratory. *J Dent Educ* 1985; **49**: 653–655.

414 Wakefield CW. Laboratory contamination of dental prosthesis. *J Prosthet Dent* 1980; **44**: 143.

415 Kahn RC, Lancaster MV, Kate W. The microbiologic cross-contamination of dental prosthesis. *J Prosthet Dent* 1982; **47**: 556.

416 Green GS, Johnson RH, Shively JA. Mimea opportunistic pathogens. *J Am Mental Assoc* 1965; **194**: 163–166.

417 O'Connell CJ, Hamilton R. Gram negative rod infections II. *Acinetobacter* infections in general hospital. *NY State J Med* 1981; **81**: 750–753.

418 Iwarson S. Post-exposure prophylaxis for hepatitis B: active or passive? *Lancet* 1989; **2**: 146–147.

419 Baker JL. What is the occupational risk to emergency care providers from the human immunodeficiency virus? *Ann Emerg Med* 1988; **17**: 700–703.

420 Kuhls TL, Cherry JD. The management of health care workers' accidental parenteral exposures to biological specimens of HIV seropositive individuals. *Infect Control* 1987; **8**: 211–213.

Appendix

Scrub liquids and creams

pH—iso-med: 3% w/w hexachlorophane. Sterling, Winthrop House, Surbiton on Thames, Surrey KT6 4PH.
Hibiscrub: 20% v/v chlorhexidine digluconate solution BP. ICI Ltd, Alderley, Macclesfield, Cheshire.
Videne: 7·5% w/v povidone-iodine. Beta Medical Products Ltd, 9 Arkwright Road, Astmoor Industrial Estate, Runcorn, Cheshire.
Betadine: 7·5% w/v povidone–iodine. Napp Laboratories Ltd, Hill Farm Avenue, Watford WD2 7RA.
Zalclense: 23% potassium fatty acid soap with 2% Irgasan DP300 (Registered trademark of Ciba–Geigy AG (contains 0·75% chlorinated phenol)). Sterling Industrial, Chapeltown, Sheffield S30 4YP.
Hibisol: 0·5% chlorhexidine digluconate in 70% isopropyl alcohol. (ICI)
Invisible skin+ : Akhab Europe, Groenmarkt 26T, 2413 AL, The Hague, Netherlands.
Skin Friend cream: CEM BVBA, Eedenstaat. 1/1, B2340, Beerse, Belgium.

Disinfectants

Glutaraldehyde preparations
Asep: Galen Ltd, Craigavon, Co. Armagh, Northern Ireland.
Asep Extra Life: Galen Ltd, Craigavon, Co. Armagh, Northern Ireland.
Cidex: Johnson and Johnson Ltd, Dental Products Division, 260 Bath Road, Slough, Bucks SL1 4EA.
Cidex Long Life: Johnson and Johnson Ltd, Dental Products Division, 260 Bath Road, Slough, Bucks SL1 4EA.
Totacide: Tenneco Organics Ltd, Rockingham Works, Avonmouth, Bristol BS11 0YT.
Totacide 28: Tenneco Organics Ltd, Rockingham Works, Avonmouth, Bristol BS11 0YT.

Hypochlorite preparations
10% (10 000 ppm) solution hypochlorite
Chloros: ICI, Runcorn, Cheshire.
Domestos: Lever Brothers, Lever House, 3 St James Road, Kingston upon Thames KT1 2BA.

Dichloroisocyanurate preparations
Presept: Surgikos: Johnson and Johnson Ltd, Dental Products Division, 260 Bath Road, Slough, Bucks SL1 4EA.

Gloves

Ansell Gammex: (Latex) Smith and Nephew Medical Ltd, Romford, Essex.
Biogel D: (Latex) Regent International Ltd, Cambridge.
Puritee: (Latex) Searle Medical Products Ltd, High Wycombe, Bucks.
Microtouch: (Latex) Surgikos Ltd, Edinburgh.
Triflex: (Polyvinyl chloride) Travenol Laboratories Ltd, Thetford, Norfolk.
Healthco disposable latex examination gloves: (Latex) Healthco International, Boston, USA.
Glads procedure gloves: (Latex) Molnlycke UK Ltd, Barnstaple, England.
Peha-Soft disposable examination gloves: (Latex) Paul Hartmann AG, Heidenheim, GFR.
Roeko Rexam examination gloves: (Latex) Roescheisen GmbH, GFR.
Surgikos Microtouch latex medical gloves: (Latex) Johnson and Johnson Ltd, Slough, England.
Featherlite latex medical procedure gloves: (Latex) Regent LRC Products, London England.
Kimguard vinyl gloves: (Vinyl) Kimberley Clark Corp., Maidstone, England.

Heavy duty industrial or household gloves

The 'Marigold' range: LRC Products Ltd, North Circular Road, London E4 8QA.

Autoclaves and accessories

Suitable autoclaves
2000: Eschmann Equipment Ltd, Lancing, West Sussex.
Aesculap: Glover Dental Supplies, Shrewbury SY1 3NF.
Betaclave: J & S Davies Ltd, Potters Bar, Hertfordshire EN6 3EE.
Little Sister II: Surgical Equipment Supplies, London (Manufacturer).
Sterifix: Nesor Products, Pentonville Road, London N1 9HR.
TST strips, sensor sheets, Brown Steriliser control tubes: Albert Brown Ltd, Abbey Gate, Leicester LE4 0AK.
KaVo Steril Indicator: Kavo Dental, Raans Road, Amersham, Bucks HP6 6JL.

'Safe' containers and safety devices

Burn-bin: Metal Box Co. Ltd, Stoke Street, Clayton, Manchester M10 4QX
Cinbin: Labco Ltd, Marlow Bottom Road, Marlow, Bucks.
Sharp-safe Bins: Frontier Medical Products, North Blakeweir Industrial Estate, Crosskeys, Gwent.
Safeguard: Dentanurse, Talgarth, Powys.
Sharpak: DRG, Dixon Road, Bristol, BS4 5QY.
Sharpbin: DRG, Dixon Road, Bristol, BS4 5QY.
Septodont Disposi Needles: Deproco Ltd, 60 Fleet Street, London, EC4Y 1JU.
Safe Air: Carbolite Furnaces, Poole BDH12 4NN.

Hepatitis B vaccine (recombinant)

Engerix B: Smith Kline and French, Mundells, Welwyn Garden City, Herts AL7 1EY.

Useful addresses

Health Equipment Information No. 185, July 1988: DH (leaflets), PO Box 21, Stanmore, Middlesex HA7 1AY.
The Associated Offices Technical Committee: St Mary's Parsonage, Manchester M60 9AP.
The Independent Engineering Insurers' Committee: 57 Ladymead, Guildford GU1 1DB.

6

Legislation Related to Occupational Hazards, Health and Safety, and Employment Protection

Any employment, including dentistry, is subject to statutory contract and common law duties. Control of hazards to dental and other staff, and to patients, is clearly a moral obligation of the employer and is also a legal obligation under the law of contract and the common law principle of negligence. A wide range of statutes and regulations may also be applicable (*see* p 262).

Relevant legislation

In Britain, knowledge of and compliance with the requirements of the Health and Safety at Work etc Act (1974) is required in dental practices, particularly where there is a laboratory on the premises (fig. 6.1)[1] and knowledge of the Factories Act 1961 is also required by independent dental laboratories. All persons at work, whether employers or self-employed, are covered by the Health and Safety at Work etc Act, with the exception of domestic servants in a private household. The Act will, no doubt, seem to many to be another tiresome piece of bureaucracy that has little relevance to them. Indeed, for those who have sufficiently spacious accommodation and who apply reasonable common sense regarding the safety of their staff, patients and equipment, there is little to worry about. However, those with a large staff and a rapid flow of patients, or those whose accommodation is cramped and lacking adequate staff facilities, could get into difficulties. Employers must keep abreast of current legislation (Health and Safety [Information for Employers] Regulations 1989). It is worth bearing in mind that prosecution for contravention of any of the requirements of the Act is usually in a Magistrates'

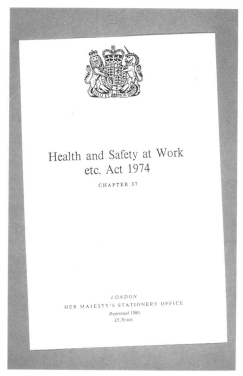

Fig. 6.1   The Health and Safety at Work Etc Act 1974 was a major turning point in occupational health.

Court and can attract a fine of £2000 or more, as well as a good deal of worry and waste of time. There is also the possibility of payment of compensation if injury or damage is involved.

The British laws that may affect dental staff are mainly the Health and Safety at Work etc Act and the Employment Protection Act. The Occupiers' Liability Act (1957), Employers' Liability (Compulsory Insurance) Act (1969), the Consumer Protection Act (1987) and, in some instances, the Factories Act (1961) and Fire Precautions Act (1971) must also be complied with and the dental practitioner must, in particular, know and comply with regulations related to radiation safety, cross-infection control and control of substances hazardous to health.[1-4]

In general terms, both premises and the activities therein must be safe to both employees, patients and visitors. If, through lack of care, somebody is injured or something is damaged, the dentist is likely to have to pay compensation, and this will apply (vicarious liability) regardless of whether the employer or employee is responsible. It is no longer possible to disclaim responsibility, even when an obvious disclaiming notice or document is posted—these are not valid in British law. There is a special responsibility if children are on the premises and due thought should be given to avoiding the sort of accidents to which they are especially prone. Doors containing breakable glass are an obvious example. Employers must therefore keep abreast of relevant current legislation, and ensure that they take out adequate insurances. It is also wise to take out public liability insurance in respect of the work premises and any domiciliary visits.

The Health and Safety at Work etc Act is an 'enabling Act', providing a framework of law under which various Regulations can be made by the Secretary of State for Employment, although they are usually drafted by the Health and Safety Executive (HSE) or Health and Safety Commission (HSC). Regulations are published in statutory instruments (SI).[2-4]

European Community Law is starting to take effect in the UK, not least, recently, in relation to protection against ionising radiation and to the Council Directive 80/1107/EEC related to risks from exposure to chemical, physical and biological hazards at work.

In the UK, the General Dental Services Committee of the BDA has agreed to support Family Practitioner Committee (FPC) and Health Board inspection of dental practices, and one of the functions of the proposed Dental Practice Advisers (DPAs) is to inspect surgeries. It has been agreed with the Department of Health that the acceptability of the following will be addressed:

(1) Suitability of equipment and instruments;
(2) Standard of decoration;
(3) Confidentiality of patient records;
(4) Adequacy of reception/waiting areas;
(5) Adequacy of toilet facilities;
(6) Compliance with Ionising Radiation Regulations;
(7) Control of cross-infection;
(8) Maintenance of compressors;
(9) Maintenance of autoclaves;
(10) Maintenance of anaesthetic equipment;
(11) Adequacy of emergency resuscitation arrangements;
(12) Adequacy of waste disposal arrangements;
(13) Secure handling and storage of drugs.

On the credit side, clinical dental staff in the National Health

Service (NHS) can claim compensation for illnesses related to occupation, as a result of the NHS Industrial Injuries Regulations (SI 1974 No. 1547). This benefit must be claimed, it will not be paid automatically, but can give up to 80% of normal income during illness or injury. However, the guidelines must have been complied with. For example, if the dentist has contracted hepatitis, such a claim is more likely to be successful if he or she has been vaccinated against hepatitis B and has adequate cross-infection control in the practice.

Recent regulations require the reporting to enforcing authorities (Health and Safety Executive) of injuries, cases of disease and dangerous events at work (Reporting of Injuries, Diseases and Dangerous Occurrences Regulations SI 2023 1985, ISBN 011 058 0230. London: HMSO, 1985. *See* Chapter 3). These regulations do not apply to accidents related to dental treatment *per se*, but would apply, for example, to a patient who tripped and broke a leg. Such accidents should be notified, by telephone if possible, with the minimum delay, and must be confirmed in writing within 7 days on Form F2508 (from HMSO).[2]

Health and Safety at Work etc Act, 1974

The Health and Safety at Work etc Act, hereafter referred to as the Act, aims particularly to secure the health, safety and welfare of those at work, the general public from risks to their health and safety arising from activities of workpeople, to control the safekeeping, use and handling of dangerous substances, and to control the emissions of noxious or offensive substances (including radiation) into the atmosphere. The Health and Safety at Work etc Act (1974) consolidated many of the provisions previously included in The Factories Act (1961) and the Offices, Shops, and Railway Premises Act (1963), but the earlier Acts remain in force. As noted above, apart from those in private domestic employment, the Act applies to all employers, employees and the self-employed, and provides statutory protection over and above common law protection. Recent regulations of importance in dentistry include the Ionising Radiation Regulations (1985); Classification, Packaging and Labelling of Dangerous Substances (1984) and Control of Substances Hazardous to Health (1988) Regulations. The BDA Advice Sheet 19 gives an overview of the Act in relation to dental practice, and salient points are discussed below.

Administration

The Secretary of State for Employment is empowered by the Act to make health and safety Regulations and either to replace or extend existing Regulations made under other statutes. He/she is advised by the Health and Safety Commission (HSC) and, although they may act on their own initiative, they must consult HSC before enacting any new Regulations or adopting Codes of Practice. Both the Secretary of State and the HSC must consult appropriate bodies such as trade unions or employers' associations before framing proposals for new or revised legislation. Although *Approved Codes of Practice* are meant to give *guidance* and not to have the force of law, a court of law might well, in criminal proceedings, expect a Code to have been observed. *Guidance Notes* have no status in law but can be extremely useful for advice.

The Health and Safety Executive (HSE) is responsible for enforcing the Act's provisions, although certain of these duties have devolved on local authorities, especially where activities are 'non-industrial'. The Health and Safety Inspectors of the HSE are responsible for ensuring these regulations are observed. The HSE also have an Employment Medical Advisory Service (EMAS; fig. 6.2). More detailed information can be obtained from leaflets, especially HSE16, which are free of charge, and from the Health and Safety Executive,* or from any local office of HSE or often from the Small Firm's Centres at the Department of Employment, Manpower Services Commission Job Centres, Citizens Advice Bureaux, and Chambers of Commerce. They include (fig. 6.2):

HSC1 Some legal aspects and how they affect you.
HSC2 The Health and Safety at Work etc Act outlined.
HSC3 Advice to employers.
HSC4 Advice to the self-employed.
HSC5 Advice to employees.
HSC6 Writing a safety policy statement; advice to employers.
HSC7 Regulations, approved codes of practice and guidance literature.
HSC8 Safety Committees.
HSC9 Time off for the training of Safety Representatives.
HSE4 Short guide to the Employers' Liability (Compulsory Insurance) Act 1969.

---

*Details may be found at the end of the chapter.

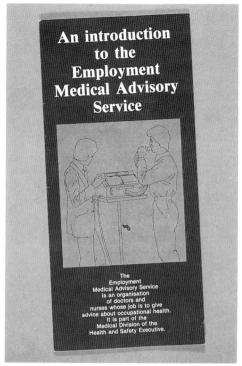

An introduction to the Employment Medical Advisory Service

The Employment Medical Advisory Service is an organisation of doctors and nurses whose job is to give advice about occupational health. It is part of the Medical Division of the Health and Safety Executive.

Fig. 6.2   The Employment Medical Advisory Service can give advice on occupational health.

HSE5 An introduction to the Employment Medical Advisory Service.

HSE11 Requirements for reporting injuries and dangerous occurrences at work.

HSE16 The Law on Health and Safety at Work. Essential facts for small businesses and the self-employed.

HSE17 Requirements for reporting cases of occupational disease.

IND/G 14L Securing compliance with health and safety legislation at work. How it is done and how it affects you.

IND/G 58L Employer's checklist (available free from 0742 752539; or 051 951 4381; or 071 229 0870).

IND/G 57L Employer's guide (ISBN 0 11883 993 4 available from HMSO).

The Act as it affects employers

Employers are obliged to ensure *as far as is reasonably practicable* the

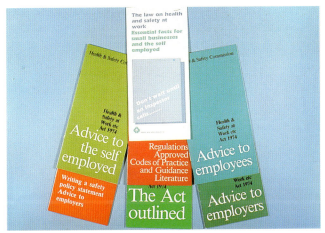

Fig. 6.3 Useful guidelines to the workings of the Health and Safety at Work Etc Act.

health, safety and welfare of their employees whilst at work. The employer has a similar duty to anyone who may be affected by the activities or placing of his/her business (fig. 6.4). As a self-employed person (whether or not he/she is also an employer), a dentist or technician also has a duty to conduct his/her undertaking in such a way that neither he/she nor any other persons who may be affected are thereby exposed to risks to health and safety.

In more specific terms, a dentist or dental laboratory owner has the same responsibilities under the Act as a dentist who has a laboratory (or other non-domestic activities) on the premises. All of the provisions apply to businesses, and common law places a duty on the employer to provide a safe working environment for even a single employee. The dentist should therefore notify his business to the Health and Safety Executive or local authority and:

(1) Provide and maintain plant and a system of work that is safe and without risk to health and safety. Equipment such as the dental unit, autoclave, radiography units and items such as the receptionist's chair or electric typewriter and laboratory equipment of various types should not therefore be dangerous.

(2) Arrange a safe system of using, handling, storing and transporting substances such as chemicals, drugs, mercury and inhalational anaesthetics. Any pressure vessel (such as an autoclave) or air receiver must be inspected annually and this must be confirmed by an engineering certificate.

(3) Provide all necessary information, instruction, training and super-

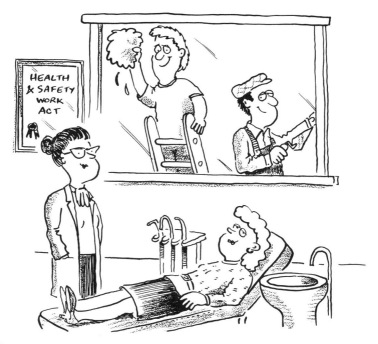

Fig. 6.4 Staff, tradesmen and patients are all covered by the Health and Safety at Work etc Act.

vision as required to ensure the health and safety at work of his/her employees. The employees should, for example, know about the risks of cross-infection, radiation and the use of drugs, chemicals and machinery.

(4) Maintain any place of work under his/her control in a condition that is safe and without risk to health, and provide safe entrances and exits.

(5) Provide and maintain a safe working environment.

(6) Conduct his/her practice in such a way as to also protect those *not in his/her employment* from risks to their health and safety. This includes not only patients, but also visitors, anyone employed to undertake repairs or maintenance, and all who may reasonably be considered to be at risk, such as those who pass by the premises. As an extreme example, an employer has been held responsible for cases of Legionnaire's disease contracted by passers-by from the effluent of an air conditioning plant. More relevant to dentistry are deaths under

anaesthesia. The dental surgeon, if responsible, may be found professionally negligent and lose his/her right to practice. Alternatively, and in addition, he/she may be found negligent and have to face trial. Furthermore, he/she has theoretically or in practice committed an offence under the Health and Safety at Work etc Act.

(7) Give such information as may be necessary to persons not in his/her employment on any aspect of the way the practice is conducted that might adversely affect their health or safety. For example, contractors should be warned about disposal of sharps, infected waste or chemicals.

There is now an approved poster (ISBN 011 7014 24 9) to comply with the Health and Safety Information for Employees Regulations, 1989. There is the alternative possibility of handing out approved leaflets. One or the other must be used. In either case, the name and address of the enforcing authority and the Employment Medical Service should be completed.

Safety policies

Persons who employ five or more employees must formulate a Safety Policy and bring it to the personal notice of their staff (*see* p 260 for an example). Ideally, each employee should be given a copy and sign a receipt that it has been received and understood.

The first part of the Safety Policy should be a general declaration of the employer's intention to provide a safe and healthy working environment, suitably amplified by his/her duties under the Act. The name of the person ultimately responsible for fulfilling the Policy (usually the principal or a designated partner or, in a laboratory, the owner), and date of formulation, must be noted. The nominated safety representative (see p 242) should be specified in the Safety Policy. Employees must also be reminded of their obligations under the Act; the Policy should be formulated after consultation with the people concerned, and it may be sensible to give each a copy of the leaflet HSC5 (see above).

The second part of the Safety Policy statement should be more specific and should cover particular hazards relating to control of cross-infection, drug and inhalational anaesthetic safety, radiography, handling of mercury and other chemicals, service supplies to equipment, pressure vessels, machinery, and so on (*see also* Control of Substances Hazardous to Health).

The employer is responsible for the training of his/her staff so that all can satisfactorily participate in the implementation of the Safety Policy. In-service training may be the most practicable and appropriate way to implement the Safety Policy. An Accident Book should be kept in all dental premises and *must* be kept where ten or more persons are employed (Social Security [Claims and Payments] Regulations; and Social Security Act 1975). Use of the HMSO Accident Book facilitates compliance with the Regulations.

The HSE produces a useful booklet: 'Our Health and Safety Policy Statement' (ISBN 011 8855 10 7).

The Act as it affects employees

The Act imposes a statutory duty over a common law duty. Employees must take reasonable care of themselves and others who may be affected by their acts or omissions at work. They must also cooperate with the employer and any other person upon whom the Act imposes a duty to see that it is complied with. The employee must not intentionally or recklessly interfere with or misuse anything provided in the interest of health, safety or welfare in pursuance of the relevant statutory provisions. Failure to comply with the Act may be grounds for dismissal.

The Act as it affects manufacturers and suppliers

Designers, manufacturers, suppliers or importers of equipment or substances used in dentistry must also ensure, as far as is reasonably practicable, that their products do not threaten safety or health. They must carry out appropriate testing and inspection and provide all necessary information relating to the purpose for which the equipment is intended, along with instructions regarding its safe use. Those who install and maintain equipment have a similar obligation (Direct Product Liability).

Enforcement of the Act

Enforcement of the law can be or may seem to be capricious, but legislation to minimise hazards in the workplace must be complied with. It seems likely that the Health and Safety Inspectorate will have their hands full dealing with considerably more hazardous industries than dental practices or laboratories, but if a practice has a troublesome patient or employee who complains to the HSE, then difficulties might arise. This has recently happened in relation to cross-infection. A relatively brief account of the process of enforcement will now follow.

The inspector for a dental practice or hospital is usually an HM Inspector of Factories. A Health and Safety Inspector may enter work premises at any reasonable time. However, if he/she considers that a dangerous situation exists, he/she can enter at any time. He/she has the right to examine premises, documents, substances, systems of work and equipment and he/she may seize equipment or render it harmless. He/she may also take measurements, samples, photographs and seek information. It is an offence to obstruct an inspector in the course of his/her statutory duties.

An inspector can, where necessary, serve either (a) an Improvement Notice or (b) a Prohibition Notice, or (c) prosecute.

An improvement notice is served upon the person who, in the opinion of the inspector, is contravening a relevant statutory provision. It specifies the provision that is being infringed, the reasons why the inspector believes this to be so, and the time allowed for remedial action.

A prohibition notice is issued when there is considered to be a risk of serious personal injury. It is served upon the person performing or controlling the dangerous activity and its effect is either immediately to stop the activity until remedial action has been taken or, if the inspector considers there is no immediate danger, to allow time to remedy the situation.

Appeals

Those who have been served with either an Improvement or a Prohibition Notice have a right of appeal to an Industrial Tribunal, provided that the appeal is lodged with the Central Office of Tribunals within 3 weeks (21 days) of the notice being served. Upon the lodging of an appeal the operation of an Improvement Notice is suspended until the matter is decided, but a Prohibition Notice can only be suspended if the Tribunal so orders, at a specially convened sitting before the main hearing. The Tribunal may decide to affirm or cancel the notice and this decision can be appealed against within 7 days, but only on the following grounds.

(1) Error on the part of the tribunal staff.
(2) A party did not receive notice of the proceedings.
(3) Absence of a party entitled to be heard.

(4) New evidence has been obtained that could not have been discovered before, or, in the interests of justice, requires a review.

Appeals to the Divisional Court and finally to the Court of Appeal are also possible.

Inspection of dental practices

For over 10 years there has been a programme of inspection of dental premises and, according to the BDA, these inspections are normally carried out by appointment (although notice is not obligatory) and take up to 45 minutes. Obvious hazards that have been the focus of attention are x-radiography, radiography equipment, general anaesthetics, mercury, and, more recently, cross-infection equipment, procedures and safety training. Potentially explosive and flammable materials also receive attention.

Penalties for contravening the Act

It is an offence liable to prosecution to contravene any of the general duties under the Act, any regulations made under it, or to ignore the serving of any notices.

Summary conviction (in a Magistrate's Court) attracts a fine of up to £2000. Conviction on indictment (before a Crown Court) can result in a fine of unlimited amount or imprisonment for a term of up to 2 years, or both. If, having been convicted of an offence, the perpetrator allows it to continue, he is liable to a fine of up to £50 for each day of its continuation.

Whilst a civil action cannot be taken solely as a result of the Act being infringed, a person who suffers injury or damage may still sue for negligence.

Safety Representatives and Committees

Recognised trade unions have the right to appoint safety representatives from among the employees at a place of work, and the recognised unions include the BDA, NALGO and USDAW. Safety representatives should have been in the practice or laboratory's employment for a minimum of 2 years, or have been in similar employment for that time, and be at least 18 years of age. No statutory liability additional to that of any other employee falls upon safety representatives.

Safety representatives should, among other things, investigate potential hazards, make representations to employers and represent the staff in dealing with the Inspectorate. Two safety representatives may request an employer to establish a safety committee, which acts as a focus both for staff participation in the prevention of hazards and for staff and employer cooperation. Employers must consult safety representatives on matters relating to the implementation of the appropriate health and safety regulations.

The extent to which the unions will insist on their rights in the case of dental practices or laboratories is unclear. Detailed regulations are found in the Statutory Instrument, HMSO, No. 500, 1977.

Radiation protection legislation

Dentists must ensure that they, their staff and patients are not exposed to unnecessary radiation (fig. 6.5). All radiography sets must conform to specified safety standards (*see* Chapter 4); all involved in

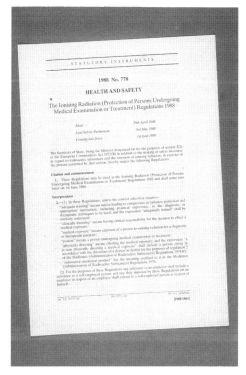

Fig. 6.5 The protection against ionising radiation is covered by recent regulations made under the Health and Safety at Work Etc Act (Ionising Radiation Regulations 1985, 1988).

their use should be aware of the hazards, and all should adopt practices that minimise the dangers. The Nuclear Inspectorate has the responsibility for monitoring radiation safety and has the right to inspect dental surgeries where there is radiography equipment.

Most modern radiography equipment complies with safety standards, since the Health and Safety at Work etc Act places an obligation on manufacturers, importers and suppliers in this respect.

An employer (including a self-employed person) must comply with the *Ionising Radiations Regulations 1985* (Statutory Instrument 1985, No 1333) and must cooperate with other employers if there is any possibility of irradiation of any employee of the other party. The employer must notify the Health and Safety Executive 28 days before he/she intends (for the first time) to work with ionising radiation. He/she must also inform the Executive of any change in the name and address of the practice.

Employers must restrict exposure of employees and other persons to ionising radiation and must designate as a Controlled Area any area where an employee can be exposed. Local operating rules such as the Family Practitioner Committee (FPC) *'Basic rules in dental radiography'* should be displayed, and a named person with appropriate knowledge should take day-to-day responsibility for ensuring compliance with the rules and for overseeing radiation safety. This will usually be the dentist. Anyone using radiography equipment should be appropriately trained, and women should be warned of the possible hazard to the foetus.

The reader is advised to study the following relevant literature which is consistent with the provisions of the European Council Directive (EC Directives 80/836 and 84/467 Euratom);

(1) The Ionising Radiations Regulations 1985, No. 1333. London: HMSO, 1985.

(2) The Ionising Radiation (Protection of persons undergoing medical examination or treatment) Regulations 1988, (Statutory Instrument No. 778). London: HMSO, 1988.

(3) Guidance notes for the protection of persons against ionising radiations arising from medical and dental use. 1988, ISBN 085951 299 1. London: HMSO, 1988 (published by the National Radiological Protection Board in conjunction with the Health Departments and the Health and Safety Executive).

(4) Radiation protection in dental practice. (Standing Dental Advisory Committee, 1988).

Walls

Solid structural walls of brick or concrete but not thin partitions will attenuate ionising radiation.

Monitoring (see also Chapter 4)

Radiography equipment should be regularly maintained, checked annually and receive a thorough radiological check at least once every 3 years. If the dose is unlikely to exceed 15 mSv*/year (1·5 rems/ year), health surveillance and monitoring are not required by law; most dentists and their staff fall into this category. Monitoring *should* be carried out if the individual workload exceeds 150 intra-oral or 50 panoramic films each week.

The personal monitors used in the UK for x-rays and gamma rays, are the badge film monitor and the thermoluminescent dosimeter (TLD). The latter is normally lithium fluoride with traces of titanium and magnesium and can measure radiation exposure dose. Monitoring in these ways is convenient and cheap and, if nothing else, it is reassuring to confirm the low level of exposure. Advice on monitoring can be sought from The National Radiation Protection Board (NRPB) Personnel Monitoring Service, Chilton, Didcot, Oxon OX11 0RQ.

Aspects of legal responsibility and employment rights in relation to cross-infection

Dental employers have ethical and legal responsibilities with respect to cross-infection control. The Health and Safety at Work etc Act and Control of Substances Hazardous to Health (COSHH) regulations have clear applicability, but also the GDC Notice, and NHS General Dental Services Regulations 1973 (para 1 of Terms of Service) advise that dental surgeries should be furnished with appropriate equipment and that treatment should be provided with suitable instruments that may be inspected by a dental officer. Finally, the patient may also, under the laws of tort, claim negligence against a dentist if they

---

Gray: Unit of absorbed dose giving 1 Joule/kg in any material.
Sievert: Dose equivalent in biological effect to 1 Joule/kg of 250 Kv x-rays (Gray × RBE).
RBE: Relative biological effectiveness is the ratio of number of Grays of two radiations which give the same biological effect on the same material in the same time.
    A postal service is available from the NRPB at a cost of £48·75, for testing the radiography equipment and film development efficiency. Parameters tested include Kv output, filtration, beam size and timer.

believe they have been avoidably harmed as a consequence of inadequate control of cross-infection.

In view of the ease with which hepatitis B can be transmitted, it would be difficult to defend a case where a patient acquired the infection after treatment in a practice where the sterilisation techniques were less than perfect. A patient has recently successfully claimed for damages after apparently acquiring hepatitis B in a practice where it was found that the hygienist's sterilisation technique was faulty. It would also be indefensible for a dentist or any clinical dental staff member, known to be a carrier particularly of the HBe antigen, to continue in practice unless effective cross-infection control measures were in force (Chapter 5).

There is often even greater anxiety about transmission of HIV, the AIDS virus, even though there is little evidence of this having happened during dental practice (but *see* p 169). The GDC has therefore issued a statement (13 January 1988) to the effect that:
'(1) Dentists who suspect that they have been infected by HIV, should seek medical advice and follow any consequent recommendations regarding modification of their practices necessary to protect their patients.

(2) Dentists who know or suspect that they are HIV-positive and who jeopardise the well-being of their patients by failing to obtain appropriate medical advice or by failing to act on such advice, are behaving unethically. Such behaviour may raise the question of professional misconduct.'

Infected staff are unlikely to transmit microbial agents to others if cross-infection control measures are effective, and this is not therefore generally regarded as a reason for treating an HIV or other virus-infected job applicant or employee any differently from others. This is discussed in a Department of Employment and Health and Safety Executive booklet '*AIDS and employment*' (1986).

Employees have statutory rights against unfair dismissal (see below) which are not reduced if the individual is infected (HSE, 1986), although an HIV-positive dentist may, as noted above, need to modify his/her practice (General Dental Council, 1988: *see* Chapter 5).

Legal responsibilities in control of substances hazardous to health

Microbiological, chemical and other hazards are covered in law by the Control of Substances Hazardous to Health (COSHH) Regulations 1988, discussed in Chapter 3.

Monitoring and other health and safety records

The Control of Substances Hazardous to Health Regulations 1988 (COSHH) impose the obligation to minimise exposure to hazardous substances. This implies that there should be monitoring of hazardous substances where this is possible (for example mercury). Although COSHH regulations do not cover ionising radiation, this should also be monitored.

The dentist has a duty to share the results of the health monitoring with the specific employee concerned and must inform the employee if a maximum exposure limit has been exceeded (COSHH Regulation 12.2). The results of monitoring the health of other persons should not specify the person's name to their colleagues.

Personal records of health and safety measures should be kept for at least 30 years (COSHH) to 50 years (Ionising Radiation Regulations 1985).

Other relevant health and safety legislation

All surgeries and laboratories must be covered by occupier and employer liability indemnity insurance. This is a statutory requirement under the Occupier's Liability Act 1984 and the Employers' Liability (Compulsory Insurance) Act 1969.

Occupier's Liability Act 1957 and 1984
This requires the occupiers of premises to take reasonable care that visitors have the safety benefits of such essentials as adequate lighting, safe stairways, and safe floor coverings.

Employers' Liability (Compulsory Insurance) Act 1969
Dental employers must insure against employee's claims for injury or illness, and display an up-to-date certificate of insurance in the practice or laboratory premises.

The Electricity at Work Regulations 1989

These regulations necessitate the use of only correctly qualified and indemnified persons for examining and repairing all electrical systems. It is in order, however, for others to undertake simple repairs to plugs, fuses, and so on.

Consumer Protection Act 1987

This Act imposes liability for damage caused wholly or partially by a defect in a product, upon the producer, importer, or anyone purporting to be manufacturers (Direct Product Liability). A dentist or technician selling second-hand equipment may be liable, although this does not apply if the product is more than 10 years old. The Act does not cover articles which have been wilfully misused or modified by the purchaser.

Factories Act 1961

The Health and Safety at Work etc Act covers much of the needs of the Factories Act but the latter is summarised here because of its particular relevance to dental laboratories.

Heating, ventilation and extraction

An adequate room temperature (60°F after the first hour) must be maintained. Air-conditioning will keep the temperature constant, heating it during the winter and cooling it in the summer.

Good ventilation is essential, as surgeries tend to become humid or steam-filled because of the autoclave and may be contaminated with mercury vapour or inhalational anaesthetics as well as the typical dental practice volatiles such as eugenol. Laboratories also tend to get steam or smoke-filled. Air extraction is necessary wherever there are dusts such as from dental alloys, plaster, ceramic or pumice (HSE guidance note EH 44 1984) or fumes such as from monomer or cyanide from plating baths. Burn-out furnaces should have smoke-extractors.

Overcrowding

Rooms must not become so overcrowded as to endanger health. A minimum of 400 cubic feet of space (not counting any area more than 14 feet from the floor) per worker is needed.

Staff facilities

Adequate staff facilities such as a cloakroom for hanging outdoor clothes, coats, jackets, etc, lockers for personal effects, and a room in which to make hot drinks and eat refreshments must be available. Within a small practice, employing perhaps only one technician, a shared facility with the dental surgery assistant will suffice, but where the practice or laboratory is larger, with three or more employees, separate cloakroom and refreshment areas should be provided.

Dangerous materials and equipment

All dangerous equipment and materials must be clearly marked and the onus is on the employer to ensure that every member of staff is trained to use the machinery and dangerous materials and that these must be as far as possible safe, and without risk to health. All machinery should be fenced, and, in particular, centrifugal casting apparatus should be guarded. Suitable safety equipment should be provided (fig. 6.6). Equipment prone to an explosive risk such as the compressor or autoclave must, under the Factories Act, be inspected by an engineer surveyor at 26-month intervals.

Also, from the 1st of July 1994 the Pressure Systems and Transportable Gas Containers Regulations 1989 will require a written scheme of examination to be prepared by a competent person for each pressure vessel. This will include details of the nature and frequency

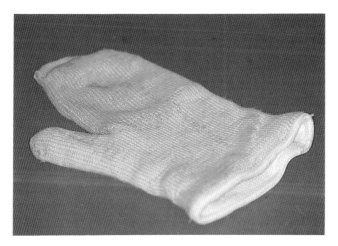

Fig. 6.6   Heat resistant gloves, or tongs, must be used for handling hot material in the laboratory.

of the examination required. It is not too early for dentists to arrange for written schemes to be prepared and implemented. Gas bottles must be stored outside the working area; acids and cyanide solutions should be kept apart and stored in a fume cupboard. Dangerous drugs must be stored in an appropriate locked receptacle and it is wise also to store poisons and medicines in a locked container.

Children and animals should never be left unattended in a practice or laboratory (fig. 6.7).

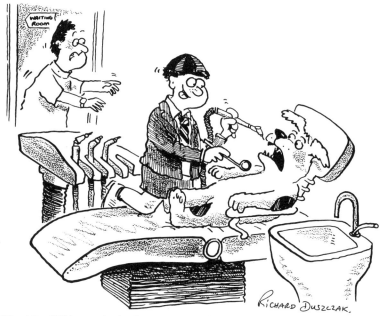

Fig. 6.7   Children and animals must not be left unattended in a practice or laboratory.

Accidents
A record must be kept of any major accident or dangerous event which must also be reported to the Factories Inspector. It is also wise to keep an unofficial record of minor accidents.

Notices
The Factories Inspector can advise about the various notices that have to be displayed under the Act.

Fire precautions

Minimisation of fire hazards has been discussed in Chapter 3. Safety precautions include the need to make known the procedures to be followed in the event of a fire. Written fire procedure notices must be displayed (Table 6.1).

There must be adequate means of fire escape and fire extinguishers for flammables, such as polymers and monomers, and for electrical and general combustibles (figs 6.8 and 6.9). Smoke detectors are useful safety devices. Fire escape routes and exits must be clearly and appropriately marked and unobstructed (figs 6.10 and 6.11).

A fire certificate will be necessary if more than 20 persons are employed, or more than 10 persons are working anywhere other than on the ground floor. The Fire Precautions Act 1971 deals with fire escapes, fire fighting equipment and other fire precautions. The owner of the premises is responsible for fire doors and escapes; the tenant is reponsible for fire extinguishers and blankets. The local Fire Brigade can give advice and are usually very helpful, and it is best to

Table 6.1 Fire safety

In addition to having a fire policy and instructions, make absolutely sure that you:

(1) install smoke detectors;
(2) know where the nearest fire alarm is;
(3) know where the nearest fire-fighting appliances are kept, have them regularly maintained and know how to use them;
(4) know the fire escape route;
(5) if you hold a position of responsibility, know what your special duties are in the event of fire;
(6) know where the Fire Assembly Point is.

In the event of a fire:
(1) Anyone detecting smoke or a smell of burning should investigate immediately and raise the alarm.
(2) Take extinguishers to the scene of the fire, then—*not before*—operate and direct the jet into the seat of the fire.
(3) If the fire is not controllable with the equipment available, shut all doors and windows in the room or area in which the fire is discovered.
(4) On hearing the alarm, remove patients from immediate danger and await instructions from the senior person in charge.
(5) All staff without direct responsibilities and all available staff not on duty and not having specific fire duties should proceed to the Fire Assembly Point, as indicated on fire instruction notices, and act as instructed by the senior person present.

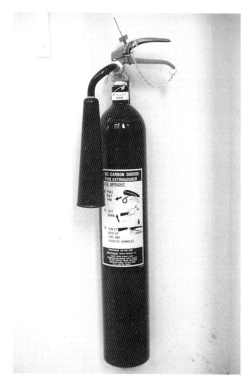

Fig. 6.8   Fire extinguishers are obligatory in any premises and should be regularly maintained.

ask the Local Authority Fire Prevention Officer to visit informally and advise as necessary.

First-aid

A first-aid box must be kept and regularly maintained (minimum contents are laid down in the Factories Act). The first-aid box should contain nothing but first-aid requisites and be readily accessible. It should contain sterile eye dressings and an eye bath, as well as an assortment of dressings, bandages and antiseptics. In most practices, except the smallest, it would probably be appropriate for one employee to have special responsibility for first-aid and for the first-aid box, after receiving suitable training. Training should include first-aid measures for the main types of accident (burns, cuts and lacerations, eye injuries, electric shock, fractures and sprains), as well

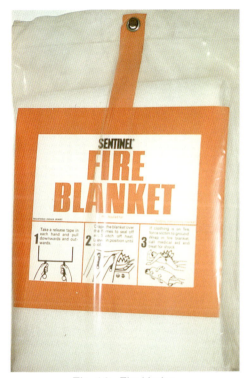

Fig. 6.9   Fire blanket.

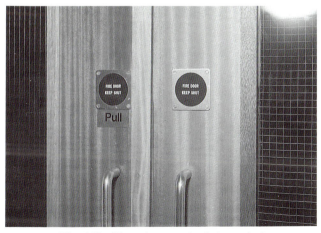

Fig. 6.10   Fire exits must clearly be marked.

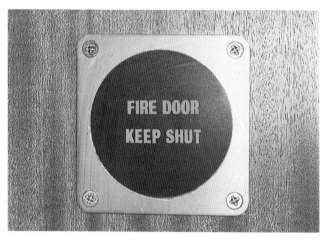

Fig. 6.11   Fire doors must be kept closed.

as treatment for shock. The St John's Ambulance Brigade handbook would be a suitable training manual. The Employment Medical Advisory Service can advise on health at work and first-aid.

Cleanliness
The surgery and laboratory must be kept clean and free from dirt, plaster, etc; all benches and floors should therefore be swept and cleaned in the evening. The walls and ceiling should be washed every 14 months and redecorated every 7 years, according to the Act. To keep the surgery and laboratory in good condition, however, a maximum of about 2 years would be preferable.

An adequate supply of drinking water and cups must be provided, as well as reasonable washing facilities for each gender if there are more than five male and female employees.

Trades Unions
In the UK, most dental technicians are in the Union of Shop, Distributive and Allied Workers (USDAW) or the Manufacturing Science and Finance Union (MSFU), although some are in the Gold and Silversmith Union, Association of University Teachers (AUT), or Confederation of Health Service Employees (COHSE).

Employment protection

Employers must take note of the laws on equal opportunities (see below). They would be well advised to read the British Dental Association guidance sheet[5] and the excellent review on employment law by Muir.[6]

Employment Protection (consolidation) Act 1978

This Act aims to protect employees against unfair dismissal or redundancy practices as well as giving the right to maternity leave for certain employees. The self-employed are not usually protected by this Act. The Employment Act (1982) amended this Act.

In general terms, fair or acceptable reasons for dismissal relate to the incapability of the employees to carry out the work for which they were employed, misconduct, or redundancy. Dismissal is also justified if to carry on work would mean that the employee was breaking the law in some way, for example by embezzling money from the practice, or if safety codes are broken. Unfair or unacceptable reasons for dismissal would be if the person was dismissed on the transfer of a practice or laboratory, because of race or pregnancy, or because of Union activities.

An employee who feels that dismissal is unfair may consult the Arbitration, Conciliation Advisory Service (ACAS) or Industrial Tribunal, provided they have a contract of employment and (except where race or pregnancy is the reason given for dismissal) have been employed continuously by the employer for a period of 2 or more years.

Most of the information relevant to this Act is contained in a series of pamphlets issued by HMSO on behalf of the Department of Employment and available from Job Centres, employment offices or unemployment benefit offices (fig. 6.12). These include:
(1) Written statement of main terms and conditions of employment.
(2) Redundancy consultation and notification.
(3) Employee's rights on insolvency of employer.
(4) Employment rights for the expectant mother.
(5) Suspension on medical grounds under health and safety regulations.
(6) Facing redundancy?—Time off for job hunting or to arrange training.

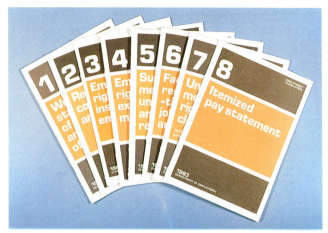

Fig. 6.12   Useful pamphlets on employment, for employers and employees.

(7) Union membership rights and the closed shop including the union labour only provisions of the Employment Act 1982.

(8) Itemised pay statement.

(9) Guarantee payments.

(10) Employment rights on the transfer of an undertaking.

(11) Rules governing continuous employment and a week's pay.

(12) Time off for public duties.

(13) Unfairly dismissed?

(14) Rights to notice and reasons for dismissal.

(15) Union secret ballots.

(16) Redundancy payments.

Employers should consult the British Dental Association Advice Sheets and those with problems related to the Act should consult ACAS.

The Act does not demand a written contract of employment, but it is advisable to have one. The main terms must be set out within 13 weeks of the start of employment. Both the name of the employer (or employing organisation) and employee must be stated, as well as the date when employment began; the rate, method and intervals at which remuneration is to be received, together with any benefits; the hours of work; holidays and holiday pay; any sick pay or pension schemes; notice; job title; disciplinary rules; and the name of the person to whom an employee can apply if dissatisfied with any disciplinary decision. Any formal changes in conditions of service should be notified within 4 weeks, and it is useful also to review working arrangements from time to time since custom and practice may change and can readily assume force.

Equal opportunities and the law

Laws which affect the right of every person to equal opportunity at work include the following:

The Disabled Persons Employment Acts 1944 and 1958
This law provides for employment opportunities for disabled persons.

Equal Pay Act 1970
This law makes it illegal to give rates of pay to women different from those to men who are doing equal work of equal value.

Sex Discrimination Act 1975
This law makes it illegal to discriminate against either a woman or a man on the grounds of their sex or marital status.

Race Relations Act 1976
This law makes it illegal to discriminate against a person on the grounds of colour, race, nationality or ethnic or national origins.

Rehabilitation of Offenders Act
This law governs discrimination against those with a criminal record.

These laws apply to recruitment of staff, terms and conditions, opportunities for promotion, and so on, and cover both direct and indirect discrimination. The former covers cases where there is less favourable treatment on grounds of, for example, race or sex. Examples might include applying higher educational or personal standards to black applicants than to white applicants or permitting male employees to enrol on day-release courses but not women. These examples are in addition to the more obvious cases where people are refused a job or a promotion because they are black rather than white or female rather than male.

Direct discrimination can be perpetrated even when no hostility is shown to a victim. An example is someone who acts on the basis of stereotyped views, such as the belief that all married women with children are liable to be absent without notice or that all married women without children will soon leave and so are not worth recruiting to jobs requiring in-service training.

Indirect discrimination can be perpetrated when women or members of minority ethnic groups are apparently treated equally, but a condition is applied which has the effect of excluding a significantly higher proportion of them than of white males. For example, a rule requiring residence in this country for a given number of years might be more difficult for members of minority ethnic groups to comply with; a rule requiring applicants to be between 17 and 28 would be more difficult for women to comply with because so many women are not in the labour market during those years for family reasons. Requiring unnecessarily high academic qualifications or experience, or setting unnecessarily rigid rules on the hours during which the work must be performed, may be indirectly discriminatory.

Unlike direct discrimination, indirect discrimination is capable of being justified. It is therefore not unlawful *if* the employer can show that the condition being challenged was *necessary* in the circumstances. It is not enough to show that it was merely convenient.

These laws are quite complicated and it is not possible here to do more than give a general outline. However, the main responsibility of an employer is to provide equal opportunities. Employees also have responsibilities not to discriminate unfairly in the way services are provided. If involved in recruiting and/or managing other staff, there must not be unfair discrimination, and one must not, in any way, encourage others to practice unfair discrimination. Sexual harassment and racial harassment are forms of discrimination, and must be avoided. There should never be victimisation of any person who has complained of discrimination or harassment, or has given information to support such a complaint, and one must not be influenced to behave in a discriminatory fashion by the views of other employees or members of the public.

Summary

(1) The Health and Safety at Work etc Act applies to dental practices and the dental surgeon (the employer) must act on its requirements.
(2) Regulations of particular importance apply to protection against radiation and to substances hazardous to health.

(3) Precautions must be taken to prevent accidents and to ensure all aspects of safety not merely for staff and patients, but also for anyone entering the practice or even (exceptionally) others.

(4) Control of cross-infection also comes within the scope of the Act.

(5) A Safety Policy should be formulated and brought to the notice of all staff.

(6) A Health and Safety Inspector may visit a practice as necessary and may do so without notice.

(7) In addition to the Health and Safety at Work etc Act, the Factories Act which has additional requirements for the health and well-being of employees also applies to dental laboratories.

(8) The Factories Act includes such matters as heating and ventilation, prevention of overcrowding and precautions against fire and accidents of any type.

(9) The Employers' Liability Act requires the employer to take out adequate insurance against employees' claims for accidents or illnesses acquired at work.

(10) The Employment Protection Act protects employees against unfair dismissal or discrimination. Claims of unfair dismissal can be troublesome and time-consuming for the employer.

(11) A precise and carefully worded Job Description is essential when taking on staff; a written contract is also desirable. These documents may protect the employer if there is a claim for unfair dismissal.

(12) A beneficial aspect of the Health and Safety at Work etc Act is that the dental surgeon may be able to obtain compensation for illnesses such as hepatitis B acquired at work, although only if reasonable precautions have been taken.

References

1 Health and Safety at Work Etc Act (1974). London: HMSO.
2 Reporting of Injuries, Diseases and Dangerous Occurences Regulations, 1985.
3 Ionizing Radiations Regulations 1985 and 1988.
4 Control of Substances Hazardous to Health Regulations 1988.
5 British Dental Association. Health and Safety at Work, 1982. Advice Sheet Number 19.
6 Muir J. Practice staff; terms of contract of employment. *Br Dent J* 1988; **165**: 342–343.

Appendix 1

Health and Safety at Work

Statement of Practice Policy

The practice of .... attaches great importance to the health, safety and welfare of employees, and asks all staff to help in maintaining a working environment which is as safe as possible for everyone, including patients, in the practice.

The practice will take all reasonable steps to maintain premises, equipment and work systems so that they are without risk to health. All appropriate regulations and codes of practice will be observed. At the same time, employees have a duty to take reasonable care of their own and others' health and safety, and to cooperate with the practice in the maintenance of a safe workplace.

Staff will be instructed in safety procedures as part of their general instruction in practice working procedures. However, there are certain basic safety rules to which special attention is drawn:

(1) Report all accidents (including spillages and sharps injuries, etc) to .... immediately, whether or not they involve personal injury.

(2) Maintain rigorous personal hygiene. Surgery staff must wear gloves before handling any instruments or materials used in the mouth.

(3) Take care in the handling of all substances used in dentistry, whether or not a specific hazard has been pointed out to you. Minimise the possibilities of ingestion, inhalation or contact with skin.

(4) Make full use of any protective clothing provided.

(5) Never touch electrical equipment with wet hands.

(6) Never run in the practice.

(7) Always stand at least 2 metres away from and behind the x-ray tube when radiographs are being taken.

(8) If a sharp instrument is dropped, do not try to catch it.

(9) If in doubt about how to use materials or equipment, read the instructions carefully.

(10) If still in doubt, ask ....

The practice intends to keep safety matters under regular scrutiny with a view to identifying hazards and taking appropriate remedial action. Employees' suggestions will be welcomed and should be made to .... , who is responsible for the coordination of measures to secure safety at work in the practice.

NB. See also the BDA Advice Sheet on Health and Safety Law for the Dental Practice or an example policy from the Dental Laboratories Association (see below).

Appendix 2

Factory Inspectorate address list

Area	Address and Telephone No.
South West	Inter-City House, Mitchell Lane, Victoria Street, Bristol BS1 6AN.Tel: 0272 290681.
South	Priestly House, Priestly Road, Basingstoke RG24 9NW.Tel: 0256 473181.
South East	3 East Grinstead House, London Road, East Grinstead, West Sussex RH19 1RR. Tel: 0342 326922.
London South	1 Long Lane, London SE1 4PG. Tel: 071 407 8911
London North	Maritime House, 1 Linton Road, Barking IG11 8HF. Tel: 081 594 5522.
East Anglia	39 Baddow Road, Chelmsford CM2 0HL. Tel: 0245 284661.
Northern Home Countries	14 Cardiff Road, Luton, Bedfordshire LU1 1PP. Tel: 0582 34121.
East Midlands	5th Floor, Belgrave House, 1 Greyfriars, Northampton NN1 2BS. Tel: 0604 21233.
West Midlands	McLaren Building, 2 Masshouse Circus, Queensway, Birmingham B4 7NP. Tel: 021 200 2299.
Wales	Brunel House, 2 Fitzalan Road, Cardiff, CF2 1SH.Tel: 0222 473777.
Marches	The Marches House, Midway, Newcastle under Lyme, Staffordshire ST5 1DT. Tel: 0782 717181.
North Midlands	Birbeck House, Trinity Square, Nottingham, NG1 4AU.Tel: 0602 470712.

South Yorkshire and Humberside	Sovereign House, 40 Silver Street, Sheffield S1 2ES.Tel: 0742 739081.
West and North Yorkshire	8 St Paul's Street, Leeds, LS1 2LE. Tel: 0532 446191.
Greater Manchester	Quay House, Quay Street, Manchester M3 3JB. Tel: 061 831 7111.
Merseyside	The Triad, Stanley Road, Bootle, Merseyside L20 3PG. Tel: 051 922 7211.
North West	Victoria House, Ormskirk Road, Preston PR1 1HH. Tel: 0772 59321.
North East	Arden House, Regent Centre, Gosforth, Newcastle upon Tyne NE3 3JN. Tel: 091 284 8448.
Scotland East	Belford House, 59 Belford Road, Edinburgh EH4 3UE. Tel: 031 225 1313.
Scotland West	314 St Vincent Street, Glasgow G3 8XG. Tel: 041 204 2646.

Appendix 3

Statutes and Regulations that may apply in dentistry

Companies Act 1989.
Control of Substances Harmful to Health Regulations 1988.
Council Directive 15 July 1980. (8018361 Euratom).
Council Directive 3 September 1984 (8414671 Euratom) amend 1 above.

Employers' Liability (Compulsory Insurance) Act 1969.
Employers' Liability (Defective Equipment) Act 1969.
European Economic Community, Council Directive July 25 1985.

Fatal Accident Act 1976.
Fire Precautions Act 1971.
Health and Safety (Information for Employees) Regulations 1989.

Industrial Training Act 1964.
Ionising Radiations Regulations 1985.
Limitation Act 1980.
National Health Service (General Dental Services) Regulations 1973.

National Health Service Act 1946.
Occupiers Liability Act 1984.
Offices, Shops and Railway Premises Act 1963.
Public Health (Recurring Nuisances) Act 1969.
Reporting of Injuries, Diseases and Dangerous Occurrences Regulations 1985.

Social Security Act 1975.
The Boiler Explosions Acts 1882 and 1890.
The Consumer Protection Act 1987.
The Control of Substances Hazardous to Health Regulations 1988.

The Dentists Act 1984
The Electricity at Work Regulations 1989.
The Factories Act 1961.
The Health and Safety (Enforcing Authority) Regulations 1989.

The Health and Safety (Enforcing Authority) Regulations 1977.

The Health and Safety at Work etc Act 1974.
The Industrial Tribunals (Improvement and Prohibition Notices Appeals) Scotland Regulations 1974.

The Industrial Tribunal (Improvement and Prohibition Notices Appeals) Regulations 1974 for England and Wales.

The Law Reform (Personal Injuries) Act 1948.
Trade Union and Labour Relations Act 1974.

Health and Safety Executive: Baynards House, 1 Chepstow Place, London W2 4TF. Tel: 071 229 0416/0870.
NRPB Personal Monitoring Service: Chilton, Didcot, Oxon OX11 0RQ. Tel: 0235 834590.
Dental Laboratories Association: Chapel House, Noel Street, Nottingham NG7 6AS.

7

Medicolegal hazards

Medicolegal hazards are (obviously enough) of a quite different nature from the risks already discussed, although the physical risks to patients especially, can give rise to claims against the dental surgeon. Indeed, the effects of litigation may be not too dissimilar to those of physical injury or illness for the dental surgeon, namely to take him/her away from work for varying periods while the matter is being thrashed out, possibly involve him/her in expense or loss of earnings for varying periods, add considerably to the mental stresses imposed on him/her and, at worst, may deprive him/her of both occupation and livelihood if it results in erasure of his/her name from *The Dentists Register*.

Some of the medicolegal hazards that may be faced by dentists will be discussed here, but clearly it is not possible to be comprehensive in the space available and it is well worth reading *Law and ethics in dentistry*[1] and *The prevention of complications in dental surgery*.[2] Changes in the law since these books were written are usually indicated in the annual reports of the medical defence organisations.

Fortunately, the current risk of being involved in litigation resulting from the practice of dentistry in Britain, is relatively small and considerably less than for a doctor. This is partly the reason for the considerably lower cost of medical defence societies' subscriptions for dentists compared with doctors. The defence societies provide an invaluable shield between the dental surgeon and the litigant, with the result that few cases—probably little more than 1%—come to court. In the United States, on the other hand, the dental surgeon has to deal directly with an insurance company, which can refuse cover with minimal justification. Patients are virtually or even actively encouraged to sue health professionals by the existence of free contingency litigation and by the size of many of the awards that are made.

Despite the protection provided by the defence organisations, the threat of litigation is a source of anxiety and usually has a heavy cost in terms of time which could otherwise be spent on productive work. Although the costs of legal representation and any awards that are made are covered by the defence societies' subscriptions, there is still the possibility, in cases of professional misconduct, that the dentist's name could be erased from *The Dentists Register* and the right to practise lost. Furthermore, it is clear that the frequency and size of litigation claims is rapidly increasing.

It is hardly necessary, therefore, to say that every effort should be made, as far as humanly possible, to avoid the risk of litigation.

General aspects of the dentist/patient relationship

It has to be accepted that, although the majority of patients seeking dental treatment are easy enough to get on with, there are a few who have been termed 'heartsink' patients,[3] whilst Gerard and Riddell[4] have analysed the types of behaviour of difficult patients who put stress on a practice. Although these are patients of a medical practice, most dentists will sooner or later have experience of similar types. These patients present a constant stream of complaints for which there is no discoverable organic cause. Gerard and Riddell[4] have suggested that these difficult patients fall into groups such as the following.

Family problems
The partners of an unhappy marriage may compete for attention and claim to be more worried about the other partner. Both may constantly complain that none of the treatments provided offer any benefit and in effect visit their hostility to one another on the doctor.

Punitive behaviour
The patient takes a close interest in medical matters and hopes to corner the doctor to show him to be wrong.

Excessive personal involvement in the patient's problems
Sympathy with a patient's serious genuine problems can lead to a dependent relationship, as a result of which objective assessment and management deteriorate.

Incompatibilities in culture and belief
A typical example quoted by Gerard and Riddell[4] is of a mother who persists in treating a child with severe asthma with homeopathic remedies, but is forced to accept conventional treatment when the child is *in extremis*. Antagonism is thus created between doctor and patient because of the disparity in their beliefs.

Medical complexity
The doctor may be made to feel inadequate by a patient with a complex or obscure illness and who has multiple expert opinions and may possibly even know more about the illness than the doctor.

Medical connections
Doctors, dentists and nurses or their families, can have excessive expectations about how they should be treated and create anxiety in the doctor or dentist that he/she may not come up to those expectations or that something may go wrong.

Manipulative patients
Patients with unusually sweet and flattering manners may, outside of the surgery, do their best to undermine the reputation of the doctor in the minds of other patients or doctors. Disruption of a practice can result.

Inevitably, many patients show several of these characteristics and are exceedingly difficult to manage, perhaps especially those who are manipulative and need to feel a sense of power over the doctor or dentist. Gerard and Riddell[4] also make very practical constructive suggestions as to how to manage these problems. However, it is likely to be considerably more difficult and probably undesirable for the dentist in such cases, to delve into family problems and intimate family secrets.

In addition to the different types of problem patients, who are otherwise healthy, there are also those who are depressed or disturbed in other ways, but are able to express their troubles only in terms of physical symptoms such as sore tongue or atypical facial pain. To dismiss such complaints as 'imagination', to get into arguments about their nature, or to suggest baldly that the patient needs psychiatric help is to invite trouble.

In practice it appears that many, perhaps even the majority of litigation claims, in the US in particular, are not truly the result of negligence, but rather the result of exasperation with the doctor or dentist. This in turn results from too casual or peremptory an approach to the patient's complaints, or even actual rudeness. The other major problem is that practitioners' records are often inadequate and there is too little to support the clinician's claims about what was said or what treatments were given. It is no oversimplification to say that (difficult though it may sometimes be) most medicolegal trouble could be avoided if the dental staff:

(1) are always pleasant to patients, maintain a friendly relationship with them and try to listen to and discuss their problems as fully as possible;[5]

(2) explain the nature of procedures to be carried out, and (within reason) the main risks, including the possibility that the treatment may not necessarily be completely successful in overcoming a particularly difficult problem. This especially applies to the provision of dentures and to tooth extraction which are common sources of medicolegal problems (see below);

(3) keep complete records not merely of work done but also of advice given in difficult cases.

Cynics might also add that it is prudent to carry these precautions to their limit when the patients are solicitors, barristers or their clerks, who have unusually ready access to litigation, and barrack room lawyers. However, a competent dentist practising to high standards should have no need to fear such patients.

The defence organisations

In the UK, these are the Medical and Dental Defence Union of Scotland (MDDUS), the Medical Defence Union (MDU) and the Medical Protection Society (MPS). The main objectives of the organisations are:

(1) To protect, support and safeguard the characters and interests of members.

(2) To provide unlimited indemnity against damages and costs (including settlements out of Court) awarded against a member in a case undertaken on his/her behalf and falling within the jurisdiction of home and overseas courts (but not cases arising from practice in the USA).

(3) To give advice and assistance with regard to any questions or problems affecting members' professional character or interests,

whether directly or indirectly (including the terms and conditions of service in salaried appointments and under the NHS).

(4) To defend members in cases where legal proceedings involving questions of professional principle or status are brought against them.

(5) To initiate proceedings for the protection of the professional interests of members.

(6) To take all proper proceedings to repress malpractice.

(7) To expose and bring to justice persons who may commit offences under any of the Acts relating to medical and dental practitioners, and also persons who may be concerned in making or supporting fraudulent or unjustifiable claims or charges against members.

Complications of dental practice

Potential sources of trouble include the following:
   Professional negligence;
   Professional misconduct;
   Breaches of National Health Service terms of service;
   Responsibilities under the Health and Safety at Work etc Act (*see* Chapter 6);
   Problems with employees or partnerships.

Professional negligence

Almost any complication of dentistry may be construed by an aggrieved patient as negligence. The possible complications of dental practice are also more numerous than might be expected. Killey and Kay,[2] for example, quote cases resulting from crushing patients' fingers, cuts or burns to lips and tongue, eye injuries, plaster squeezed into an old gunshot wound of the palate, swallowing parts of a mouth mirror, inhalation of inlays, reamers or teeth, swallowing the air turbine, dislocation and fractures of the jaw, assault (slapping the cheek of an hysterical child, or extractions without proper consent), a fire started and burns sustained by a patient during induction of anaesthesia, inhalation of a fragment of broken forceps, broken needles left in the tissues, extraction of the wrong tooth, accidental injection of antiseptics, corrosives and even of lighter fuel, failure to record teeth extracted as agreed by the patient, performing extractions on the wrong patient or on the wrong side of the mouth, swallowing a denture, severing the Achilles tendon and fracturing a foot during anaesthesia, deaths from inhaled throat packs or teeth, allegedly inadequate anaesthesia, failure to recognise bilateral dislocation of the mandible, burning with a hot water bottle, osteomyelitis after extractions, burns from faulty radiographic equipment, infection following an intravenous anaesthetic, and deaths from accidental inhalation of CO_2 and from intravenous and inhalational anaesthetics.

More recent examples, some of which have had to be settled at enormous cost, include the following taken at random from the Medical Protection Society's Annual Reports:

(1) Bell's palsy following an inferior dental block injection.

(2) Failure to take radiographs and to diagnose widespread dental caries in a child.

(3) Failure to diagnose and treat periodontal disease.

(4) Failure to keep a record of having informed a patient that roots had been retained after extractions.

(5) Failure to take an adequate medical history, and alleged triggering of epilepsy by prilocaine.

(6) Swallowing a prophylaxis brush which had not been properly fixed to the handpiece.

(7) Damage to the inferior dental nerve by endodontic treatment without radiographs.

(8) Injection of trichloroacetic acid with which the surgery assistant had filled a syringe in mistake for glycerine.

(9) Unsatisfactory dental implants.

(10) Ear and nerve damage resulting from mandibular condylotomy.

(11) Transmission of hepatitis B due to inadequate instrument sterilisation.

(12) Failure to give antibiotic prophylaxis against infective endocarditis.

In the past at least, the most common causes for complaints were for faulty dentures and for complications of extractions, particularly third molars. Such troubles should be avoidable if a dental surgeon does not attempt any procedures beyond his competence, and, equally important, explains the possible complications to the patient. Informed consent must be obtained for operative treatment. Nevertheless, there are patients for whom no denture is satisfactory, and in many cases it is impossible to find adequate criteria for a 'satisfactory' denture.

Negligence is usually defined as a 'failure to exercise reasonable skill and care' or 'omission to do something which a reasonable man or woman, guided by those considerations which ordinarily regulate the conduct of human affairs, would do, or something which a prudent and reasonable man or woman would not do'.

The interpretation of 'reasonable skill and care' depends on the situation. Every practitioner is expected to possess a certain degree of skill and to exercise care to the same standard as that exercised by the majority of his/her colleagues. However, he/she is not expected to possess the skill of the specialist, (unless he/she is one); equally, it would not be exercising 'reasonable care' if treatment were attempted which should be provided by a specialist, unless there are abnormal circumstances that warrant such action.

Reasonable skill and care must be exercised whether the patient be NHS, private, *or even being treated gratuitously.*

For a claim of negligence to succeed, it has to be proved that:
(1) The dentist owed a 'duty of care' to that patient in the prevailing circumstances.
(2) There was a breach of that duty.
(3) Damage was sustained as a result.

Time limits for actions in negligence
These are fixed by the Limitations Acts of 1939 and 1963, the Law Reform (Limitation of Actions) Act 1954 and by the Law Reform (Miscellaneous Provisions) Act 1971. These stipulate that, in cases involving personal injury arising from negligence, or breach of contract, an action must be started within 3 years of the incident from which the cause of the action arose (or, with the leave of the Court, within 3 years of when the Plaintiff became aware, or ought to have become aware, of a cause of action).

Res ipsa loquitur
This is a legal maxim which translated means 'the thing speaks for itself' and may be pleaded by the plaintiff in certain circumstances where the very nature of the incident is sufficient to suggest a lack of care. If the plea is accepted, then the onus is on the defendant to prove that he/she is not guilty of negligence but that some agency outside his/her control was responsible for the damage occasioned to the patient.

Vicarious liability
According to law, a master (employer) can be held responsible for any negligence on the part of a servant (employee) committed whilst

performing a duty of his employment; this is 'vicarious liability'. A dentist can thus be held responsible for all acts and omissions both of his/her lay and professional staff, *whether or not the member of staff involved was acting according to instructions given.* However, every individual still remains liable for his/her own acts and thus a claim in negligence could be brought against the servant, the master, or both.

A case has arisen where the principal of a practice was held responsible for a case of infective endocarditis after a locum tenens had failed to follow the instructions in the patient's notes and, as a consequence, failed to give prophylactic antibiotics.

Incorrect treatment
Incorrect treatment may give rise to allegations of negligence. These mistakes usually arise from the treatment of the wrong patient, the wrong side or the wrong tooth, and from failing to examine the patient and the record card adequately immediately before treatment.

Extractions
Difficulties can arise with the extraction of teeth both during and after operation unless the dentist:
(1) Obtains informed consent for the extractions and the use of anaesthesia.
(2) Gives the necessary pre-operative instructions.
(3) Takes pre-operative radiographs if any difficulties are anticipated.
(4) Ensures that only the correct teeth are extracted.
(5) Checks extracted teeth to determine whether they are complete. If incomplete, then the patient should be told (and this recorded) and a decision taken on whether or not to operate further.
(6) Checks that the number of teeth extracted corresponds with the treatment plan. If a tooth appears to be missing, the mouth should be searched and if this fails to reveal the missing tooth, abdominal and thoracic radiographs must be considered.
(8) Takes radiographs if a root has been fractured.
(9) Provides adequate post-operative attention.
(10) Advises the patient about post-operative care and where to contact the operator, out of hours, in the event of an emergency.

It is remarkably easy, in a busy practice with a full waiting room, to make a mistake with extractions. It is essential first to confirm the identity of the patient, then to check, with the patient's dental chart, precisely which teeth have to be extracted and that informed consent has been given both to the extraction and to the type of anaesthesia proposed. The kind of mistakes which have led to legal complications have been mentioned earlier.

Third molar surgery, in particular, is an area where unexpected complications are all too common. The possible medicolegal consequences of such operations have been reviewed by Haskell,[6] who points out that mere impaction of a third molar is not in itself an indication for its removal and that the operation should be attempted *only* when there is a firm indication for so doing.

A Consensus Development Conference on the removal of third molars[7] in 1979 also came to the conclusion that there was little evidence for the benefit of removal of third molars solely to prevent or relieve overcrowding of anterior teeth but that third molars should be extracted only if there was evidence of irreversible disease.

A large follow-up study on 11 598 patients with 3702 impacted but asymptomatic third molars which had remained untreated for an average period of 27 years, showed that the only significant complications were development of dentigerous cysts in 0·8%, periodontal ligament damage and bone loss distal to the second molar in 4·5%, or pressure resorption of the latter in 4·8%. There was no major increase in complications with increasing age. By contrast, 8·8% of 636 treated patients had complications, including one fracture of the mandible, as a result of the extractions.[8]

Even more important as a source of medicolegal claims and as a possible cause of fatal accidents, are the complications of general anaesthesia, as discussed later.

Antibiotic prophylaxis against infective endocarditis
One of the more common types of claim recently, has been for failure to provide antibiotic prophylaxis against infective endocarditis. This is often made particularly difficult for the practitioner by obsolete instructions, given to the patient by the family doctor or by the cardiologist, that *all* dental procedures should have antibiotic cover. It has been difficult for the dental practitioner to argue against such 'expert' advice, but this problem should be manageable by adherence to the advice given in the *Dental Practitioners' Formulary*. Although no antibiotics can be guaranteed to prevent infective endocarditis in a susceptible person, adherence to authoritative recommendations is

regarded as consistent with fulfilling the practitioner's professional obligations.[9]

Unfortunately, dental extractions happen to have been the first identified cause of bacteraemias in healthy persons, over half a century ago, and hence a possible cause of infective endocarditis. Although dental operations precede only 10% to 15% of cases of infective endocarditis, old ideas die hard and a cardiologist is likely to ascribe the disease to dental treatment, even if the events are purely coincidental or caused by bacteria not normally found in the mouth.

Another difficulty arises when a patient gives a history of having had rheumatic fever. Even in the few cases where this history can be substantiated, only approximately 30% of the patients will have sustained cardiac damage. In such cases, the patient can be referred to a cardiologist to confirm whether there is any heart disease; alternatively, the standard antibiotic prophylaxis can be given, even though in the majority of cases it would be unnecessary. It is particularly important, therefore, to inform the patient of possible risks from reactions to the antibiotic.

General anaesthesia and sedation

General anaesthesia and so-called sedation when an intravenous barbiturate is used (actually this is of course intravenous anaesthesia), are among the most dangerous procedures in dentistry. Most deaths in the dental surgery have resulted from these anaesthetics. Since the dental conditions for which these anaesthetics are given are not usually in themselves life-threatening, any significant morbidity, much less any mortality, from anaesthetics is unacceptable.

There is undoubtedly a need for general anaesthesia in dentistry, but only on relatively rare occasions. The indications have been clearly stated by the Joint Subcommittee on Dental Anaesthesia. The chief source of trouble is when the operator acts as anaesthetist. If a death results in these circumstances, not only are criminal charges possible, but erasure from *The Dentists Register* is a virtually inevitable consequence of the General Dental Council (GDC) disciplinary proceedings.

Operator anaesthetists frequently used to (and some still do) use an intravenous barbiturate, such as methohexitone. The latter is not merely an extremely powerful anaesthetic agent, but also a potent respiratory depressant and this property has probably been the main cause of deaths in the dental chair.

The other major hazard is that of obstruction of the airway and recently a case has resulted from a death under general anaesthesia, administered for provision of restorative work. Although the anaesthetic was administered by a medical colleague, neither an endotracheal tube nor an adequate throat pack had been inserted.

Deaths in the dental chair are likely to lead to an inquest and may occasionally result in a charge of manslaughter—a criminal charge.

Intravenous sedation with diazepam or midazolam is, by comparison, remarkably safe though, as discussed below, deaths have resulted during midazolam use. These benzodiazepines are only mild respiratory depressants and overdose may not have any serious consequences apart from delaying recovery. However, if sedation is enhanced by giving, in addition, an opioid such as pentazocine, then respiratory depression is greatly increased and can be fatal. Therefore, even intravenous sedation needs to be in expert hands.

The GDC have amended their *Notice for the guidance of dentists* and indicated the absolute minimum conditions acceptable for the administration of sedation (*see* p 304).

Contravention of these requirements may result in erasure from *The Dentists Register*. This has happened in a recent case, where a patient died after administration of midazolam alone. A leading article[10] noted that four deaths associated with midazolam (mainly given for conscious sedation) as well as 14 causes of other serious complications had been reported to the Committee on Safety of Medicines by November 1987.

Possible reasons for greater dangers from the administration of midazolam than from diazepam, are that midazolam is a considerably more potent drug and in sufficient dosage can produce general anaesthesia. Rapid administration of diazepam can cause apnoea, but this is transient. Rapid administration of midazolam, by contrast, may cause apnoea which persists long enough to be harmful. In addition, there is a suspicion, as yet unconfirmed, that the muscle relaxant effect of midazolam may be sufficient to weaken respiratory effort.

Recommended precautions are that, in view of wide inter-individual variation in response to midazolam and the greater sensitivity of the elderly to this drug, administration should be slow and carefully titrated to the response. Supplemental oxygen should also be given to compensate for the decreased saturation associated with administration of midazolam.

A postal survey carried out in the UK[11] showed that, in 1986, 20% of responding dentists carried no specific means of administering oxygen in an emergency and that about 37% of those using intravenous sedation did not possess emergency airways. Since only 40% of dentists replied to the questionnaire, it is highly likely that many more lacked resuscitative equipment.

There is a case for having, in the emergency box, the benzodiazepine antagonist flumazenil, to counteract overdosage or idiosyncratic responses, particularly to midazolam. In the case of diazepam, which is longer-acting than midazolam, it should be noted that flumazenil, has only a brief action, but it does not appear necessary to give it repeatedly until recovery is complete.

Benzodiazepine-associated fantasies
Several allegations of assault while under sedation, particularly with midazolam, have been made by women.[12] Absence of a trained assistant is, as mentioned earlier and noted on p 304, in contravention of the GDC's recommendations. Moreover, absence of such an assistant as a witness, also makes it difficult for the dentist to prove to the patient or the General Dental Council that there was no sexual interference.

Inhalational sedation with nitrous oxide and oxygen is generally safe (provided that consciousness is not lost), and is now the most widely used sedation technique according to the survey by Shirlaw *et al.*[11] Nitrous oxide and oxygen (relative analgesia), or intravenous sedation, together with local analgesia have considerably diminished the need for general anaesthesia for most patients, including many of those who are exceptionally nervous.

One area of doubt is whether nitrous oxide should be given during pregnancy. Nitrous oxide, as discussed in Chapters 1 and 3, depresses vitamin B12 metabolism. For adults, this effect is not significant after administration of nitrous oxide for less than 6 hours, but although there is as yet no direct evidence of foetal damage from nitrous oxide alone, some studies have suggested an increased rate of foetal loss in women who had had operations under general anaesthesia during pregnancy. With the increasing awareness among the public of the risk of congenital abnormalities or stillbirths which may result from administration of drugs, complications of this kind after anaesthesia (even if coincidental) could be a source of troublesome litigation.

Those who consider themselves expert operator–anaesthetists, and particularly those who persist in using intravenous barbiturates such as methohexitone or unconventional mixtures of drugs, should take note of a case in California, where there were no fewer than three deaths at the hands of a dentist, who administered a cocktail of methohexitone and other drugs. *The dentist was found guilty of second degree murder and sentenced to 15 years' imprisonment.* There have also been cases of dental manslaughter in Britain.

Another complication of anaesthesia which might, among other effects, form a medicolegal hazard is that of hepatitis after administration of halothane (Chapter 3). The risk is greatest after repeated administrations and this drug should not be repeated after an interval of less than 6 months. To do so, or to fail to take a history of previous administrations, with resulting hepatitis, could lead to claims for negligence.

Dentures
Many allegations of unsatisfactory treatment arise from the provision of dentures. The supplying of dentures comes under the Supply of Goods (Implied Terms) Act 1973, which means that a practitioner has a duty to produce 'goods' (dentures) suitable for the purpose for which they were intended and complying with the terms of the 'contract' agreed with the patient. Failure to achieve these requirements can result in either a failure to obtain the quoted fee or a successful claim by the patient for reimbursement of any fees already paid.

Providing treatment contrary to one's clinical opinion
Persuasive patients occasionally induce an unwise practitioner to provide treatment contrary to his/her clinical opinion and later allege negligence and/or refuse to pay the agreed fees. When such treatment has failed, it can be impossible to prove that 'reasonable skill and care' were, indeed, exercised.

Use of radiographs
Many dental conditions cannot properly be diagnosed without radiographic evidence. Failure to obtain radiographs can, if there is consequential damage to the patient, be deemed a failure to exercise 'reasonable skill and care'. The same applies if the radiographs are insufficient or unsuitable, under or over-exposed, incorrectly angled

or badly positioned, so as to prove of poor diagnostic value. Of course, the question of radiation safety is important (*see* Chapter 4).

Situations which normally require the addition of radiographic evidence include:

(1) Diagnosis of unerupted teeth (especially in orthodontic cases).

(2) Proposed extraction of misaligned or impacted teeth.

(3) Before and during provision of endodontic treatment.

(4) Assessment of the suitability of teeth to be crowned or used as bridge abutments.

(5) Detection of retained roots when such are suspected following a history of difficult extractions.

(6) Investigation of a source of infection.

(7) Suspected facial fractures or head injuries.

Consent

Evidence of consent is essential protection for the practitioner when a claim is made against him/her. In the absence of valid consent, even perfectly satisfactory treatment can be regarded as an assault. Obviously, the signing of a proper consent form indicating that the patient understands the implications of what is to be done, is virtually essential before a general anaesthetic is given.

The MPS booklet *Consent, confidentiality and disclosure of medical records* is a valuable guide to this sometimes complex issue. Only the main principles can be discussed here. Consent can be verbal or even implied. The fact that the patient has come (for example) with toothache to the dentist, implies that he wants something done about it. In most cases, satisfactory treatment is given and even if the patient's consent is not specifically asked for, no trouble results. Even so, it is always wise to describe the nature of the proposed treatment and a mumbled 'OK' will constitute consent. However, it is also possible for such a patient to make a claim even years after the event, so that a signed consent form is a valuable document confirming that the patient had agreed to receive appropriate treatment. The consent form, to be valid, should also indicate that the patient was informed of any likely risks. The general consent form recommended by the Medical Protection Society has proved to be satisfactory.

Informed consent

For consent to be valid it must be 'informed consent'; in other words the need for treatment and the form it will take must be *understood by the patient.* The practitioner must therefore give all appropriate information and in such terms that the patient is clear about the implications. Questions posed by the patient should be answered truthfully.

The nature of informed consent is a complex issue. The information must be sufficient for the patient to make a rational choice of whether or not to accept the proposed treatment. At the same time, it is clearly not possible to explain the nature of every possible complication of treatment (as some of the examples quoted earlier have shown) and this is not required by English law. Moreover, some patients have actually complained that they do not wish to be frightened by being told of too many possible complications.

The nebulous concept 'judgement' is therefore required if the dentist is to tell the patient enough, but not too much, about the risks of treatment. What information is to be given is a matter of the dentist's discretion, but its nature and in what terms it is given can still be challenged in court. It should also be borne in mind that dental treatment is rarely essential for the patient's survival and could frequently be regarded as being little more than cosmetic in nature. Serious complications from such treatment are therefore less acceptable than when dealing with a life-threatening emergency.

Any form of treatment (even an examination, or the taking of a radiograph) if carried out without the consent of the patient (or some person legally competent to give consent on his behalf) is an assault and, as such, may lead to legal action. However, the interest of the patient is always paramount, and the treatment of a true *emergency* should be based on clinical rather than legal considerations—nevertheless, only do that which is immediately essential. Consent must be obtained freely after explanation of the need for the procedure to be carried out. Consent obtained by duress (force, fear or fraud) is invalid.

Consent may be implied or expressed. The fact that a patient has made an appointment and elects to sit in the dental chair is implied consent to *an examination*, but nothing more. However, a specific verbal request to 'take this tooth out' clearly is expressed consent to the operation, although not to any particular form of anaesthesia. The advantage of having a third person present is obvious, since in any dispute as to what was said and agreed, it would be otherwise merely the patient's word against the dentist's. Make and keep good clinical records, including what was said to the patient.

Written consent is best, as it can be proved. It is particularly important to obtain this, either from the patient or from some other person competent to give it, when any procedure involves a special risk or when a general anaesthetic or sedation is to be given. Express permission should be obtained for anything other than dental examinations and for the withdrawal of blood for diagnostic purposes. For more complicated diagnostic procedures such as biopsy and for the various forms of endoscopy and isotope scans, written permission is best obtained, as for surgical operations. Written consent should refer to *one specific procedure*. 'Blanket' permission on admission to hospital to cover any subsequent procedures over any length of time, is inadequate.

Written consent should be obtained on a special form and witnessed in writing by a third, disinterested party. It is important to point out that the procedure may not be carried out by any particular dentist or doctor.

Finally, examination or treatment of female patients by male dentists should invariably be made in the presence of a female nurse or receptionist or, failing that, a female relative. *This is imperative when general anaesthetics or sedatives are being administered.*

Who can give consent

Adult patients. Conscious, mentally sound adults (persons over 16 years of age) give consent themselves (ages differ under Scottish law).

Adults unable to give consent. Mentally handicapped adults are in the same position as minors (see below) and permission is obtained from guardians, or the officer in charge of the institution in which they reside if no relatives are available.

Certified psychiatric in-patients compulsorily detained in an institution, may give their own consent to treatment if they are able to comprehend the nature of the procedure. If not, consent provision in the Mental Health Act 1983 may apply. Interestingly, the relatives have no legal standing in the matter.

Consent for routine treatment of *unconscious* adults is obtained from close relatives. In acute emergencies, when no relative is readily available, consent is justifiably dispensed with, but care must be taken that surgical procedures do not go beyond the minimum required to save life.

Minors. In England and Wales, Section 8 of the Family Law Reform Act (1969) fixes the age of consent at 16. If the treatment required by an adolescent is extensive or drastic, or requires a general anaesthetic then, except in the case of emergency, the dentist would be wise to consult the parents, having first informed the patient that he intends to do so.

The Act does not remove the power of the parents to give consent for treatment for anyone under the age of majority (ie under 18 years). For a patient under the age of 16 years, the consent of a parent or guardian should be obtained, although those under 16 can give valid consent if they understand the issues. Sometimes the permission of the person in *loco parentis* (such as the headmaster of a residential school) is obtained; however, if the situation constitutes an emergency, this is not absolutely necessary.

Where the parent or guardian of a minor refuses consent for an urgent diagnostic or therapeutic procedure, the dentist's position is governed partly by personal ethics and partly by law. This situation usually arises from religious objections, notably Jehovah's Witnesses, in respect of blood transfusion. Where transfusion or other procedures are held to be life-saving, the doctor or dentist may proceed according to his/her own conscience (and trust that the courts will support that view) or he/she may seek the help of the Children's Officer of the Local Authority. An emergency court can be convened at the bed-side at any time and a Magistrate may authorise the removal of the child's custody from the parents to a 'fit person', (usually a Children's Officer) who then gives consent to the procedure.

The Department of Health have directed that this mechanism be abandoned and if the doctor or dentist acts in good faith in urgent circumstances, his decision will be upheld against the parents' objections.

Emergencies. Consent is implied for life-saving measures, such as clearing an airway. However, any related, but less urgent problems, should be dealt with later, when consent can be obtained.

Examinations for medicolegal purposes. Examinations carried out at the request of a third party, may be to the potential detriment of the patient and therefore *consent* must be obtained from the patient or another competent person. No third party such as the police can authorise an examination without the patient's consent.

Express consent should always be obtained from the patient in these cases, since he may not have come voluntarily and, therefore, implied consent cannot be assumed. A third party should always be present when oral consent is obtained, and should witness in writing, a written form of consent.

The *victim* of alleged criminal actions, especially sexual assault, is another candidate for examinations requested by the police. Such examinations are usually carried out by a retained Police Surgeon, but, in an emergency or where none is available, any other practitioner may be requested to carry out the examination.

A person, accused or otherwise, has the right to be examined by a dentist of his or her own choice.

No employer has the right to force a dental examination upon an unwilling employee.

It has been normal practice for all children in State schools to be examined dentally. If parents refuse consent they should arrange for their own practitioner to conduct an alternative examination.

The effect of consent to a hazardous procedure
If a practitioner is aware that a certain operation carries a particular risk of damage to his/her patient, he/she must inform the patient accordingly when obtaining consent. The practitioner who attempts such an operation without informing the patient of the known hazard places him/herself at a much greater risk of subsequent legal action than when *informed* consent is obtained. If the expected damage materialises, the patient may, despite the informed consent given, attempt to sue the practitioner for negligence. To succeed in such a claim, the patient needs to prove that, although aware of the risk, the practitioner still failed to exercise *reasonable skill and care*, either in the manner of his/her operating, or even by attempting the operation him/herself instead of arranging for a more experienced colleague to undertake it.

Prevention of harm to patients
Apart from complications of treatment, other accidents are occasionally unavoidable, often through no fault of the practitioner. As discussed earlier (*see* Chapter 6), there are numerous hazards in the

premises apart from those directly associated with the practice of dentistry, many of which are quite unpredictable. In the event of any such incident, however, the practitioner's immediate duty is to care for his/her patient, to minimise the possibility of any more damaging effects.

As a general rule, the dentist should not admit any liability or offer compensation to a patient after such an accident. Obviously, however, there are some situations when a patient should be told of a mistake and an obvious example is the incorrect extraction of a tooth. Again, no offer of compensation should be made, but the practitioner's defence society must be informed immediately. The practitioner's duty to his/her patient remains, however, and regardless of circumstances, all possible clinical steps should be taken to alleviate the condition he/she has produced.

Confidentiality

The patient is entitled to information about his/her illness, within limits determined by the dentist, who alone can decide what measure of information should be disclosed. Conversely, a dentist's strict duty to his/her patient is not to disclose such information to any other person (including a relative), except those properly entitled to receive it. Naturally, the parents or guardians of small children are entitled to full disclosure, but as the age of a young person approaches 16 years, the position alters. The consent of a young person between 16 and 19 should be obtained before disclosure is made to the parents. Where a sensible, well-orientated young person even of 14 years is concerned, the doctor or dentist must judge for him/herself whether the patient's reluctance to allow disclosure to the parents should be honoured.

The Data Protection Act 1984 should be borne in mind. In brief, the effect of this act is that any personal information held *on a computer* must be accessible to that person. Failure to release any of this personal information can lead to a complaint to the Data Protection Registrar or proceedings by the complainant in a court or tribunal or both. Handwritten information, it should be noted, does not come under this Act.

Professional confidences

Professional confidences may be broken only under one of the following conditions. Your medical defence society should be consulted in most cases beforehand:

(1) Consent of the patient to disclosure of relevant information;
(2) As a statutory duty laid down by law (eg Misuse of Drugs Act 1971);
(3) By order of a Court of Law;
(4) In the interests of the community (an especially contentious concept).

Disclosure of medical or dental records

(1) As a general rule, records should be released only to another practitioner and should not be released to a lay person without good cause.
(2) In hospital, the notes of any NHS patient belong to the hospital authority and not to the practitioner in charge.
(3) Where any legal action concerning negligence of dental or nursing staff is concerned or even suspected, records should not be allowed into the hands of solicitors without prior consultation with the defence society (but see (7) below).
(4) Records should not be given to employers, insurance companies or their representatives without the consent of the patient (or his/her immediate relatives, if he/she is mentally incapacitated or deceased).
(5) In cases not concerning the reputation of the dentist or hospital, no reasonable request for records should be refused from solicitors or insurance companies dealing with compensation claims, etc, providing the patient's consent has been obtained.
(6) Although patients have right of access to their records, the records should not normally be given to the patient if the information therein would be harmful to his/her own interests; nevertheless, the Data Protection Act must be adhered to.
(7) The only absolute authority that obliges release of records is a court order for 'discovery' of such documents. However, recent changes in the law have made it easier for lawyers to obtain records, even where a case has not yet been set down for trial. Thus, solicitors can now peruse clinical records to see if there might be sufficient grounds to bring a legal action.
(8) Dubious requests should be referred to the medical defence society.

Privileged communications

Confidences or defamatory statements divulged by the doctor or dentist are liable to civil action unless there is indemnity from civil action, given by law in two degrees.

Absolute privilege is that which applies to any statements made in a Court of Law (or Parliament) and extends to statements made to solicitors or barristers in the course of preparation for a Court hearing. Nothing said in these circumstances can be used as grounds for an action for slander.

Qualified privilege. Outside a Court of Law, certain breaches of confidence or defamatory statements by a doctor or dentist may be protected if certain conditions are observed. The statement must not be malicious and must be made in good faith to a party having a duty to receive it.

Reports to the police

A dental practitioner may be approached by the police for information relating to a patient. Before any statement is given, the reasons for the request should be ascertained and then the unwritten rules of 'confidentiality' should be considered.

The most common situations which give rise to such approaches are:

(1) A check on the whereabouts of a suspected person on a particular day and time.

(2) To obtain evidence of an assault by a person other than the practitioner.

(3) To obtain dental identification of an unconscious or deceased person, or one suffering from loss of memory.

(4) Through the use of forensic odontology to establish the guilt or otherwise of persons suspected of murder or assault, coupled with the infliction of bites.

(5) A complaint received by the police that the practitioner had assaulted a patient (bodily or indecently).

The reasons for the requested information must determine the practitioner's decision to assist or not to assist without the permission of the patient (parent or guardian in the case of a minor). Where the identification of a deceased person is involved, a practitioner should have no hesitation in assisting the authorities, as many processes of law, helpful to relatives, cannot be put into operation until death has been legally established.

Requests by the authorities for the dental records to identify victims killed in air crashes and other major disasters, and victims of death by accident or suicide should also be honoured.

No persons, except in very special circumstances (Road Traffic Act, 1972; see below) *has* to make a statement to, or reply to questions from, the police. When a practitioner accepts that his duty is to cooperate with the police he might be well advised to inform the latter that he will provide a written statement. Verbal statements made on the spot can be unfortunately phrased and thereby misconstrued. A written statement made in the practitioner's own time can be checked and double-checked before submission. This is particularly important when clinical details of injuries received by a patient need to be incorporated.

Road Traffic Act 1972
Section 168 of this Act provides that where the driver of a vehicle is alleged to be guilty of certain traffic offences, the person keeping the vehicle (the owner) or *any other person* 'shall if required give any information which it is in his or her power to give and may lead to the identification of the driver' (includes a person riding a cycle).

Notification of police. There are times when the practitioner may feel inclined to notify the police about the actions of a patient. In general, unless the patient gives consent, the practitioner should make no effort to notify the police unless:

(1) There is the possibility of repetition of grave illness or even death, such as might follow from the persistent activities of a professional abortionist, using septic methods.

(2) Where evidence of attempted poisoning exists, further medical proof should be obtained, and attempts made to persuade the patient to consent to disclosure. It has been suggested that any approach to the authorities in such a case should be via a private interview with a senior police officer or Chief Constable.

(3) A more common circumstance is in connection with injuries to children which are suspected of being inflicted by the parents (child abuse). The decision to break professional confidence in such circumstances can be most difficult, but is vital if further injury and even the death of a child is to be averted. Careful records, including photographs, should be kept. The opinion of a doctor or paediatrician should be obtained and where a decision is made, the doctor should seek the assistance of specialised officers in child welfare (Inspectors of the National Society for Prevention of Cruelty to Children and Children's Officers) rather than approach the police.

Ethical relations with colleagues

The greatest care should be taken when dealing with a patient, not to criticise or denigrate the professional ability of another, even by innocent implication. Differences of opinion over diagnosis and treatment are legitimate, but should be conveyed in a way which will not undermine the patient's confidence in the other practitioner. Where there is a significant difference of opinion, this should be settled by direct contact between the two practitioners, not via the patient.

Treatment in practice

Where the patient of another practitioner attends a second practitioner for diagnosis or treatment, the patient should be advised to return to his/her own practitioner. If he/she refuses, the best course is to contact the original dentist and settle the matter in a way which arouses no professional controversy. Under the NHS, a patient may change dentists at will.

Treatment in hospital

In the case of an in-patient in hospital, the dental officer to the institution should carry out the dental treatment demanded by the patient's general condition. If further dental treatment is necessary, nothing should be done to influence the patient's free choice of dentist.

In the case of a patient attending the out-patient department, the dental officer to the institution should advise on any dental treatment necessitated by the patient's general condition; if treatment is necessary, nothing should be done to influence the patient's free choice of dentist. It is unethical for a hospital dental officer to use his position to influence patients to consult either him/herself or a colleague in a private capacity.

In all cases, where treatment in hospital is given to a patient referred by another practitioner, full information concerning that treatment should be passed on to the patient's own practitioner (and without undue delay). There should be no undue extension of supervision, after the patient has been discharged, and the patient should be returned to the care of his/her own practitioner within the limits of the individual case and the complexity of the treatment. This emphasises the need for early and full communication between hospital and the general practitioner, so that appropriate treatment may be continued by the latter.

Dichotomy
The practitioner's choice of consultant should be determined solely by his/her opinion on the suitability of the specialist to advise in the given case, and not to any personal association, especially in the matter of a fee. Dichotomy is not only unethical, but constitutes a bribe in contravention of the Prevention of Corruption Act. Whether criminal proceedings arise or not, the practice might lead to disciplinary proceedings before the GDC.

Complaints by patients
Verbal complaints from patients should be dealt with as tactfully as possible. Where the patient's comments suggest poor quality of treatment, the matter should be referred to the medical defence society. Written complaints should be referred, *unanswered*, to the medical defence society.

Breaches of NHS terms of service—Dental Service Committee
Dental surgeons working within the NHS are under contract to their Family Health Services Authority (FHSA). Under this contract, the dentist is required (among other considerations) to employ a proper degree of skill and attention in his/her work and provide such treatment as the patient is prepared to undergo, to maintain oral health. In addition, of course, he/she should not make any claims for work that he/she has not done, or claim for work excluded by the provisions of the Scale of Fees.

Any complaints are normally dealt with by the Dental Service Committees (DSCs) set up by the local FPCs. However, Noar[13] has pointed out that the Schanschieff report recommends that allegations of overtreatment should be dealt with by the FPC itself, rather than by the Local Dental Committee.

A Dental Service Committee consists of a lay chairman, three dentists appointed by the Local Dental Committee and three lay persons appointed by the FPC.

Complaints about poor quality of dental treatment or overtreatment may come from patients or from the Dental Practice Board

(DPB). The statutory time limits are that the complaint should be made within '6 months after the completion of treatment or within 13 weeks after the matter which gave rise to the complaint came to the complainant's notice'.

If the complaint justifies formal investigation, the FPC will write to the practitioner asking for written observations about the complaint to be submitted within 28 days. However, *before* any such report is submitted, the dentist is strongly advised to consult his medical defence society.

Unless the complaint is trivial in nature, an oral hearing is then usually held and provides an opportunity for both the complainant and the dental surgeon to present their cases. However, if the complaint is found to have been justified, the Dental Services Committee can recommend to the FPC one of several possible alternatives. These are:

(1) That the dentist be warned to comply more closely with his/her Terms of Service.

(2) To deduct from the dentist's remuneration, a sum to cover any reasonable expenses incurred by anyone as a result of the breach of Terms of Service.

(3) To make a further financial withholding from the dentist's remuneration.

(4) To determine a period during which everything except examinations or emergency treatment, must be submitted for prior approval by the DPB.

(5) To carry out an enquiry by the National Health Service Tribunal to consider whether the dentist should remain on the Dental List.

Clearly, complaints to the FPC must be taken seriously. Moreover, if the case is regarded as sufficiently serious and results in the withholding of at least £750, the case may also be referred to the General Dental Council to consider whether the dentist has been guilty of professional misconduct. If so, the consequences can be even more serious.

Misconduct

Professional misconduct
In so far as they apply to dental practice, dental practitioners, like doctors, should abide by:

(1) The Hippocratic Oath (p 306).

(2) The Declaration of Geneva (p 307).

(3) The International Code of Medical Ethics (p 308).

(4) The Declaration of Lisbon regarding the Rights of Patients (p 309).

The terms of these documents are given in full in the Appendices, but there are many aspects of the International Code of Medical Ethics (1983) which may not apply to the practice of dentistry. Nevertheless, relevant to the publicity recently given to overprescribing (usually unnecessary restorative work or orthodontics), this document specifically states: 'A physician shall not permit motives of profit to influence the free and independent exercise of professional judgement on behalf of patients'.

It is also important to emphasise here the rights of the patient, and to note in particular, the following:

(1) The patient has the right to choose a physician (or dentist) freely.

(2) The patient has a right to be cared for by a physician who is free to make clinical and ethical judgements without any outside interference.

(3) The patient has a right to accept or refuse treatment *after receiving adequate information.*

Curiously, the phrasing of this Declaration does not seem specifically to indicate that the patient should receive adequate information about the nature of treatment advised and its possible consequences, but it is undoubtedly desirable that a patient should sign an adequate consent form for any dental procedure where there is any significant element of risk. If unforeseen complications arise, lack of a signed consent form may complicate the medicolegal consequences.

The sustaining of a charge of professional misconduct is particularly harmful to the dental surgeon, as it can lead to withdrawal of Registration by the General Dental Council and loss of livelihood. Professional misconduct includes both unprofessional behaviour towards patients, such as sexual or non-sexual assault, and also criminal offences. The latter include both those related to and those unrelated to dentistry. In the former category is defraudment of the Dental Practice Board. In the latter category are obvious types of criminal behaviour, including such offences as unlawful possession of drugs, theft and driving under the influence of drink or drugs.

It is also worth remembering that failure to pay the annual Registration Fee (even if not deliberate), can lead to erasure from *The*

Dentists Register. Indeed, there has been an increase in the number of dentists and hygienists who have been instructed to cease practising by the GDC as a result of not being registered in the current *Dentists Register* or *Hygienists' Roll*. In at least one case, the dentist had failed to pay his annual retention fee, merely because he had failed to notify the GDC of his change of address and had not, as a consequence, received his renewal notice. As a result, he had to face the charge of unlawful practice in a Magistrate's Court. He was fined and had to pay part of the prosecution's costs, even though it was accepted that his offence was not wilful but merely due to inefficiency. The offence of carrying out dental practice when the person's name does not appear in the current *Dentists Register* is punishable on conviction by a fine of up to £1000.

Although complaints may be dealt with initially by such bodies as the Dental Services Committees or the GDC, this may not be the end of the matter. Some offences, such as unlawful possession of drugs or failure to pay the annual retention fee for *The Dentists Register* (even if not wilful) can lead to criminal proceedings. It should also be noted that criminal convictions other than minor motoring offences, are automatically reported to the GDC, who are likely to initiate disciplinary procedures to establish whether the facts also give rise to the charge of serious professional misconduct and, if so, to take appropriate action (fig. 7.1).

Expert opinions and the dental report

Actions for negligence depend not merely on the patient's allegations, but usually also on the support of this claim by the opinions, obtained by the patient's solicitor, from other dentists or doctors, who are regarded as experts in the area of dentistry concerned. This however assumes, but alas it is not always the case, that so-called 'experts', who are often professors or consultants in dental subjects, keep abreast of their subject.

General dental practitioners can also be asked to produce an expert report on treatment by another practitioner. The subject of the Dental Report has been dealt with in detail by Hill,[14] who points out that such reports have the following components:

(1) A statement by the patient of the details of the dental treatment.
(2) A statement of the nature of the patient's complaint about this treatment.
(3) A medical history where relevant.

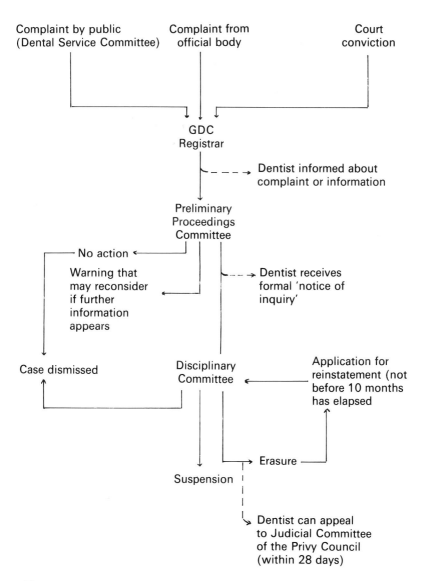

Fig. 7.1 Disciplinary procedures of the General Dental Council (*see also* p 300).

(4) Details of clinical and other investigations, such as radiographs.

(5) An opinion as to whether or not this treatment could or could not be regarded as satisfactory *under the circumstances.*

As Hill[14] points out, the practitioner making the report should only apply standards that would be applicable to his/her own work. He/she should avoid the term 'negligence' in the report. The term 'negligence' should only be used if, in the dentist's opinion, the work fell below the standard expected of a reasonable dentist of similar training, skill or experience. In civil law, 'negligence' does not mean neglect or moral blameworthiness. The dentist should also resist attempts by the solicitor to persuade him/her to estimate the price of replacing unsatisfactory work.

Preparing a report is a time-consuming business and frequently also generates a considerable amount of correspondence. The practitioner can therefore request an appropriate fee for the use of this time and expertise.

Difficulties with employees or partners (*see also* Chapter 6)

There have been numerous complaints of unfair dismissals by employees. In one such case, an angry dentist had also thrown a steriliser lead at his receptionist and raised a bruise on her head. Although a settlement was made out of court, this could have led to a private prosecution for common assault as well as to a police prosecution for common assault and for assault occasioning actual bodily harm.

In other cases, there have been complaints of sexual harassment, and sometimes the case has been complicated by emotional involvement between the dentist and the employee. Whether or not such cases are dismissed, the Medical Protection Society points out that the hearings of Industrial Tribunals are not private. The result may be that the press report the case in excessive detail and cause the dentist (who may be innocent) considerable embarrassment. This can damage his/her professional reputation, and the case may be drawn to the attention of the GDC. In addition, attendances at the Tribunal cause loss of time from the practice and other irritations.

Because of the risk of charges of unfair dismissal and even greater problems if the employee claims that this was due to racial discrimination, enormous care must be taken when choosing a new employee or in providing adequate evidence of, for example, embezzlement when dismissing an employee.

An example of how complex a case of a claim for unfair dismissal can become, was described recently by the Medical Protection Society who were able to help their member. A DSA/receptionist claimed unfair dismissal after repeated warnings for poor time-keeping. The Society's solicitors, however, successfully argued that the Tribunal had no jurisdiction to consider the application, because the plaintiff had been in the dentist's employment for less than 2 years. Although she had been employed by him at a previous practice, there had been a gap between the two jobs and hence a break in the continuity of the employment.

In addition, the Tribunal indicated to the nurse that she could claim unfair sex discrimination because of pregnancy. In such a claim, the 2 years' continuous employment conditions did not apply. However, this was successfully countered by the argument that for the nurse to claim sexual discrimination, it would be necessary, in a business with fewer than five employees, for her to provide evidence of victimisation by the dentist. Such a claim would have to show that (in effect) positive steps had been taken to prevent her from being treated equally under the Equal Pay Act or Sex Discrimination Act and that she was treated less favourably than any other employee in the circumstances.

In another case, a dentist dismissed a receptionist after complaints about her overbearing manner to patients. A member of staff had also left because of her rudeness and antagonism. The dentist accordingly spoke to the receptionist about these complaints and, later, sent a letter of dismissal. The receptionist brought an application for unfair dismissal. The dentist was advised that (a) he had acted precipitately and that a proper warnings procedure should have been followed in such a case; (b) he should have allowed the receptionist more time to act on his complaints and (c) he had damaged his case by giving the receptionist a good reference. The probability of the Tribunal finding against the dentist was therefore high and, on the advice of the defence society, the case was settled out of court by the dentist.

Employment Law—recent trends
The Medical Protection Society encourages practitioner employers to obtain a copy of the ACAS Code of Practice. Indeed, it is highly advisable to do so. Among other points, this code emphasises the need to set out, in a contract of employment, the type of conduct that would lead to dismissal or summary dismissal (*see also* Chapter 6).

Examples of such conduct include theft, persistent absences without explanation and abusive or insubordinate behaviour. It is also necessary to follow a proper warnings procedure, to take immediate action to investigate any alleged misconduct and then allow the employee to put his or her side of the case.

The courts have, incidentally, confirmed that the test of whether an employee was fairly dismissed for theft depended on whether the employer has genuine reasons to believe that the employee was guilty when dismissed. A later acquittal of the employee by a criminal court does not necessarily cause the dismissal to be unfair, since criminal courts have to apply totally different standards of proof and, in particular, that the crime was committed 'beyond reasonable doubt'.

Other difficulties with employees could arise from failure to comply with the Health and Safety at Work etc Act (*see* Chapter 6) or to supply a contract of employment, including an adequate job description, within the statutory period.

Partnerships
It is common for dentists to practise together without any formal, written agreement. This frequently works well, but can have unfortunate consequences. Problems can also result from entering into a formal agreement without adequate consideration of the terms. For example, a newly-qualified practitioner was unable to escape the consequences of an onerous and unreasonable partnership agreement he had signed and which penalised him financially.

Defence societies do not intervene in disputes between partners or between partners and their assistants or associates, but may offer valuable advice when there are disputes between professionals and may be able to help with arbitration or conciliation procedures. The Medical Protection Society also publishes a helpful booklet (*Considering partnership*), which sets out the main questions that must be answered when entering into a partnership.

Fitness for practice

The Health Committee of the GDC has jurisdiction over dentists whose fitness to practise is seriously impaired by their physical or mental condition. Moreover, the Health Committee has had to direct the Registrar to suspend the registrations of several dentists whose fitness to practise was found, after investigation, to be seriously impaired.

Fitness to practise would be impaired particularly by alcoholism or dependence on other drugs, and, under such circumstances, the Health Committee can recommend that a practitioner should undergo treatment or remain under medical supervision. Continued registration of a dentist can also be conditional upon compliance, for a period of up to 3 years, with other requirements considered by the Committee to be necessary in the interests of the public or of the dentist him/herself. Such requirements might be that the dentist should only work with a colleague, or should only undertake certain types of work.

Dependence on drugs

In mentioning this problem, aspects of which have already been discussed in Chapters 1 and 3, it is important to remember that alcohol is the most widely abused drug. In addition, benzodiazepines and anaesthetic agents, particularly nitrous oxide, can be abused by dentists.

Drug abuse is not merely a possible cause of loss of right to practise; the drug-dependent dentist can also cause considerable problems for patients, staff, family and professional colleagues, as discussed later.

Very little is known about what leads to drug dependence. There appears to be a small genctic component to alcoholism, but more important, intolerable stress and easy access to drugs (particularly alcohol) increase the likelihood of abuse. Knowledge about drugs and their ill-effects seems to offer no protection and there is reason to believe that the incidence of drug abuse by doctors and dentists is higher than by comparable groups of the population.

Little is known about the level of drug abuse by dentists in the UK, but some information is available from the US, as discussed in Chapter 1. Occasionally, cases come to light as a result, for example, of accidents to patients, or police cases when a dentist has been found to be in illegal possession of drugs. Cases only rarely appear before the GDC; those that do probably represent only the tip of the iceberg.

Offences stemming from drug abuse

The hazards to the dentist's right to practise as a result of drug abuse stem from:

(1) Unfitness to practise as a consequence of abuse;
(2) Illegal possession of controlled drugs;
(3) Illegal prescribing or falsifying prescriptions;
(4) Other criminal offences (such as lethal car accidents) secondary to drug abuse.

At one time, a doctor was virtually automatically struck off the Register if found to be drunk in charge of a motor vehicle. This has happened when the vehicle was stationary and the doctor was not even in the driving seat. In view of the possibility of random breath tests for motorists, and the greatly increased public concern about drunk drivers, even greater care must be taken by the doctor or dentist not to break the law in this way.

As one of the prices that doctors and dentists therefore have to pay for belonging to professions, in the true sense of the word, is that there are greater than normal restraints on their behaviour. Thus, for a non-professional, it is not necessarily an offence to be drunk at work, provided that he is not disorderly. Doctors and dentists, by contrast, if drunk when dealing with patients, could rightly be regarded as unfit to practise and have their right to practise limited or removed.

Abuse of anaesthetic agents
A special hazard for dentists and anaesthetists is that of nitrous oxide abuse. Nitrous oxide has similar properties to morphine and related drugs, but is not a Controlled Drug. The main way by which nitrous oxide abuse among dentists has come to light is as a consequence of neurological damage resulting from long-term inhalation (*see* Chapters 1, 2 and 3). The main safety factor with nitrous oxide abuse by dentists is that its inebriating effects wear off rapidly, and they are unlikely to be so unwise as to continue sniffing the gas in their patients' presence. By contrast, nitrous oxide sniffing by anaesthetists during long operations has lead to anaesthetic deaths or irreversible brain damage among patients, as a result of the anaesthetist's drowsiness.

Other inhalational anaesthetics have been abused almost since they were first introduced. A remarkable illustration of this risk was the 'ether revels' that were a well recognised phenomenon in nineteenth century America, despite the strongly puritanical ethos of the period and despite the pungent odour and irritating character of the drug. The risk of abuse of such substances as halothane or enflurane by dentists seems to be small but should not be dismissed. Unlike nitrous oxide, these fluids can easily be carried by the addict and surreptitiously abused. In America, for example, a nurse who was admitted to hospital for hypertension was found to have renal calcinosis and skeletal sclerosis due to fluoride intoxication. This was secondary to abuse of methoxyflurane (an antecedent of enflurane) which she sniffed from a soaked handkerchief even after admission to hospital.

Habits such as this in a dentist could readily lead to charges of unfitness to practise and referral to the Health Committee of the GDC. In addition, there can be serious risks to health. The neurological damage from prolonged abuse of nitrous oxide has been mentioned, while abuse of halothane could lead to severe hepatitis or even fatal liver damage (Chapter 3).

Illegal prescribing
This is another aspect of drug abuse. An illustrative example is a dentist who had become dependent on Distalgesic (which contains the opioid dextropropoxyphene); he lost the right to practise as a result of putting a false name on a prescription to obtain additional supplies of this drug for himself. Erasure from *The Dentists Register* followed this offence, even though Distalgesic was not a Controlled Drug.

Measures to deal with drug abuse among dental staff
There is understandable concern in the US, particularly about drug dependence among health professionals. In view of the regularity with which so many Britons follow American habits and fashions, and indeed have slavishly followed the American patterns of drug abuse, it seems prudent to note the American Dental Association's Report (Chemical Dependency (sic) and Dental Practice)[15] which describes the problems of dealing with drug dependence among dentists (*see* Chapter 1).

Statements in the ADA Report, from dentists who had become hopelessly dependent on nitrous oxide, cocaine and alcohol, and the opioid oxycodone, give some idea of the destructive effects of these habits on dental practice and family life. As the ADA Report points out, those who are drug-dependent become incapable of realistic perception of their abnormal behaviour and therefore of seeking help. Frequently also, the family and professional colleagues protect the addict from the consequences of his/her habit and thereby maintain the state of dependence. Unlikely though this may sound, there has been, in the past at least, a curious sympathy for the alcoholic. Moreover, the family and colleagues are likely to fear the emotional disturbance or hostility from the addict in response to any suggestion that help is needed and to any efforts to obtain such help. Colleagues also dislike the idea of betraying another professional. Nevertheless, in addition to the risk to the drug-dependent dentist's right to practise, his/her erratic behaviour can cause considerable problems to partners or other colleagues and can endanger patients and the reputation of a practice.

Signs that a dentist may be drug-dependent include increasing withdrawal from family or social activity, erratic attendance at or unexplained absences from work, deterioration in the quality of work, accidents (often minor but increasingly frequent) and deterioration in personal hygiene and mode of dress. In addition, whispers of irregular behaviour may reach a colleague from social contacts, or there may be complaints from patients who wish to transfer to another member of the practice. It is essential, therefore, to persuade the drug-dependent dentist to seek sympathetic expert help, which ensures anonymity and confidentiality. Such help is available through an organisation such as the Medical Protection Society or professional self-help groups, as advertised in professional journals. Such help should be sought before there are any truly disastrous consequences.

In view of the seriousness and dimensions of this problem, a special group, the Doctors' and Dentists' Group, has been set up to provide informal personal help to alcoholic or drug-dependent doctors and dentists, and their families.

Help with health problems
The Sick Dentist. The General Dental Services Committee (GDSC) have a sick dentist scheme (p 310). Help is obtainable through the Local Dental Committee secretary, BDA Branch or Section secretaries, or Family Practitioner Committee (FPC) administrators (fig. 7.2). A British Doctors' and Dentists' Group (BDDG) is now available for advice on alcohol or drug abuse*.
The Health Committee of the General Dental Council. The Dentists' Act 1984, gives the GDC jurisdiction in cases where the fitness to

---

*Details can be found at the end of the chapter.

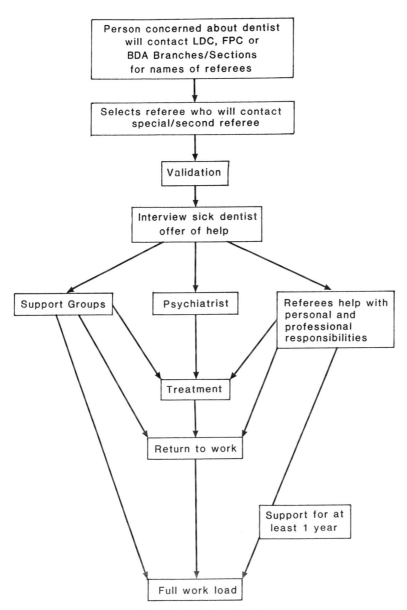

Fig. 7.2 Sick Dentist's scheme.

practise of a dentist is seriously impaired by reason of his physical or mental condition. The Act requires the GDC to make rules to govern the consideration of such cases and to establish a Health Committee to which the cases must eventually be referred. The rules, made after consultation with professional bodies, are approved by the Privy Council as the Health Committee (Procedure) Rules 1984.

When the GDC receives information suggesting that the fitness to practise of a dentist may be seriously impaired, the information is first considered by the President or another member of the GDC appointed for the purpose. If he/she is satisfied from the evidence that the dentist's fitness to practise is seriously impaired, the dentist is then informed accordingly and invited to agree within 14 days to submit to examination by at least two medical examiners. These medical examiners are chosen by the President from panels of examiners nominated by professional bodies. Examiners are nominated in all parts of the United Kingdom, so that examinations may be arranged locally if this is considered appropriate. It is also open to the dentist at this stage both to nominate other medical practitioners to carry out the examination and report to the President on his/her fitness to practise and to submit observations or other relevant evidence with regard to this. The dentist should also consult a medical defence society and, if a member, the British Dental Association (BDA).

Where a dentist agrees to submit to examination, the medical examiners are asked to report on his/her fitness to engage in practice, either generally or on a limited basis and on the management of his/her case, which they recommend. Where the dentist refuses to be medically examined, or the medical examiners report unanimously that the dentist is not fit to practise at all, or only to a limited degree, the President may invite the dentist to attend a meeting of the Health Committee. The same applies in the case of a difference of opinion among the medical examiners, but it appears to the President that the dentist may not be fit to practise except to a limited degree. Cases may occasionally be referred to the Health Committee by the Preliminary Proceedings Committee of the GDC or Professional Conduct Committee of the GDC, where a dentist has been convicted or is alleged to have committed serious professional misconduct, but it appears to either Committee that the dentist's fitness to practise may be seriously impaired by reason of a physical or mental condition.

The Health Committee meets in private and, in most cases, the principal evidence before it consists of the reports of the medical examiners. Its proceedings are regulated by set rules and are of a judicial nature. The Health Committee is assisted both by a legal assessor and by medical assessors. The medical assessors are chosen by the President, with regard to the physical or mental condition which is alleged to impair the dentist's fitness to practise, from panels nominated by professional bodies.

The Health Committee may, if it thinks fit, either adjourn consideration of a case or proceed to determine whether the dentist's fitness to practise is seriously impaired; it may impose conditions upon his/her registration for a period not exceeding 3 years or suspend registration for a period not exceeding 12 months. Cases where conditions have been imposed or a dentist's registration has been suspended are reviewed by the Health Committee from time to time.

There is a right of appeal to the Judicial Committee of the Privy Council against a direction of the Health Committee, but only on a question of law.

The Misuse of Drugs Act 1971

In addition to the risk of the dentist becoming dependent on drugs, there is also the risk of his/her supplying, knowingly or unknowingly, drugs to another dependent person. Controlled Drugs covered by the Misuse of Drugs Act 1971 are drugs whose use can lead to dependence (addiction); the main groups are morphine and similar drugs (opioids), most barbiturates and stimulant drugs such as cocaine and amphetamine.

Offences under the Misuse of Drugs Act are criminal offences. The main examples are supplying such drugs without any medical indication (namely for the purposes of abuse) and possession of these drugs without the legal provisions for doing so and for personal use.

The dentist can legally prescribe any of these drugs where there is a genuine clinical indication. Pethidine, for example, could be justifiably prescribed for post-operative pain and it is even permissible to prescribe it for a known addict if there is a genuine clinical indication. However, to do this the prescription has to be in a specified form in the practitioner's own handwriting and known to the pharmacist. The prescription is not repeatable and *must* incorporate the words 'for dental treatment only'.

Within the terms of the NHS, the only Controlled Drugs currently prescribable are pethidine and pentazocine. However, any Controlled Drug can be prescribed *when there is a clinical indication for doing so and at the patient's expense*. However, there is hardly ever any justification for so doing.

The dentist can also keep a stock of Controlled Drugs (providing that the conditions for obtaining and storing them, and keeping the necessary records, are fulfilled) if he/she feels there is a clinical need. It is allowable, for example, to keep morphine in stock for emergency treatment of myocardial infarction in the dental surgery, or of cocaine for occasions when local anaesthesia is ineffective. This may happen particularly in apicectomies.

In practice, the nuisance of having to fulfil the regulations is probably great enough to discourage most practitioners from using or stocking any of these drugs. In addition, keeping a stock brings with it the risk of thefts by or for addicts, and the consequent attention of the police.

Civil and criminal cases

It may be helpful to indicate the nature of the differences between these two types of cases. Civil cases arc usually of no interest to the GDC. Criminal convictions, on the other hand, usually precipitate a disciplinary enquiry at the very least.

Cases dealt with by civil law are those offences which adversely affect the private rights of individuals. Actions for alleged negligence, breach of contract, divorce or libel are examples of civil law. Civil cases are dealt with in the County Courts or in the High Court of Justice (usually the Queen's Bench Division for alleged negligence). A jury is called only for special reasons, such as actions for libel. If the plaintiff succeeds in a civil case, the defendant (the dentist) may be required to give compensation for up to £5000 in a County Court or a larger amount in the High Court.

Criminal charges typically involve the police. Minor offences are tried in a Magistrates' Court, without a jury, while major offences are tried in the Crown Court. Criminal offences which a dentist might commit in relation to dental practice are common or indecent assault on a patient, fraud (particularly against the National Health Service) or theft, misuse of drugs, serious evasions of income tax or practice without his/her name appearing in *The Dentists Register*. Criminal negligence, such as the death of a patient in the chair as a consequence of gross and reckless conduct, would also bring about a criminal charge. Criminal and civil law may overlap in certain cases and criminal negligence is an example of an offence which has somewhat ill-defined boundaries. In essence, it is the practice of dentistry of such a kind as to be without any regard to the professional duties due to a patient and resulting in severe injury or even death.

The death of a patient in the dental surgery or allegedly resulting from dental treatment or anaesthesia is considered initially by a coroner. A coroner is a barrister or solicitor, or a registered medical practitioner of at least 5 years' standing, who may also have either of these legal qualifications. If the coroner finds that the death was not from natural causes, or if there is any doubt about the matter, then an inquest is convened in the coroner's court. In Scotland, however, these matters are dealt with in the sheriff's court, as a fatal accident enquiry. If there is any suspicion of manslaughter, a jury may be called and if the findings are against the dentist, criminal proceedings may be initiated against him by the police or the Director of Public Prosecutions (the Procurator Fiscal in Scotland). An informative section on inquests is included in the MPS booklet *Pitfalls of practice*.

It should be noted that these statements apply mainly to England and Wales and that procedures are slightly different in Scotland.

Conclusions

This chapter makes no pretence to being comprehensive, but is intended to emphasise the variety of medicolegal problems that can involve the unlucky or careless practitioner. The chances of being involved in litigation may be small but are real enough to necessitate taking every precaution to avoid it. A little time spent in reading the annual reports of the defence societies and any of their relevant booklets is well worthwhile. Other required reading includes the publications relating to the Health and Safety at Work etc Act and the rights of employees, as discussed in Chapter 6.

The surest way of keeping out of trouble is to maintain the highest standards of clinical and ethical practice at all times. Improvements in the standard of delivery of care is the key to reducing the hazards and the numbers of complaints and claims. Continuing education is also extremely important. The dental practitioner who fails to keep him/herself informed may live to regret having failed to take the trouble.

304   OCCUPATIONAL HAZARDS TO DENTAL STAFF

References

1   Seear J. *Law and ethics in dental practice.* Bristol: Wright, 1975.
2   Killey C, Kay LW. *The prevention of complications in dental surgery.* 2nd ed. Edinburgh: Churchill Livingstone, 1977.
3   O'Dowd TC. Five years of heartsink patients in general practice. *Br Med J* 1988; **297**: 528–530.
4   Gerard TJ, Riddell JD. Difficult patients: black holes and secrets. *Br Med J* 1988; **297**: 530–532.
5   Grace M. The importance of good communication. *Med Protect Soc Ann Rep* 1987; **95**: 49–52.
6   Haskell R. Medico-legal consequences of extracting lower third molar teeth. *Med Protect Soc Ann Rep* 1986; **94**: 51–52.
7   Consensus development conference summaries; removal of third molars. National Institute of Health 1979; **2**: 65.
8   Stanley HR, Alattar M, Collett WK, Stringfellow HR, Spiegel EH. Pathological sequelae of 'neglected' impacted third molars. *J Oral Pathol* 1988; **17**: 113–117.
9   Cawson RA. Infective endocarditis as a complication of dental treatment. *Br Dent J* 1981 **151**: 409.
10 Leading article. Midazolam—is antagonism justified? *Lancet* 1988; **2**: 140–142.
11 Shirlaw PJ, Scully C, Griffiths MJ, Levers BGH, Woodwards RTM. General anaesthesia, parenteral sedation and emergency drugs and equipment in general dental practice. *J Dent* 1986; **14**: 247–250.
12 Brahams D. Benzodiazepine sedation and allegations of sexual assault. *Lancet* 1989; **2**: 1339–1340.
13 Noar SJ. Dental Services Committee. *J Med Defence Union* 1986; Spring: 14–15.
14 Hill TR. The Dental Report. *Med Protect Soc Ann Rep* 1986; **94**: 53–56.
15 Peters AC. Council on Dental Practice: Chemical dependency and dental practice. *J Am Dent Assoc* 1987; **114**: 509–515.

Appendix 1

General Dental Council

Amendment to the Notice for the Guidance of Dentists approved by the Council at its meeting on 9 May 1989, to replace paragraphs 12 to 16 of the Notice dated May 1988.

General Anaesthesia and Sedation

(1) Where a general anaesthetic is administered, the Council considers that it should be by a person other than the dentist treating the patient, who should remain with the patient throughout the anaesthetic procedure and until the patient's protective reflexes have returned.
(2) This second person should be a dental or medical practitioner

appropriately trained and experienced in the use of anaesthetic drugs for dental purposes. As part of a programme of training in anaesthesia, the general anaesthetic may be administered by a dental or medical practitioner under the direct supervision of the said second person.

(3) Where intravenous or inhalational sedation techniques are employed, a suitably experienced practitioner may assume the responsibility of sedating the patient, as well as operating, provided that as a minimum requirement a second appropriate person is present through the procedure. Such an appropriate person might be a suitably trained dental surgery assistant or dental auxiliary, whose experience and training enables that person to be an efficient member of the dental team and who is capable of monitoring the clinical condition of the patient. Should the occasion arise, he or she must also be capable of assisting the dentist in case of emergency.

(4) For these purposes, the following definition of simple sedation should be understood to apply: 'A technique in which the use of a drug or drugs produces a state of depression of the central nervous system enabling treatment to be carried out, but during which communication is maintained such that the patient will respond to command throughout the period of sedation. The drugs and techniques used should carry a margin of safety wide enough to render unintended loss of consciousness unlikely'.

(5) Neither general anaesthesia nor sedation should be employed unless proper equipment for their administration is used and adequate facilities for the resuscitation of the patient are readily available, with both dentist and staff trained in their use. Resuscitation is very much a matter of skill and timing and dentists must ensure that all those assisting them know precisely what is required of them, should an emergency arise, and that they regularly practise their routine in a simulated emergency against the clock. The Council considers it essential that the equipment necessary for basic life support, including suction apparatus to clear the airway, oral airways to maintain it and positive pressure equipment with appropriate attachments to inflate the lungs with oxygen, must be immediately to hand and ready for use in the operating room.

(6) A dentist who carried out treatment under general anaesthesia or sedation without fulfilling these conditions would almost certainly be considered to have acted in a manner which constitutes serious professional misconduct. *May 1989*

Appendix 2

The Hippocratic Oath

The Hippocratic Oath, probably dating from about the fifth century BC, has been translated thus:

'I swear by Apollo Physician, by Asclepius, by Health, by Panacea and by all the gods and goddesses, making them my witnesses, that I will carry out, according to my ability and judgement, this oath and this indenture. To hold my teacher in this art equal to my own parents; to make him partner in my livelihood; when he is in need of money to share mine with him; to consider his family as my own brothers, and to teach them this art, if they want to learn it, without fee or indenture; to impart precept, oral instruction, and all other instruction to my own sons, the sons of my teacher and to indentured pupils who have taken the physician's oath, but to nobody else. I will use treatment to help the sick according to my ability and judgement, but never with a view to injury and wrong-doing. Neither will I administer a poison to anybody when asked to do so, nor will I suggest such a course. Similarly I will not give a woman a pessary to cause abortion. But I will keep pure and holy both my life and my art. I will not use the knife, not even, verily, on sufferers from stone, but I will give place to such as are craftsmen therein. Into whatsoever houses I enter, I will enter to help the sick and I will abstain from all intentional wrong-doing and harm, especially from abusing the bodies of man or woman, bond or free. And whatsoever I shall see or hear in the course of my profession, as well as outside my profession in my intercourse with men, if it be what should not be published abroad, I will never divulge, holding such things to be holy secrets. Now if I carry out this oath, and break it not, may I gain for ever reputation among all men for my life and for my art; but if I transgress it and forswear myself, may the opposite befall me'.

Appendix 3

The Declaration of Geneva

In 1948 the recently formed World Medical Association (WMA) produced a modern restatement of the Hippocratic Oath, called the Declaration of Geneva. It was amended by the WMA in 1983 and states:

'At the time of being admitted as a Member of the Medical Profession:

I solemnly pledge myself to consecrate my life to the service of humanity;

I will give to my teachers the respect and gratitude which is their due;

I will practise my profession with conscience and dignity;

The health of my patient will be my first consideration;

I will respect the secrets which are confided in me, even after the patient has died;

I will maintain by all the means in my power, the honour and the noble traditions of the medical profession;

My colleagues will be my brothers;

I will not permit considerations of religion, nationality, race, party politics or social standing to intervene between my duty and my patients;

I will maintain the utmost respect for human life from its beginning, and even under threat I will not use my medical knowledge contrary to the laws of humanity;

I make these promises solemnly, freely and upon my honour.'

Appendix 4

The International Code of Medical Ethics

The English text of this code produced by the World Medical Association, is as follows (1983 revision)

Duties of physicians in general
A physician shall always maintain the highest standards of professional conduct.

A physician shall not permit motives of profit to influence the free and independent exercise of professional judgement on behalf of patients.

A physician shall, in all types of medical practice, be dedicated to providing competent medical service in full technical and moral independence, with compassion and respect for human dignity.

A physician shall deal honestly with patients and colleagues, and strive to expose those physicians deficient in character or competence, or who engage in fraud or deception.

The following practices are deemed to be unethical conduct:

(a) Self advertising by physicians, unless permitted by the laws of the country and the Code of Ethics of the National Medical Association.
(b) Paying or receiving any fee or any other consideration solely to procure the referral of a patient or for prescribing or referring a patient to any source.

A physician shall respect the rights of patients, of colleagues, and of other health professionals, and shall safeguard patient confidences.

A physician shall act only in the patient's interest when providing medical care which might have the effect of weakening the physical and mental condition of the patient.

A physician shall use great caution in divulging discoveries or new techniques or treatment through non-professional channels.

A physician shall certify only that which he has personally verified.

Duties of physicians to the sick
A physician shall always bear in mind the obligation of preserving human life.

A physician shall owe his patients complete loyalty and all the resources of his science. Whenever an examination or treatment is beyond the physician's capability, he should summon another physician who has the necessary ability.

A physician shall preserve absolute confidentiality on all he knows about his patient even after the patient has died.

A physician shall give emergency care as a humanitarian duty unless he is assured that others are willing and able to give such care.

Duties of physicians to each other
A physician shall behave towards his colleagues as he would have them behave towards him.

A physician shall not entice patients from his colleagues.

A physician shall observe the principles of the 'Declaration of Geneva' approved by the World Medical Association.

Appendix 5

Rights of the Patient (Declaration of Lisbon)

In 1981, the World Medical Association adopted a Statement on the rights of the patient. Known as the 'Declaration of Lisbon', it reads:

'Recognising that there may be practical, ethical or legal difficulties, a physician should always act according to his/her conscience and always in the best interest of the patient. The following Declaration represents some of the principal rights which the medical profession seeks to provide to patients.

Whenever legislation or government action denies these rights of the patient, physicians should seek by appropriate means to assure or to restore them.

(a) The patient has the right to choose a physician freely.

(b) The patient has the right to be cared for by a physician who is free to make clinical and ethical judgements without any outside interference.

(c) The patient has the right to accept or to refuse treatment after receiving adequate information.

(d) The patient has the right to expect that his physician will respect the confidential nature of all his medical and personal details.

(e) The patient has the right to die in dignity.

(f) The patient has the right to receive or to decline spiritual and moral comfort, including the help of a minister of an appropriate religion.

Appendix 6

The Sick Dentists Scheme
(Courtesy of Mr J. Mee)

The objectives of the scheme are to:

(1) Identify dentists suffering the effects of addiction to alcohol or drugs (or other relevant conditions);

(2) Validate reports received in confidence with the utmost care;

(3) Persuade the sick dentist by a prescribed system of confrontation that he/she has an illness and must accept help in order to recover;

(4) Assist the sick dentist with the practical problems that will be encountered in maintaining his/her practice and family during treatment and recovery until professional competence is restored;

(5) Assist the recovering dentist in formulating a life-style that will be conducive to continuing uninterrupted recovery.

The outline scheme is illustrated in figure 7.2. A member of the family, staff, a colleague or others concerned about the health of a GDP first contacts the LDC Secretary, BDA Branch or Section Secretary or FPC Administrator to obtain the names, addresses and private telephone numbers of four Regional referees.

The four Regional referees are from a list of nominees, one from each LDC, by the Regional LDC where this exists or, if not, the GDSC. The four referees should be reasonably spread throughout their Region. The basic requirement of a referee is a desire to help, but in a quiet unpublicised manner that cannot be construed as moralistic. In addition, the referee should be:

(1) a good listener and strong motivator;
(2) aware of contemporary attitudes and not influenced by outdated ones;
(3) drawn from the senior end of the profession, either recently retired or close to doing so;
(4) well known and respected at local level and therefore not likely to be viewed as one who would profit from another's misfortune;
(5) fit, active, mobile and ready to travel considerable distances at short notice;
(6) respected for his/her common sense and judgement.

Having obtained the names of the four Regional referees, the person concerned about the health of the dentist decides which one to approach. Only one referee should be approached. The referee, when contacted, will confirm the confidential nature of the information being given, seek identification of the person making the report and the nature of the particular problem giving rise to their concern. The chosen referee will contact BDA Headquarters for the name of a 'special' referee who will be a recovering alcoholic/addict. The British Doctors and Dentists Alcoholic Group has agreed to nominate referees to this confidential list of 'special' referees.

The two referees then interview the person who first reported the dentist, seeking information from which to assess the cause of their concern and whether the condition of the dentist is giving rise to any of the problems outlined above. They will be assured that strict confidence of the report is guaranteed and that the sick dentist will not be informed of the source. To assist in validation of the report, it will be necessary to ask whether anyone else is aware of the problem and if so to interview them.

Having conducted a thorough validation exercise and satisfied themselves of the credibility of the report, the referees should then arrange to visit the sick dentist. At this point the sick dentist's medical practitioner should be identified, appraised of the situation and the procedures in hand and invited to cooperate. If it is established that the problem is not alcohol/drug related, the 'special' referee will withdraw from the case and a second, general referee will be appointed by the first referee. Full instructions and advice on how to approach and deal with a sick colleague will form part of the special information package for referees which will have restricted distribution. It must be understood that each case will need to be treated on its own merits by the acting referees, who in their turn would use their initiative as the case develops in its own way.

In cases of addictive diseases, the referees will arrange contact between the sick dentist and local support groups (Alcoholics Anonymous, British Doctors and Dentists Alcoholic Group, etc). These groups will provide continuing support during treatment and recovery. The referees will also provide help with personal and professional responsibilities during the period of treatment and early recovery. The type and degree of help required will vary according to the type of practice. In all cases, the referees will have ready answers to such questions as 'what about my practice and family income if I take time off for treatment?' The dentist must be persuaded that it is to his/her advantage to lose a few weeks' work in the knowledge that if he/she can get rid of the problem, his/her income should automatically increase. If left to his/her habit, the financial position will continue to deteriorate to the inevitable conclusion.

Treatment of addictive diseases may require that the dentist stops work to receive in-patient therapy. All cases vary, but 4 to 6 weeks' absence from practice is to be anticipated as an average period of time for treatment. Support should be offered to encourage the dentist to meet with a psychiatrist or other appropriate clinician.

Where the problem is alcoholism or drug abuse, it is important that the psychiatrist has special experience of these diseases. It is also preferable that the psychiatrist is from the same area as the dentist, so that he/she can be available for follow-up monitoring, arrange in-patient hospital care where appropriate and liaise with the sick dentist's GMP. A list of specialist psychiatrists will be available to referees.

If the dentist agrees to seek help, the psychiatrist should make a verbal report on the outcome to the referees. The referees should continue to keep in contact with the dentist during treatment and early recovery, providing help with his/her personal or professional responsibilities. The dentist should generally be supported for at least one year after treatment, or for a period of time considered necessary by the referees and psychiatrist.

Appendix 7

Glossary of abbreviations

ACAS	Arbitration, Conciliation, Advisory Service
ADA	American Dental Association
AIDS	Acquired immune deficiency syndrome
ANUG	Acute necrotising ulcerative gingivitis
ARC	AIDS-related complex
B cells	B lymphocytes
BCG	Bacillus Calmette Guerin
BDA	British Dental Association
BDDG	British Doctors' and Dentists' Group
BS	British Standard
BW	Bitewing (radiograph)
CD4	Cluster of differentiation 4
CDC	Centers for Disease Control
CMV	Cytomegalovirus
CO$_2$	Carbon dioxide
COSHH	Control of Substances Hazardous to Health
dB	Decibel
DH	Department of Health
DPA	Dental Practice Adviser
DPB	Dental Practice Board
DSA	Dental surgery assistant
DSC	Dental Service Committee
EBV	Epstein-Barr virus
EC	European Community
ECNL	Equivalent continuous noise level
ELF	Extremely low frequency
ELISA	Enzyme linked immunosorbent assay
EMAS	Employment Medical Advisory Service
FPC	Family Practitioner Committee
GDC	General Dental Council
GDSC	General Dental Services Committee
Gy	Gray
HAV	Hepatitis A virus
HBIG	Hepatitis B immune globulin
HBV	Hepatitis B virus
HCV	Hepatitis C virus

HDV	Hepatitis D virus
HHV	Human herpes virus
HIV	Human immunodeficiency virus
HMSO	Her Majesty's Stationery Office
HPV	Human papillomavirus
HSC	Health and Safety Committee
HSE	Health and Safety Executive
HSV	Herpes simplex virus
HSAW	Health and Safety at Work
HSW	Health and Safety at Work
HTLV	Human T lymphotropic virus
Hz	Hertz
KS	Kaposi's sarcoma
kV	Kilovolt
LASER	Light amplification by stimulated emission of radiation
LDC	Local Dental Committee
LPA	Laser Protection Adviser
MDDUS	Medical and Dental Defence Union of Scotland
MDU	Medical Defence Union
MEL	Maximum exposure limit
MMR	Mumps, measles, rubella
MPE	Maximum permissible exposure
MPS	Medical Protection Society
MRI	Magnetic resonance imaging
mA	Milliampere
NANBH	Non-A non-B hepatitis
NdYAG	Neodymium, yttrium,aluminium, garnet (laser)
NHS	National Health Service
NMR	Nuclear magnetic resonance
NRPB	National radiation protection board
OES	Occupational Exposure Standards
OI	Opportunistic Infections
PA	Periapical (radiograph)
PCR	Polymerase chain reaction
pgl	Persistent generalised lymphadenopathy
ppm	Parts per million
RBE	Relative biological effectiveness
RPA	Radiation Protection Advisor
RPS	Radiation Protection Supervisor
RSI	Repetitive strain injury

SDAC	Standing Dental Advisory Committee
SMR	Standardised mortality ratio
Sv	Sievert
T cells	T lymphocytes
UV	Ultraviolet
VDT	Video display terminal
VDU	Video display unit
VLF	Very low frequency
VZV	Varicella-zoster virus

Index

Notes